AF901461

Francesca Milano
Antonio L. Gracco
Massimiliano Di Giosia

Dental management of Obstructive Sleep Apnea (OSA)

A Practical Manual

Foreword
Ofer Jacobowitz

edra
PUBLISHING

Original title
La gestione odontoiatrica del paziente con Sindrome delle Apnee Ostruttive del Sonno. Manuale pratico
Francesca Milano, Antonio L. Gracco, Massimiliano Di Giosia

©2019 EDRA s.p.A. – All rights reserved
ISBN: 978-88-214-4879-9

Translation and copyediting: Enago, New York City (NY), USA
Layout: Daniela Manunza

©2020 Edra Publishing US LLC – All rights reserved

ISBN: 978-1-7351497-2-1
eISBN: 978-1-7351497-8-3

- The rights of translation, electronic storage, reproduction or total or partial adaptation by any means (including microfilms and photostatic copies), are reserved for all countries.

- Photocopies for personal use of the reader can be made within the limits of 15% of each volume upon payment to the SIAE of the compensation provided by the art. 68, paragraphs 4 and 5, of the law of 22 April 1941 n. 633. Photocopies made for professional, economic or commercial purposes or for any use other than personal use can be made following a specific authorization issued by CLEARedi, Licensing and Authorization Center for Editorial Reproductions, Corso di Porta Romana 108, 20122 Milan, e-mail permissions@clearedi.org and website www.clearedi.org.

- Knowledge and best practice in this field are constantly changing: As new research and experience broaden our knowledge, changes in practice, treatment, and drug therapy may become necessary or appropriate. Readers are advised to check the most current information provided (i) or procedures featured or (ii) by the manufacturer of each product to be administered, to verify the recommended dose or formula, the method and duration of administration, and contraindications. It is the responsibility of the practitioners, relying on their own experience and knowledge of the patient, to make diagnoses, to determine dosages and the best treatment for each individual patient, and to take all appropriate safety precautions. To the fullest extent of the law, neither the Publisher nor the Editors assume any liability for any injury and/ or damage to persons or property arising out of or related to any use of the material contained in this book.

- This publication contains the author's opinions and is intended to provide precise and accurate information.

- The processing of the texts, even if taken care of with scrupulous attention, cannot entail specific responsibilities for the author and / or the publisher for any errors or inaccuracies.

- The Publisher has made every effort to obtain and cite the exact sources of the illustrations. If in some cases he has not been able to find the right holders, he is available to remedy any inadvertent omissions or errors in the references cited. All registered trademarks mentioned belong to their legitimate owners.

Edra Publishing US LLC
3309 Northlake Boulevard,
Suite 203,
Palm Beach Gardens,
FL, 33403
EIN: 844113980
info@edrapublishing.com
www.edrapublishing.com

Printed by "Printer Trento" S.r.l., Trento (Italy), September 2020

Authors

Francesca Milano
Dentist, Specialist in Orthodontics

Antonio L. Gracco
Associate Professor, Università degli Studi di Padova

Massimiliano Di Giosia
Assistant Professor, University of North Carolina at Chapel Hill Adams School of Dentistry

Simone Baiardi
DIBINEM - Department of Biomedical and Neuromotor Sciences, Alma Mater Studiorum, Università degli Studi di Bologna

Chiara Bellini
Operating Unit of Otolaryngology and Head and Neck Surgery, Ospedale G.B. Morgagni-L. Pierantoni, Forlì

Bruno Carlo Brevi
Maxillofacial Surgery Unit, Azienda Ospedaliera di Pisa

Aldo Campanini
Operating Unit of Otolaryngology and Head and Neck Surgery, Ospedale G.B. Morgagni-L. Pierantoni, Forlì

Fabio Cirignotta
Sleep Medicine Center, Neurology Unit, Azienda Ospedaliera Università di Bologna, Policlinico S. Orsola-Malpighi, Bologna

Andrea De Vito
Operating Unit of Otolaryngology and Head and Neck Surgery, Forlì-Faenza

Donald Falace
Professor Emeritus, University of Kentucky, College of Dentistry, KY Lexington, USA

Giannicola Iannella
Sense Organs Department, Sapienza Università di Roma

Oreste Marrone
Institute of Biomedicine and Molecular Immunology, CNR, Palermo

Giuseppe Meccariello
Operating Unit of Otolaryngology and Head and Neck Surgery, AUSL Romagna, Forlì-Faenza

Susanna Mondini
Centro Medicina del Sonno, Unità Operativa di Neurologia, Azienda Ospedaliera Università di Bologna, Policlinico S. Orsola-Malpighi, Bologna

Filippo Montevecchi
Operating Unit of Otolaryngology and Head and Neck Surgery, AUSL Romagna, Forlì-Faenza

Antonio Sanna
Pneumology Unit, AUSL Toscana Centro, Ospedale San Jacopo, Pistoia

Giovanni Sorrenti
Operating Unit of Otolaryngology, Azienda Ospedaliera Università di Bologna, Policlinico Sant'Orsola-Malpighi, Bologna

Luigi Taranto-Montemurro
Brigham and Women's Hospital and Harvard Medical School, Boston, Massachusetts, USA

Claudio Vicini
Operating Unit of Otolaryngology and Head and Neck Surgery, AUSL Romagna, Forlì-Faenza, Department of Biomedical and Surgical Sciences, Otolaryngology Clinic, Università degli Studi di Ferrara

Contributors

Riccardo Albertini
Operating Unit of Otolaryngology, Azienda Ospedaliera Università di Bologna, Policlinico Sant'Orsola-Malpighi, Bologna

Andrea Bargellini
Department of Orthodontics, Università degli Studi di Torino

Chiara Bellini
Operating Unit of Otolaryngology and Head and Neck Surgery, AUSL Romagna, Forlì-Faenza

Steven D. Bender
Center for Facial Pain and Sleep Medicine, Department of Oral and Maxillofacial Surgery, Texas A&M College of Dentistry, Dallas, USA

Giuseppe Caccamo
Operating Unit of Otolaryngology, Azienda Ospedaliera Università di Bologna, Policlinico Sant'Orsola-Malpighi, Bologna

Giovanni Cammaroto
Operating Unit of Otolaryngology and Head and Neck Surgery, AUSL Romagna, Forlì-Faenza

Tommaso Castroflorio
Department of Orthodontics, Dental School, Università degli Studi di Torino

Chiara Copelli
Maxillofacial Surgery Unit, Azienda Ospedaliera di Parma

Alberto Di Blasio
Maxillofacial Surgery Unit, Azienda Ospedaliera di Parma

Chiara Di Blasio
Maxillofacial Surgery Unit, Azienda Ospedaliera di Parma

Giovanni D'Agostino
Operating Unit of Otolaryngology and Head and Neck Surgery, AUSL Romagna, Forlì-Faenza

Elisabetta Firinu
Operating Unit of Otolaryngology and Head and Neck Surgery, AUSL Romagna, Forlì-Faenza

Francesco Giovacchini
Maxillofacial Surgery Unit, Azienda Ospedaliera di Parma

Riccardo Gobbi
Operating Unit of Otolaryngology and Head and Neck Surgery, AUSL Romagna, Forlì-Faenza

Irene Pelligra
Operating Unit of Otolaryngology, Azienda Ospedaliera Università di Bologna, Policlinico Sant'Orsola-Malpighi, Bologna

Ottavio Piccin
Operating Unit of Otolaryngology, Azienda Ospedaliera Università di Bologna, Policlinico Sant'Orsola-Malpighi, Bologna

Francesco Stomeo
Department of Biomedical and Surgical Sciences, Otolaryngology Clinic, Università degli Studi di Ferrara

Foreword to the English edition

The treatment of obstructive sleep apnea is fraught with many challenges as no single treatment modality suits all. Positive airway pressure, oral appliance therapy, maxillofacial and soft tissue surgery, weight loss and behavioral approaches all have an important role for sleep apnea in the current age of personalized medicine. The patient benefits when experts from a variety of disciplines such as dentistry, otorhinolaryngology, neurology, oral maxillofacial surgery, pulmonology collaborate for optimal care and learn from each other.

To this extent, Francesca Milano, Antonio Gracco and Massimiliano Di Giosia have crafted this highly practical manual, with contributions from leading Italian experts from diverse fields. It is a valuable guide not only for the sleep apnea dentist but for all medical and surgical sleep apnea specialists alike. The approach to the patient is presented methodically beginning with the symptomatology of the disorder, diagnostic criteria and challenges, clinical assessment methods and decision process for treatment. Next, the therapeutic modalities for OSA are described in detail, both medical and surgical, and how they are adapted to the patient. The last section of the book focuses in detail on practical oral appliance therapy with chapters replete with beautiful images, greatly enhancing comprehension. Finally, case studies are presented that illustrate the treatment considerations and approach to actual patients.

I congratulate the editors and distinguished authors for having participated in this great work. It will be of great value for all of us who labor to help those with sleep apnea.

Ofer Jacobowitz MD PhD FAASM
Associate Professor, Otolaryngology, Head and Neck Surgery, Sleep Medicine
ENT and Allergy Associates and Zucker School of Medicine,
Hofstra University
New York, NY

Foreword to the Italian edition

Sleep medicine has been able to achieve a leading role in the diverse horizon of healthcare disciplines.

The growing interest in this branch has been attributed to the high incidence of sleep disorders and the undeniable attraction toward a multidisciplinary approach, which ennobles medical knowledge.

In this regard, odontology experts in sleep medicine play pivotal roles as the potential initial filters for identifying pathological conditions as well as the promoters of modern and effective therapeutic hypotheses.

In the past decades, scientific publications on sleep medicine have received several important contributions from dentistry, indicating the need to establish specialized foundation courses at medical institutions.

In this regard, it is my pleasure to accept this book edited by Francesca Milano, Antonio L. Gracco, and Massimiliano Di Giosia, who have skillfully coordinated and organized the contributions of several scholars among the major Italian experts in this fascinating discipline.

The text has a very precise structure. The first chapter enables dentists to understand sleep disorders in detail, including their signs and symptoms, and the necessary tools required to make a correct diagnosis. The central part of the text describes different therapeutic hypotheses that involve pneumologists; ear, nose, and throat specialists; maxillofacial surgeons; and neurologists. Finally, the last four chapters depict the clinical dental approach, different types of dental devices, and their management. The last chapter is particularly interesting as it includes the descriptions of some clinical cases from anamnesis to the last follow-up. Here the authors aimed to thoroughly illustrate the different paths distinguishing the multidisciplinary approach adopted for patients with obstructive sleep apnea syndrome.

Antonella Polimeni
Full Professor of Odontostomatological Diseases
Sapienza Università di Roma

Foreword to the Italian edition

Dental devices have become increasingly suitable for treating patients with obstructive sleep apnea syndrome. To date, the literature has proved the efficacy of dental devices in reducing the number of respiratory events and improving the symptoms of daytime sleepiness. Furthermore, their efficacy in cardiovascular health is very promising. Studies have reported a decrease in arterial pressure, similar to that achieved with continuous positive airway pressure (CPAP), although the latter is more effective in reducing the number of obstructive sleep apnea events. The beneficial effects of dental devices can be attributed to the higher rate of patient adherence to the therapy than to CPAP.

Several types of dental devices are available in the market, and several treatment methods have been proposed by professionals. Therefore, it is necessary to identify the best clinical practice based on the most recent evidence to optimize the therapeutic results. This book provides the latest know-how details in this field.

Marie Marklund, PhD, DDS
Umeå University
Umeå, Sweden

Preface

We were keenly dedicated to drafting this text because sleep medicine is a growing field attracting increased scientific attention, and we hope our enthusiasm for this topic is captured within our book.

The pathophysiological aspects of sleep, various range of related pathologies, comorbidities, and corresponding social and economic implications are complex but fascinating, and we strive to understand and address these complexities through the lens of dental sleep medicine.

We believe that dentistry can acquire a leading role in this regard. Reportedly, more than 80% of patients with sleep-related pathologies do not receive a proper diagnosis; however, dentists with expertise in sleep medicine can easily identify such pathological conditions and encourage active participation while providing effective treatment.

Considering the diagnostic and therapeutic roles, through this book, we aimed to provide information that can serve as basis for in-depth analyses and evaluations of pathological conditions for all dentists interested in committing themselves to sleep medicine.

We believe that the text is structured so as to present three macro-areas reflecting the ideal pathway for development.

The first part of the book is dedicated to the description and diagnosis of sleep disorders. Our expert colleagues (neurologists; pneumologists; and ear, nose, and throat specialists) have brilliantly described the ideal approach to identify the pathology by providing detailed instructions on identifying the clinical signs and symptoms and interpreting the data of diagnostic tools such as polysomnography or sleep endoscopy.

The second part of the book discusses the different therapeutic options for treating sleep disorders. The obstruction site, weight, jaw conformation, and sleep position assumed by patients are crucial information. Therefore, it is necessary to determine the most suitable therapeutic options and conditions under which they can be employed. We believe that the second part of the book is fundamental to understanding the procedures, tools, techniques, and terminologies useful for multidisciplinary dialog, which defines this discipline in a unique way.

The last chapter thoroughly describes some clinical cases as well the clinical approach adopted for patients with obstructive sleep apnea syndrome from the first medical consultation to the last follow-up.

Using this information, clinicians can learn to identify patients' pathological conditions and perform careful anamnestic and clinical assessments and, if needed, interpret specific questionnaires on sleep or medical reports of CT, polysomnography, or sleep endoscopy.

We would like to thank Miss Ivonne Guzman for her valuable help in reviewing the chapters.

The Authors

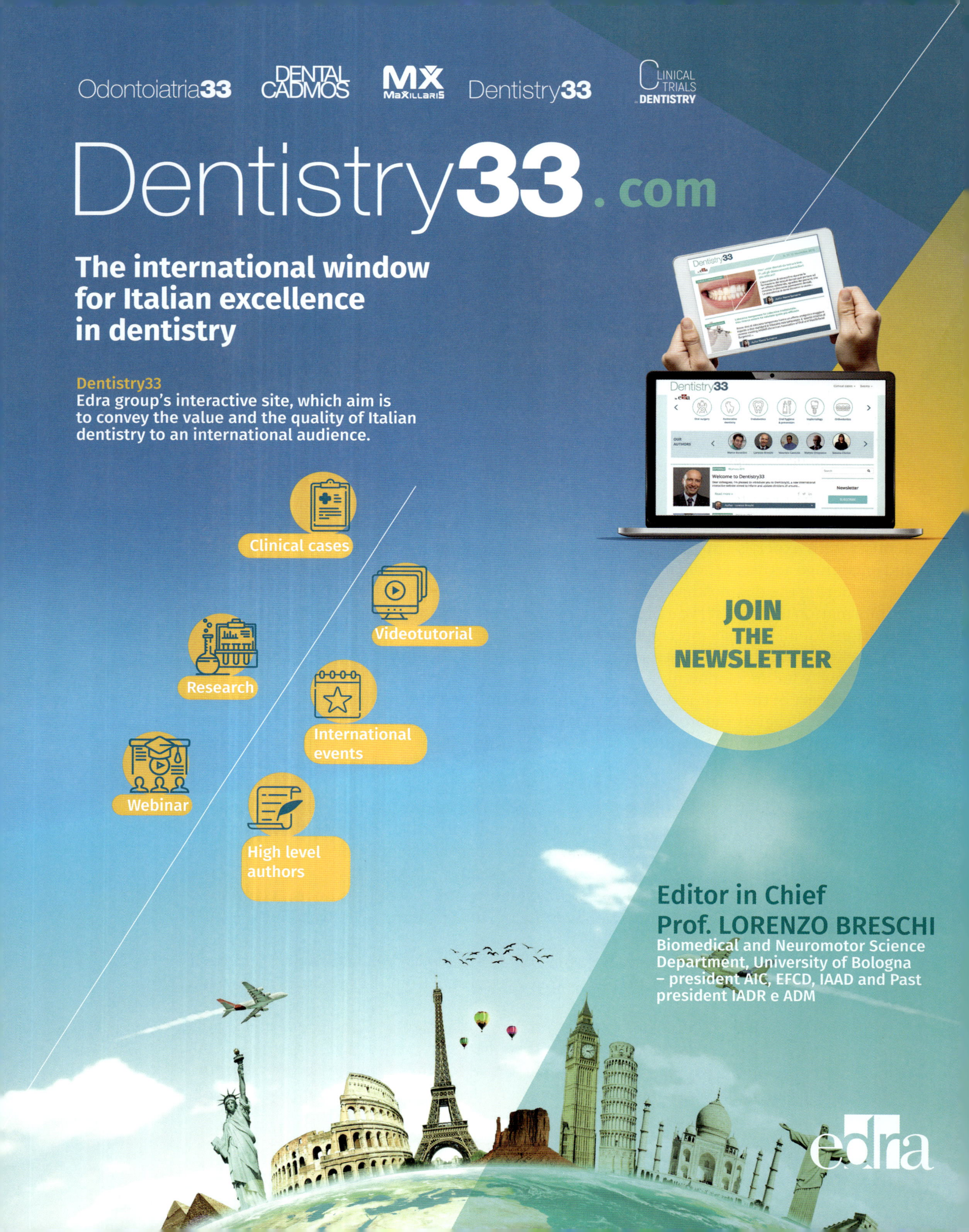
Odontoiatria33
DENTAL CADMOS
MX MAXILLARIS
Dentistry33
CLINICAL TRIALS IN DENTISTRY
Dentistry33.com
The international window for Italian excellence in dentistry
Dentistry33
Edra group's interactive site, which aim is to convey the value and the quality of Italian dentistry to an international audience.
Clinical cases
Videotutorial
Research
International events
Webinar
High level authors
JOIN THE NEWSLETTER
Editor in Chief
Prof. LORENZO BRESCHI
Biomedical and Neuromotor Science Department, University of Bologna – president AIC, EFCD, IAAD and Past president IADR e ADM
edra

Table of contents

To our families

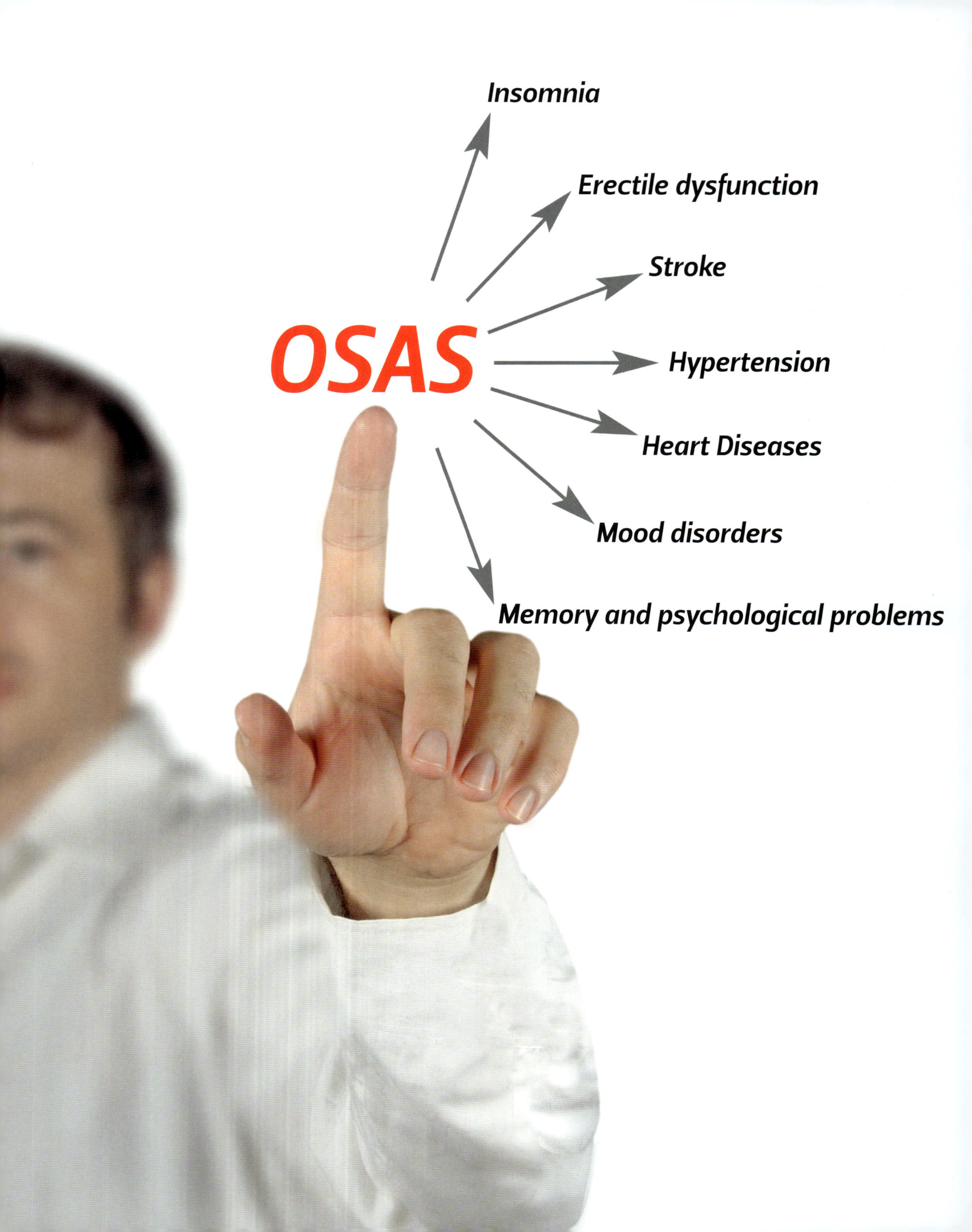
Insomnia
Erectile dysfunction
Stroke
OSAS
Hypertension
Heart Diseases
Mood disorders
Memory and psychological problems

INTRODUCTION TO OBSTRUCTIVE SLEEP APNEA SYNDROME

Oreste Marrone

Objectives

- Understanding the terminologies related to sleep medicine
- Learning the criteria for defining patients with obstructive sleep apnea syndrome (OSAS)
- Understanding OSAS etiology and pathophysiology
- Understanding the risks and complications of untreated OSAS

Definition

Obstructive sleep apnea syndrome (OSAS) is characterized by repeated episodes of respiratory disorders during which the upper airways are affected by an occlusion (obstructive apnea) or a reduction in the caliber [respiratory effort-related arousal (RERA), obstructive hypopnea] during sleep; they occur more frequently at the oropharyngeal level.

During sleep recordings, obstructive apnea is characterized by the cessation of airflow associated with movements of the chest and abdominal walls. However, central apnea is characterized by the absence of respiratory movements with no airflow, and hypopnea is characterized by an airflow reduction of at least 30%, followed by desaturation. For several years, desaturation was defined as at least 4% reduction in the oxyhemoglobin levels; however, currently, the preferable minimum threshold is 3%. In the case of sleep recordings via full polysomnography (including indications for sleep staging and identification of arousal), hypopnea can be identified even in the absence of desaturation when airflow reduction is followed by arousal. A more thorough analysis enables the classification of hypopnea as central or obstructive. RERA was initially defined as a respiratory disorder that does not satisfy the criteria for apnea or hypopnea. RERA is characterized by an increase in respiratory efforts, often following a crescendo trend, which can be detected by recording esophageal pressures; however, these efforts terminate upon arousal. Because of difficulties in performing a routine monitoring of esophageal pressures and because inspiratory efforts are usually associated with a limitation of inspiratory flow in the presence of an occlusion (refer to the Pathophysiology section below), it is currently preferable to replace the esophageal pressure analysis with an airflow morphological analysis, which can be evaluated using a nasal pressure sensor. Flattening of the inspiratory curve indicates an airflow limitation. Even if there is no perfect agreement in the number and duration of respiratory events between the identified RERA and the esophageal pressure and airflow, the differences are considered to be negligible (Ayappa et al. 2000). The common criterion for identifying respiratory events is an event duration of at least 10 seconds.

The apnea-hypopnea index (AHI) is defined as the average number of apnea and hypopnea events per hour of sleep; the respiratory disturbance index (RDI) is defined as the combined average number of apnea/hypopnea events and RERAs per hour of sleep (Berry et al. 2012); and the oxygen desaturation index (ODI) is defined as the number of artery desaturation events per hour of sleep.

OSAS is defined on the basis of clinical, polygraphic, and polysomnographic criteria.

According to the 3rd International Classification of Sleep Disorders (ICSD-3), the diagnostic criteria for OSAS are as follows:

❶ The presence of one or more of the following symptoms:

- Diurnal sleepiness, nonrestorative sleep, fatigue, or insomnia symptoms
- Waking up with a choking sensation
- Habitual snoring and/or breathing interruptions during sleep
- Diagnosis of hypertension, mood disorders, acute coronary artery disease, stroke, congestive heart failure, atrial fibrillation, or type 2 diabetes

2. Five or more obstructive respiratory events (obstructive and mixed apnea, hypopnea, or RERAs) identified per hour of sleep on polysomnography (AHI > 5) or per hour of monitoring on respiratory polygraphy

or:

3. Fifteen or more obstructive respiratory events identified per hour of sleep on polysomnography (AHI > 15) or per hour of monitoring on respiratory polygraphy

Unlike polysomnography, respiratory polygraphy has the disadvantage of underestimating the number of obstructive respiratory events per hour because the total sleep time [determined via electroencephalography (EEG)] is not recorded. In this case, the respiratory event index (REI) can be used to define the frequency of events based on the monitoring time rather than the total sleep time.

Snoring that is not associated with an RDI of ≥5 or with symptoms is defined as "primary snoring" (Iber et al. 2007).

RERAs are not always investigated because they have minor relevance and are difficult to identify in comparison with other sleep respiratory events. Often, the identification of RERAs is limited to calculating AHI. Normally, AHI and RDI differ only slightly among patients with severe sleep-disordered breathing (SDB), whereas they can differ considerably among patients with minor SDB. In such cases, RDI must be exactly estimated because a high RDI and a low AHI can help reveal the origin of symptoms suspected to be associated with SDB despite their severity in comparison with the gravity evaluated using AHI alone. The minimum RDI that was conventionally considered pathological was 5, although some studies have considered minimum RDI threshold levels of 10 or 15. High RDI threshold levels between 5 and 15 excluding the central events are considered sufficient to identify OSAS.

Epidemiology

Several studies have been published on SDB; however, these studies have not reported consistent results.

The difficulty in estimating the prevalence of SDB is mainly attributed to the differences in the modality used to sample populations and the assessment methods of respiratory events as well as the criteria and definition used to identify these events. Particularly different assessment methods have been used to identify hypopnea, which invalidates the comparability of the results reported by previous studies.

For several years, the Wisconsin Sleep Cohort Study (1993) on patients aged 30–60 years was the most important epidemiological study investigating the prevalence of OSAS. The essential criterion for identifying hypopnea was the presence of ≥4% desaturation. This study reported an AHI of ≥5 in 25% of men and 9% of women, whereas the prevalence of OSAS, defined by the association of at least five apnea/hypopnea events per hour of sleep with excessive diurnal sleepiness, was 4% in men and 2% in women (Young et al. 1993).

A recent study in Switzerland (the HypnoLaus Study; Heinzer et al. 2015) investigated the prevalence of SDB in a cohort of 2,121 patients aged between 40 and 85 years who underwent polysomnography. The scoring of respiratory events during sleep was performed using the 2012 criteria of the American Academy of Sleep Medicine, which enable the identification of hypopnea when airflow reduction is associated with a ≥3% desaturation or with arousal alone. An AHI of ≥5 was reported in 83.8% of men and 60.8% of women, whereas a diagnosis of OSAS (according to the aforementioned ICSD-3 criteria) could be established in 74.7% of men and 52.1% of women. The notably elevated prevalence values reported by the HypnoLaus Study compared with those reported by the Wisconsin Sleep Cohort Study could be attributed to the older age of patients in the HypnoLaus Study; however, the differences were particularly associated with the different criteria used to identify hypopnea and diagnose OSAS.

Unlike the differences in the prevalence values, there was a major agreement in identifying the most relevant risk factors for OSAS: male sex, obesity, and older age.

Regarding sex differences, studies performed at sleep laboratories on suspected cases of SDB have reported that OSAS was 4–10-fold more prevalent in men than in women. Nevertheless, studies on the overall population have reported that OSAS is only 2–3-fold more frequent in men that in women. The reasons for this discrepancy can be attributed to the different representations of OSAS. In the case of men, snoring is more clearly reported, whereas women tend to more frequently exhibit unspecific symptoms such as tiredness, migraine, depression, and insomnia, which are less directly attributed to OSAS (Ye et al. 2009). The main reason for the differences in the prevalence of OSAS between men and women is attributed to the fact that the typical fat distribution in men involves the upper parts of the body, which are higher risk factors than obesity. The characteristics of the upper airways may also play an adverse role in men; in particular, the larger-sized pharynx in men is associated with increases in the expansion of the upper airway region, which can lead to obstruction and thus to higher apnea incidence (Malhotra et al. 2002). The pharyngeal critical pressure, i.e., the pressure inside the upper airways at which they collapse, is generally higher in men than in women for particular a body mass index (BMI). This means that respiratory efforts are sufficient for obstruction to occur in men, whereas more intense respiratory efforts are required in women.

Obesity represents one of the most important risk factors for OSAS. OSAS is highly prevalent among individuals with a BMI of >40 kg/m2 and, according to some estimates, its prevalence rate can be >90% (Valencia-Flores et al. 2000). Nevertheless, it is unclear whether the neck and abdominal circumferences can indicate the presence of OSAS with more accuracy (Riha 2010). However, OSAS is commonly detected in individuals with normal weights, but it is more frequent in obese individuals in whom OSAS tends to be severe. Over time, the variations in BMI correlate with the variations in OSAS severity (Peppard et al. 2000). However, strong interindividual differences in the effects of weight variations have been reported, indicating that bariatric surgery does not ensure recovery from SDB in all patients (Greenburg et al. 2009).

With aging, the prevalence of OSAS in the adult population has increased gradually, and the influence of obesity on the occurrence of OSAS has considerably reduced. The increased prevalence of OSAS can be an "age-correlated" phenomenon primarily attributed to the increase in the risk factors for OSAS in older individuals, without losing the clinical characteristics typical of younger individuals. Nevertheless, the increased prevalence of OSAS in older individuals can be partially dependent on age. This would favor an increased prevalence of SDB with reduced severity. Clinical observations have revealed that older individuals are more frequently asymptomatic, whereas the prevalence of symptomatic OSAS does not increase beyond middle age (Bixler et al. 1998). Despite the unlikely appearance of severe OSAS in older individuals, there is clear evidence that OSAS can increase sleepiness and aggravate some risks factor such as stroke in older individuals (Martinez- Garcia et al. 2012).

Menopause appears to be another risk factor for OSAS. After menopause, adipose tissues tend to present a more male-like distribution in women, whereas muscular mass decreases with increases in fat mass (Resta et al. 2003). These changes result in a minor difference in the prevalence of OSAS in such women compared with that in men of the same age; however, the predisposing and protective effects of hormones on OSAS are complex and remain to be clarified.

Finally, cigarette smoking is another common risk factor for OSAS. The hypothesized mechanisms underlying this association include an increase in upper airway inflammation, a reduction in the sensitivity of the upper airway mucosa to stimuli evoking the activity of dilator muscles, and an increase in arousal that may occur because of some components of the cigarette smoke.

Pathophysiology

Upper airways do not have a rigid bone or cartilage frame, particularly at the pharyngeal level. Their patency is attributed to a complex system of dilator muscles such as the genioglossus and tensor palatine muscles. As a whole, these muscles with the ribcage and diaphragm muscles respond via reflexes to stimuli from the upper airways by modulating the intensity of their contractions.

This phenomenon occurs extremely effectively in the wakefulness state. During sleep, the reflexes influencing the pharyngeal musculature tend to cease, and the tonic activity of the pharyngeal dilator muscles as well as of almost the entire skeletal musculature decreases simultaneously (Horner 1996; Edwards and White 2011). Physiologically, the pharynx becomes more collapsible, and its caliber reduces, whereas the resistance of the upper airways increases.

To prevent an excessive reduction in the pharynx caliber, the respiratory tract induces traction in a bottom-up manner by stretching as the lungs expand, subsequently allowing the pharynx to relax during expiration (Van de Graff 1998). The larger the lung volumes are, the longer the pharynx can remain dilated. This is also a reason why obese individuals have a reduced vital capability, particularly in the supine position, and why they are predisposed to upper airway obstruction during sleep. Furthermore, the residual functional capability can be reduced during sleep, causing the traction mechanism of the pharynx to be less effective (Badr 1996).

In anatomically predisposed individuals, the reduction in the upper airway caliber due to diminished muscular activity during sleep can be exaggerated, leading to upper airway obstruction. In the case of partial obstruction, limited inspiratory airflow can be observed.

In fact, the airflow initially increases rapidly and then decreases gradually during normal inspiration. When the pharynx is partially obstructed, the airflow reaches its highest speed at the initiation of inspiration and remains nearly constant until expiration, independent of the presence of the respiratory efforts of the diaphragm and ribcage muscles. This limitation can be weak, having minimal influence on respiratory function, or it can be strong, considerably reducing ventilation. This can possibly lead to the onset of events such as RERAs, obstructive hypopneas, or, especially in deep sleep, periods of stable hypoventilation. When the upper airways are totally obstructed, the airflow ceases, leading to obstructive apnea. Partial obstruction of the upper airways tends to be associated with snoring, whereas snoring may appear only between apneic events in obstructive apnea. During partial or total obstruction, inspiratory efforts typically increase until the obstruction is alleviated. Unblocking of an obstruction generally occurs with arousal (an abrupt awakening or sleep interruption of a minimum duration normally fixed at 3 seconds), although the possibility that some obstructive episodes are resolved without cortical participation has been currently recognized (Younes 2004). When the obstruction is unblocked, brief but often marked increases in blood pressure and cardiac frequency are observed. In the case of most overt OSAS, apneic events repeat themselves in more or less long sequences, alternating with brief episodes of hyperventilation. This results in different physiological activities occurring synchronically in a cyclical trend; specifically, the respiratory function exhibits an alternate apnea and hypoventilation, increases and decreases in respiratory efforts, and increases and decreases in oxyhemoglobin saturation, which generates typical intermittent hypoxia. The cardiocirculatory effects include decreases and increases in systemic blood and lung pressures, cardiac frequency and output. This sleep is characterized by a continuous alternation of deepening or weakening and arousals (highly cyclical pattern, 📷 1.1).

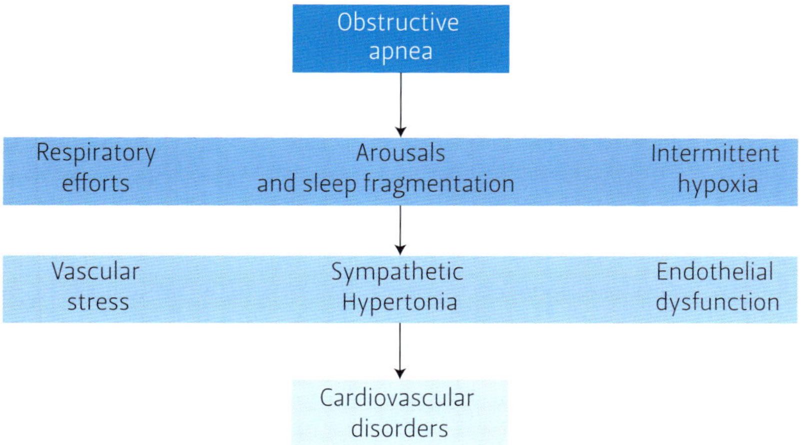

📷 1.1 Pathogenetic mechanisms underlying the association between OSAS and cardiovascular diseases.

Upper airways can collapse at different sites, including the soft palate (most frequent), the base of the tongue, pharyngeal walls, or the larynx (less frequent), particularly at the epiglottis level. Upper airway obstruction can occur through convergence of the lateral walls or concentric tightening of the upper airways. The expansion of the obstructed area varies according to individuals and sometimes even in the same individual according to episodes (Faber and Grymer 2003).

Pathoetiology

Conventionally, the pathogenesis of OSAS was distinguished according to pathogenetic anatomical and functional factors. More recently, the pathogenetic factors have been classified into four groups, each of which is identified by a letter of the PALM acronym as follows: passive critical closing pressure, arousal threshold, loop gain, and muscular responsiveness.

Passive critical closing pressure (its definition has been previously reported) is a measurement of collapsibility, and it mainly depends on anatomical factors (Gold and Schwarz 1996). Pathogenetic anatomical factors for obstruction involve reductions in the upper airway caliber. The most easily detectable factor is tonsil and adenoid hypertrophy, which is typical of pediatric OSAS. The upper airway lumen may become narrow because of hypertrophy of other soft structures (e.g., tongue, palate, and uvula) or craniofacial alterations such as mandibular retrognathism or micrognathism (Dempsey et al. 2002). In obese individuals, adipose tissues can compress the pharyngeal lumen from outside and thus shrink it. An anteroposterior elongated shape of the horizontal pharyngeal section can represent a predisposing factor for obstruction. In fact, the lateral pharyngeal walls are important constrictor muscle sites, whereas the dilator muscles mainly act in an anteroposterior direction and are thus less effective in dilating the organ laterally (Leiter 1996). While the dimensions of the horizontal pharynx section can represent predisposing factors for obstruction when they are reduced, the vertical dimensions represent a risk factor for OSAS when they are increased because of the larger expansion of the area that can be occluded (Malhotra et al. 2002). Water retention (peripharyngeal edema) and the movement of interstitial fluids in the rostral direction from the lower to the upper parts of the body after assuming a sloping position can also represent predisposing factors for pharyngeal narrowing. Edema can be problematic, particularly in the case of excessive extracellular volume (i.e., cardiac failure, kidney terminal failure) (White and Bradley 2012). A certain improvement in OSAS can be achieved by treatment with diuretics or other mechanical methods aiming to redistribute the fluids.

The arousal threshold is the stimulus necessary to induce arousal from sleep. A low threshold is typical of the several forms of insomnia, whereas a high threshold is identified in cases of excessive sleepiness. According to the most common opinion, the causes of arousal can be stimuli generated during apnea (hypoxia, hypercapnia, and particularly respiratory efforts). Arousal involves an immediate increase in the muscular activity at the pharyngeal level, allowing or facilitating the unblocking of the obstruction, the recovery of ventilation, and the restoration of the normal tension of arterial blood gases. Thus, under this viewpoint, arousal plays a beneficial role. Independent of whether arousal occurs due to respiratory efforts or occurs spontaneously, it is associated with a brief period of hyperventilation that not infrequently can lead to tension of $O2$ and particularly of $CO2$ to such a level that nullifies the output of the nervous control centers to the respiratory muscles and to those of the upper airways. In this manner, arousal can promote or perpetrate the onset of apnea (Wellman et al. 2003, 2004). Hence, a low arousal threshold favors respiratory instability and apnea (Gleeson et al. 1990, Dempsey et al. 1996). Conversely, a high arousal threshold (necessity of extremely intense stimuli for awakening), as observed in deep sleep, tends to be associated with stable sleep as well as respiration.

Loop gain is the intensity with which the system regulating the homeostasis of the arterial blood gases reacts with perturbations that alter their levels to bring them back to normal levels. It is primarily the end result of the responses of the respiratory centers to hypoxia and hypercapnia ("controller gain") and the measure by which the arterial blood gas levels change due to variations in ventilation produced by the central respiratory control ("plant gain"). When loop gain is very high, the system tends to be instable, and a type of periodic breathing may develop. In this context, both central and obstructive apnea may develop. Both controller gain and an increase in plant gain can contribute to increasing the loop gain. Controller gain is often increased in OSAS, but it is also elevated in some pathologies such as cardiac failure. Obesity is one of the causes underlying the increase in plant gain because it reduces the lung volume, leading to a decrease in the oxygen reserves in the lungs and thus amplifying the effects of variations in ventilation on the changes in oxygen reserves at the alveolar and therefore the arterial levels.

Finally, it has been reported that the upper airway dilator muscles have the ability to increase their activity in response to hypoxia and hypercapnia. This response can protect the upper airways from obstruction and, in some cases, unblock obstruction in absence of arousal.

Scarce muscular responsiveness can be caused by an alteration in the upper airway mucosa caused mainly by inflammatory mechanisms that reduce the receptor sensitivity to stimuli that are responsible for increasing the pharyngeal dilator muscles activity in a reflexive manner (Horner 1996; Petrof et al. 1996). The functionality of the pharyngeal musculature can be compromised by acquired neuromuscular diseases such as lateral amyotrophic sclerosis or congenital neuromuscular diseases such as the Charcot-Marie-Tooth disease.

Other pathogenetic hypotheses associate OSAS with systemic alterations rather than local anomalies of the upper airways. In particular, it has been proposed that obesity represents a predisposing factor for OSAS through the noxious influences of metabolic and inflammatory alterations in the regulation of respiration occurring during metabolic syndrome (Vgontzas et al. 2005). This theory is supported by the fact that in the case of suspected OSAS, an increase in the waist circumference is considered a more important index than BMI, which varies independently from the distribution of adipose tissue. Furthermore, after losing weight, a reduction in abdominal fat is more strongly correlated with a reduction in AHI than with an increase in the dimensions of the upper airways (Sutherland et al 2011).

Clinical aspects and complications

OSAS has a heterogeneous clinical presentation that varies according to the patient's age and sex in many cases. Conventionally, the diurnal and nocturnal symptoms of OSAS are distinguished in clinical practice.

The most frequent nocturnal symptom reported by patients (or by their partners or parents in the case of children) is intense snoring, which can occur during partial upper airway obstruction or in the interval between an episode of apnea and the subsequent episode when the soft structures of the upper airways vibrate. The absence of intense snoring makes the diagnosis impossible even if it is not excluded completely. Some patients have reported nocturnal awakening associated with a sense of choking. This symptom must be distinguished from acid reflux with larynx spasm and nocturnal paroxysmal dyspnea, which is more typical of nocturnal asthma and some cases of chronic obstructive pulmonary disease (COPD). Furthermore, patients may report frequent awakenings and fragmented sleep. Other symptoms reported by patients include insufficiently restorative sleep, nocturnal diaphoresis, nocturia or polyuria (probably due to the release of atrial natriuretic factors induced by apnea), and nasal congestion.

The most frequently reported diurnal symptom is excessive sleepiness; however, accumulating evidence paradoxically suggests that some patients mainly experience insomnia. Some diurnal symptoms of OSAS include morning migraine, difficulty in focusing, irritability, and mood disorders. Moreover, OSAS can be associated with decreased libido and erectile dysfunction.

The clinical relevance of OSAS also lies in the risks associated with this pathology. In the presence of OSAS, some diseases may have a more severe course and a weakened response to treatment. The number of diseases for which OSAS can represent a risk factor has gradually increased over time (■ 1.1). Studies have extensively demonstrated that OSAS increases the incidence of some diseases as well as certain disorders (e.g., cardiovascular diseases); however, little information is available regarding the association between OSAS and the risk factors for other disorders. In some cases, OSAS can also increase the mortality rate.

The association between OSAS and cardiovascular diseases is extremely strong and partly justified by the higher prevalence of OSAS in older individuals as well as in men and obese individuals. Several experimental and epidemiological studies have supported the direct role of OSAS as a cardiovascular risk factor.

The pathogenesis of cardiovascular diseases in patients with OSAS is extremely complex. It is believed that the main mediators between OSAS and cardiovascular diseases are vascular stress, hypertonia, and endothelial dysfunction, whose presence has been extensively demonstrated in OSAS.

On the basis of these alterations, which gradually appear as chronic effects of recurrent apnea, some immediate effects of obstructive apnea have been particularly represented by respiratory efforts and fragmented sleep due to

1.1 Diseases in which OSAS can represent a risk factor.

Cardiovascular diseases
Collagen diseases
Metabolic disorders and diabetes
Psoriasis
Kidney failure
Eye disorders
Chronic obstructive pulmonary disease
Epilepsy
Neoplasm
Dementia

recurrent arousal and intermittent hypoxia (Kohler and Stradling 2010). The effects of stress on intrapleural vessels and the heart can be attributed to inspiratory efforts, leading to the formation of aortic aneurysm and contributing to the onset of atrial fibrillations and cardiac failure. Sleep fragmentation is considered one of the most important causes of hypertonia in patients with OSAS; this in turn can lead to an increase in vascular rigidity and contribute to endothelial dysfunction and the onset of arterial hypertension. In addition to increasing the sympathetic tone, intermittent hypoxia may act by promoting oxidative stress conditions, stimulating the production of nuclear transcription factor NF-kB, and consequently increasing the production of inflammatory factors. The subsequent endothelial dysfunction may lead to an altered balance between factors regulating the vascular tone and those influencing blood coagulability, thus leading to increased arterial blood pressure, atherosclerotic alterations in vessel walls, and cardiovascular diseases (Budhiraja et al. 2007).

Currently, OSAS is recognized as a possible cause of arterial hypertension, particularly in younger individuals. However, it has been recently reported that OSAS exerts a significant effect on blood pressure in older patients (Bixler et al. 2000; Roche et al. 2012). Furthermore, OSAS is often responsible for nondipping arterial pressure during sleep, and it is considered one of the most common causes of drug-resistant hypertension (Kario 2009). OSAS treatment restores the normal dipping of arterial pressure during the night and improves the response to antihypertensive medication; moreover, it can reduce pressure levels. However, in this regard, the response is highly variable among individuals. Analyses of the available data in the medical literature have indicated that on an average, long-term CPAP treatment reduces arterial pressure in a statistically significant but quantitatively modest manner (Montesi et al. 2012).

The important effects of OSAS on the activity of the autonomous nervous system favor the onset of atrial fibrillation and several types of tachy-brady arrhythmia (Olmetti et al. 2008; Monahan et al. 2009). Although rare, it is possible that arrhythmia caused by OSAS acquires clinically threatening connotations (Serizawa et al. 2008).

OSAS can be associated with an increased incidence of coronary heart diseases (Gottlieb et al. 2010). Some studies have reported that OSAS can compromise the recovery capabilities of the left ventricle after myocardial infarction (Nakashima et al. 2006). Conversely, other studies have reported that the expansion of the infarcted area in patients with OSAS may be minor possibly because the chronic exposition to moderate intermittent hypoxia may result in an increase in the expansion of the collateral coronary circles (Shah et al. 2012).

OSAS is observed in most patients with stroke because it may represent a risk factor for cerebrovascular disorders and precede their occurrence or it may be an effect of the disorders that are aggravated or manifested immediately within days after the onset of stroke (Neau et al. 2002). In patients with stroke, the presence of OSAS worsens their recovery capabilities and diminishes their life expectancy (Martinez-Garcia et al. 2009).

Over time, obstructive apnea reduces the systolic and diastolic ventricular functionality both on the right and left sides and, in predisposed individuals, favors the onset of cardiac failure (Romero-Corral et al. 2007). In turn, this can cause SDB to worsen via an association with an increase of body liquids that can be responsible of edema with subsequent reductions of the pharyngeal caliber. In cases of cardiac failure, obstructive apnea often coexists with central apnea. When cardiac failure worsens, obstructive apnea tends to advances to central apnea, whereas an improvement may have the opposite effect (Ryan et al. 2010). The chronic treatment of obstructive apnea reduces the sympathetic tone and improves ventricular function (Egea et al. 2008).

The association between OSAS and chronic respiratory diseases has been defined as "overlap syndrome," although ordinarily this term indicates the association between OSAS and COPD. In patients with COPD, the consequences of OSAS can be extremely severe because SDB can manifest particularly severe characteristics and the evolution of this disease can be rapid with an early incidence of hypoxemic and hypercapnic respiratory failure, pulmonary hypertension, and decreased life expectancy (Weitzenblum et al. 2008).

Hypoxemic-hypercapnic respiratory failure can also occur in patients with obesity hypoventilation syndrome (OHS). OHS is characterized by obesity and hypercapnia during wakefulness in the absence of neuromuscular, mechanical, or metabolic alterations that can support hypoventilation. OSAS is present in the majority of patients with OHS, and if treated, it can lead to remission of respiratory failure, whereas untreated OHS can result in extremely high mortality rates (Mokhlesi et al. 2008).

Metabolic disorders that pose a risk to patients with OSAS are also observed in obese patients, particularly in patients with visceral obesity. Considering the close relationship between OSAS and obesity, the direct role of OSAS as a risk factor for metabolic alterations has often been questioned, particularly in the case of cardiovascular diseases. Currently, our understanding of pathogenetic mechanisms and observations of experimental and clinical studies suggest that OSAS represents a risk factor independent of obesity. Regarding cardiovascular diseases, the role of metabolic disorders is mainly attributed to factors such as sleep fragmentation and intermittent hypoxia. It is believed that sleep fragmentation results in an increase in sympathetic tone in addition to being associated with both insulin- and noninsulin-dependent mechanisms of glucose disposal (Stamakis et al. 2010). Intermittent hypoxia can contribute to an increase in sympathetic activity, promote the release of inflammatory factors through the major formation of NF-κB, and favor an increase in insulin resistance and the occurrence of atherogenic dyslipidemia (Levy et al. 2008). OSAS appears to occur independent of insulin resistance, and it is frequently associated with metabolic syndrome and type 2 diabetes mellitus (Pamidi and Tasali 2012). Despite some disagreement, longitudinal observations, although discordant, suggest that the incidence of type 2 diabetes mellitus has increased, at least in patients with moderate or severe OSAS (Wang et al. 2013). According to some observations, patients with OSAS exhibit higher levels of triglycerides and cholesterol in their blood serum but reduced levels of high-density lipoprotein (HDL) cholesterol (Bonsignore et al. 2012). It has been proposed that the progression of nonalcoholic hepatic steatosis is affected by inflammatory activation and dyslipidemia that is partially subsequent to an altered functioning of lipid metabolism pathways at the hepatic level (Aron-Wisnesky et al. 2012). However, the possibility of reducing metabolic alterations in OSAS by treating apnea remains controversial.

Compared with the outcomes reported for the general population, patients with OSAS have a higher mortality rate at the same age. The mortality rate is higher in patients with more severe somatic symptom disorder (SDD), and it becomes significant when AHI is >30. The mortality rate is reduced by apnea treatment (Young et al. 2008). Patients with OSAS have an increased mortality rate for cardiovascular diseases (Marin et al. 2005) as well as neoplastic diseases according to more recent studies (Nieto et al. 2012). The risk of mortality has gradually decreased since OSAS diagnosis was first reported (Lavie 2007). However, OSAS is associated with an increased risk of mortality in patients with cardiovascular diseases as well as in older individuals. It is possible that OSAS increases the risk of mortality in patients aged >50 years only by aggravating the course of coexisting diseases without increasing the incidence of new disorders (Marrone et al. 2013).

REFERENCES

Aron-Wisnewsky J, Minville C, Tordjman J, et al. Chronic intermittent hypoxia is a major trigger for non-alcoholic fatty liver disease in morbid obese. *J Hepatol.* 2012;56:225-233.

Ayappa I, Norman RG, Krieger AC, Rosen A, O'malley RL, Rapoport DM. Non-invasive detection of respiratory effort-related arousals (REras) by a nasal cannula/pressure transducer system. *Sleep.* 2000;23:763-777.

Badr MS. Effect of ventilatory drive on upper airway patency in humans during NREM sleep. *Respir Physiol.* 1996;103:1-10.

Berry RB, Brooks R, Gamaldo CE, Harding SM, Marcus CL, Vaughn BV (American Academy of Sleep Medicine). *The AASM Manual for the Scoring of Sleep and Associated Events: Rules, Terminology and Technical Specifications*, Version 2.0. www.aasmnet.org. Darien, Illinois: American Academy of Sleep Medicine; 2012.

Bixler EO, Vgontzas AN, Lin HM, et al. Association of hypertension and sleep-disordered breathing. *Arch Intern Med.* 2000;160:2289-2295.

Bixler EO, Vgontzas AN, Ten Have T, Tyson K, Kales A. Effects of age on sleep apnea in men: I. Prevalence and severity. *Am J Respir Crit Care Med.* 1998;157:144-148.

Bonsignore MR, McNicholas WT, Montserrat JM, Eckel J. Adipose tissue in obesity and obstructive sleep apnoea. *Eur Respir J.* 2012;39:746-767.

Budhiraja R, Parthasarathy S, Quan SF. Endothelial dysfunction in obstructive sleep apnea. *J Clin Sleep Med.* 2007;3:409-415.

Dempsey JA, Skatrud JB, Jacques AJ, et al. Anatomic determinants of sleep-disordered breathing across the spectrum of clinical and nonclinical male subjects. *Chest.* 2002;122:840-851.

Dempsey JA, Smith CA, Harms CA, Chow CM, Saupe KW. Sleep-induced breathing instability. *Sleep.* 1996;19:236-247.

Edwards BA, White DP. Control of the pharyngeal musculature during wakefulness and sleep: implications in normal controls and sleep apnea. *Head Neck.* 2011;33 Suppl 1:S37-S45.

Egea CJ, Aizpuru F, Pinto JA, et al. (Spanish Group of Sleep Breathing Disorders). Cardiac function after CPAP therapy in patients with chronic heart failure and sleep apnea: a multicenter study. *Sleep Med.* 2008;9:660-666.

Faber CE, Grymer L. Available techniques for objective assessment of upper airway narrowing in snoring and sleep apnea. Sleep Breath. 2003;7:77-86.

Gleeson K, Zwillich CW, White DP. The influence of increasing ventilatory effort on arousal from sleep. *Am Rev Respir Dis.* 1990;142:295-300.

Gold AR, Schwartz AR. The pharyngeal critical pressure. The whys and hows of using nasal continuous positive airway pressure diagnostically. *Chest.* 1996;110:1077-1088.

Gottlieb D, Yenokyan G, Newman A, et al., Shahar. Prospective study of obstructive sleep apnea and incident coronary heart disease and heart failure: the Sleep Heart Health Study. *Circulation.* 2010;122:352-360.

Greenburg DL, Lettieri C, Eliasson A. Effects of surgical weight loss on measures of obstructive sleep apnea: a meta-analysis. *Am J Med.* 2009;122:535-542.

Heinzer R, Vat S, Marques-Vidal P, et al. Prevalence of sleep-disordered breathing in the general population: the HypnoLaus study. *Lancet Respir Med.* 2015 Apr;3(4):310-318.

Horner RL. Motor control of the pharyngeal musculature and implications for the pathogenesis of obstructive sleep apnea. *Sleep.* 1996;19:827-853.

Iber C, Ancoli-Israel S, Chessonn A, Quan SF. *The AASM manual for the scoring of sleep and associated events: rules, terminology and technical specification s.* 1st ed. Westchester, Illinois: American Academy of Sleep Medicine; 2007.

Kario K. Obstructive sleep apnea syndrome and hypertension: ambulatory blood pressure. *Hypertens Res.* 2009;32:428-432.

Kohler M, Stradling JR. Mechanisms of vascular damage in obstructive sleep apnea. *Nat Rev Cardiol.* 2010;7:677-685.

Lavie P. Mortality in sleep apnoea syndrome: a review of the evidence. *Eur Respir Rev.* 2007;16:203-210.

Leiter JC. Upper airway shape: Is it important in the pathogenesis of obstructive sleep apnea? *Am J Respir Crit Care Med.* 1996;153:894-898.

Lévy P, Pépin JL, Arnaud C, et al. Intermittent hypoxia and sleep-disordered breathing: current concepts and perspectives. *Eur Respir J.* 2008;32:1082-1095.

Malhotra A, Huang Y, Fogel RB, et al. The male predisposition to pharyngeal collapse. importance of airway length. *Am J Respir Crit Care Med.* 2002;166:1388-1395.

Marin JM, Carrizo SJ, Vicente E, Agusti AG. Long-term cardiovascular outcomes in men with obstructive sleep apnoea-hypopnoea with or without treatment with continuous positive airway pressure: an observational study. *Lancet.* 2005;365:1046-1053.

Marrone O, Lo Bue A, Salvaggio A, Dardanoni G, Insalaco G. Comorbidities and survival in obstructive sleep apnoea beyond the age of 50. *Eur J Clin Invest.* 2013;43:27-33.

Martínez-García MA, Campos-Rodríguez F, Catalán-Serra P, et al. Cardiovascular mortality in obstructive sleep apnea in the elderly: role of long-term continuous positive airway pressure treatment: a prospective observational study. *Am J Respir Crit Care Med.* 2012;186:909-916.

Martínez-García MA, Soler-Cataluña JJ, Ejarque-Martínez L, et al. Continuous positive airway pressure treatment reduces mortality in patients with ischemic stroke and obstructive sleep apnea. A 5-year follow-up study. *Am J Respir Crit Care Med.* 2009;180:36-41.

Mokhlesi B, Kryger MH, Grunstein RR. Assessment and management of patients with obesity hypoventilation syndrome. *Proc Am Thorac Soc.* 2008;5:218-225.

Monahan K, Storfer-Isser A, Mehra R, et al. Triggering of nocturnal arrhythmias by sleep-disordered breathing events. *J Am Coll Cardiol.* 2009;54:1797-1804.

Montesi SB, Edwards BA, Malhotra A, Bakker JP. The Effect of Continuous Positive Airway Pressure Treatment on

Blood Pressure: A systematic review and meta-analysis of randomized controlled trials. *J Clin Sleep Med.* 2012;8:587-596.

Nakashima H, Katayama T, Takagi C, et al. Obstructive sleep apnoea inhibits the recovery of left ventricular function in patients with acute myocardial infarction. *Eur Heart J.* 2006;27:2317-2322.

Neau JP, Paquereau J, Meurice JC, Chavagnat JJ, Gil R. Stroke and sleep apnoea: cause or consequence? *Sleep Med Rev.* 2002;6:457-469.

Nieto FJ, Peppard PE, Young T, Finn L, Hla KM, Farre R. Sleep-disordered breathing and cancer mortality. Results from the Wisconsin Sleep Cohort Study. *Am J Respir Crit Care Med.* 2012;186:190-194.

Olmetti F, La Rovere MT, Robbi E, Taurino AE, Fanfulla F. Nocturnal cardiac arrhythmia in patients with obstructive sleep apnea. *Sleep Med.* 2008;9:475-480.

Pamidi S, Tasali E. Obstructive sleep apnea and type 2 diabetes: is there a link? *Front Neurol.* 2012;3:126.

Peppard PE, Young T, Palta M, Dempsey J, Skatrud J. Longitudinal study of moderate weight change and sleep-disordered breathing. *JAMA.* 2000 20;284(23):3015-3021.

Petrof BJ, Hendricks JC, Pack AI. Does upper airway muscle injury trigger a vicious cycle in obstructive sleep apnea? A hypothesis. *Sleep.* 1996;19:465-471.

Resta O, Caratozzolo G, Pannacciulli N, et al. Gender, age and menopause effects on the prevalence and the characteristics of obstructive sleep apnea in obesity. *Eur J Clin Invest.* 2003;33:1084-1089.

Riha RL. Regional fat distribution and sleep apnea: sex makes a difference. *Sleep.* 2010;33:419-420.

Roche F, Pépin JL, Achour-Crawford E, Tamisier R, et al. (PROOF Study Group). At 68 years, unrecognised sleep apnoea is associated with elevated ambulatory blood pressure. *Eur Respir J.* 2012;40:649-656.

Romero-Corral A, Somers VK, Pellikka PA, et al. Decreased right and left ventricular myocardial performance in obstructive sleep apnea. *Chest.* 2007;132:1863-1870.

Ryan CM, Floras JS, Logan AG, et al. Shift in sleep apnoea type in heart failure patients in the CANPAP trial. *Eur Respir J.* 2010;35:592-597.

Schwab RJ, Gefter WB, Hoffman EA, Gupta KB, Pack AI. Dynamic upper airway imaging during awake respiration in normal subjects and patients with sleep disordered breathing. *Am Rev Respir Dis.* 1993;148:1385-1400.

Schwab RJ, Pasirstein M, Pierson R, et al. Identification of upper airway anatomic risk factors for obstructive sleep apnea with volumetric magnetic resonance imaging. *Am J Respir Crit Care Med.* 2003;168:522-530.

Serizawa N, Yumino D, Kajimoto K, et al. Impact of sleep-disordered breathing on life-threatening ventricular arrhythmia in heart failure patients with implantable cardiovert-er-defibrillator. *Am J Cardiol.* 2008;102:1064-1068.

Shah N, Redline S, Yaggi HK, et al. Obstructive sleep apnea and acute myocardial infarction severity: ischemic preconditioning? *Sleep Breath.* 2013 May;17(2):819-826. doi: 10.1007/s11325-012-0770-7.

Stamatakis KA, Punjabi NM. Effects of sleep fragmentation on glucose metabolism in normal subjects. *Chest.* 2010;137:95-101.

Sutherland K, Lee RWW, Phillips CL, et al. Effect of weight loss on upper airway size and facial fat in men with obstructive sleep apnoea. *Thorax.* 2011;66:797-803.

Valencia-Flores M, Orea A, Castaño VA, et al. Prevalence of sleep apnea and electrocardiographic disturbances in morbidly obese patients. *Obes Res.* 2000;8:262-269.

Van de Graaff WB. Thoracic influence on upper airway patency. *J Appl Physiol.* 1988;65:2124-2131.

Vgontzas AN, Bixler EO, Chrousos GP. Sleep apnea is a manifestation of the metabolic syndrome. *Sleep Med Rev.* 2005;9:211-224.

Wang X, Bi Y, Zhang Q, Pan F. Obstructive sleep apnoea and the risk of type 2 diabetes: A meta-analysis of prospective cohort studies. *Respirology.* 2013;18:140-146.

Weitzenblum E, Chaouat A, Kessler R, Canuet M. Overlap syndrome: obstructive sleep apnea in patients with chronic obstructive pulmonary disease. *Proc Am Thorac Soc.* 2008;5:237-241.

Wellman A, Jordan AS, Malhotra A, et al. Ventilatory control and airway anatomy in obstructive sleep apnea. *Am J Respir Crit Care Med.* 2004;170:1225-1232.

Wellman A, Malhotra A, Fogel RB, Edwards JK, Schory K, White DP. Respiratory system loop gain in normal men and women measured with proportional-assist ventilation. *J Appl Physiol.* 2003;94:205-212.

White LH, Bradley TD. Role of nocturnal rostral fluid shift in the pathogenesis of obstructive and central sleep apnoea. *J Physiol.* 2013 Mar;591(5):1179-1193. doi: 10.1113/jphysiol.2012.245159.

Ye L, Pien GW, Weaver TE. Gender differences in the clinical manifestation of obstructive sleep apnea. *Sleep Med.* 2009;10:1075-84.

Younes M. Role of arousals in the pathogenesis of obstructive sleep apnea. *Am J Respir Crit Care Med.* 2004;169:623-633.

Young T, Finn L, Peppard PE, et al. Sleep disordered breathing and mortality: eighteen-year follow-up of the Wisconsin Sleep Cohort. *Sleep.* 2008;31:1071-1078.

Young T, Palta M, Dempsey J, Skatrud J, Weber S, Badr S. The occurrence of sleep disordered breathing among middle-aged adults. *N Engl J Med* 1993;328: 1230-1235.

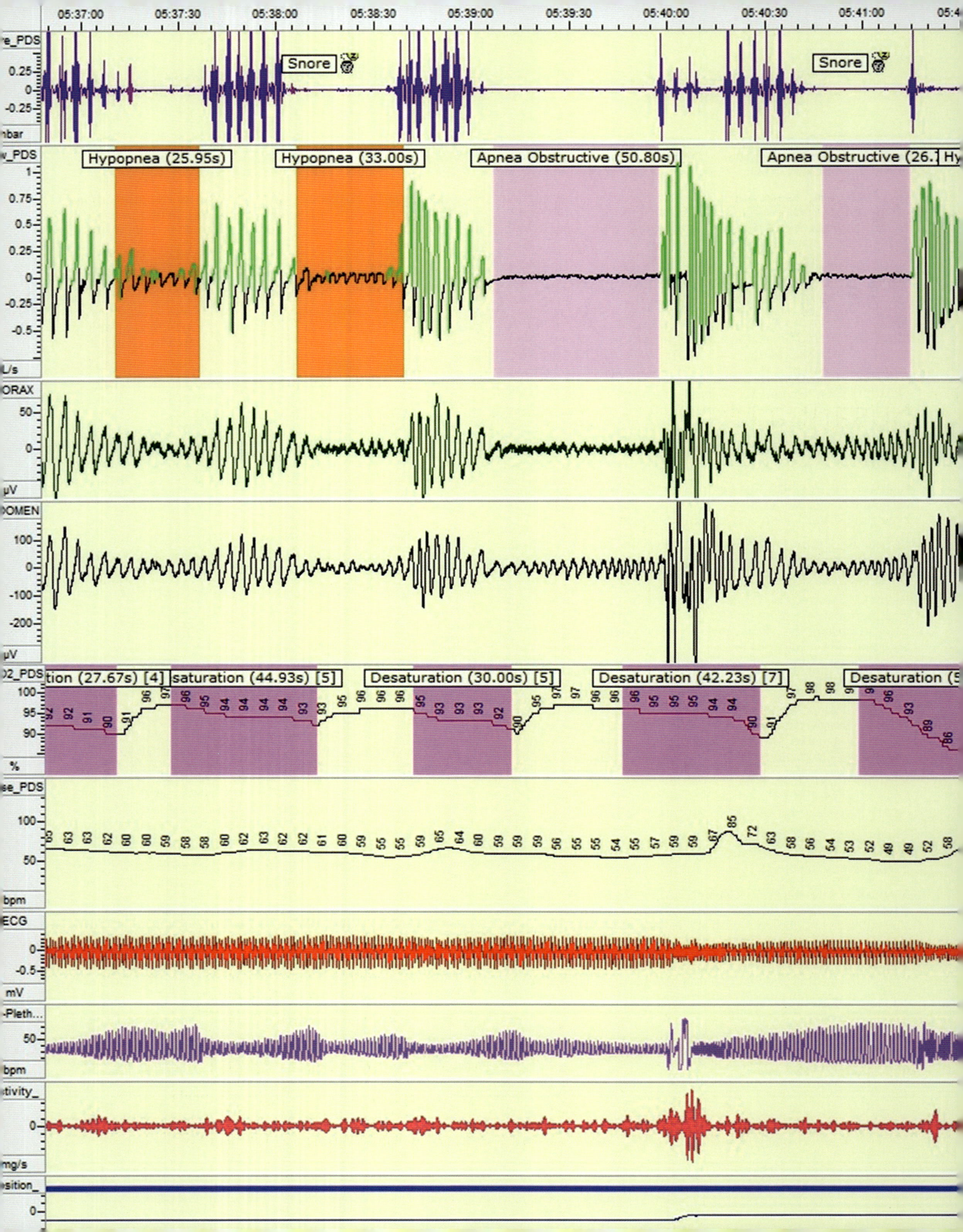

05:37:00
05:37:30
05:38:00
05:38:30
05:39:00
05:39:30
05:40:00
05:40:30
05:41:00
Snore
Snore
Hypopnea (25.95s)
Hypopnea (33.00s)
Apnea Obstructive (50.80s)
tion (27.67s) [4]
saturation (44.93s) [5]
Desaturation (30.00s) [5]
Desaturation (42.23s) [7]
ECG
L/s
µV
mV
bpm
mg/s
%

Sleep diagnosis and polysomnography

Susanna Mondini · Simone Baiardi

Objectives

- Acquiring useful knowledge about the diagnostic classification of patients with obstructive sleep apnea syndrome (OSAS)
- Learning to interpret differential diagnoses associated with obstructive sleep apnea
- Learning the differences among the available instrumental examination methods to ensure that OSAS diagnosis is made with certainty

Introduction

OSAS is a respiratory disorder that occurs during sleep and is characterized by repeated episodes of complete or partial obstruction of the upper airways (apnea or hypopnea), resulting in decreased arterial oxygen saturation (SaO_2) and microawakenings with consequences on quality of life and the cardiocerebrovascular system.

The first epidemiological cohort study conducted in the United States in the early 1990s estimated that **the prevalence of OSAS** (moderate-severe, ≥15 apneic/hypopneic events per hour of sleep) was 9% in men and 4% in women (Young *et al.* 1993). Subsequent studies on similar cohorts and longitudinal studies for 20 years have demonstrated an increase in the prevalence of OSAS: 13% in men and 6% in women aged between 30 and 70 years, particularly in young adults. This increase was attributed to an epidemic increase in obesity (Young *et al.* 2002; Peppard *et al.* 2013). More recently, a Swiss epidemiological study was performed in 2015 on a cohort of subjects of a wider age range (between 40 and 85 years; average age, 57 years; 48% men) who were only slightly overweight [average body mass index (BMI), 25.6 kg/m2]. This study was conducted with full-night in-home polysomnography, and a moderate-severe OSAS prevalence (≥15 apneic/hypopneic events per hour of sleep even without symptoms) of 23% in adult women and 49% in adult men was documented (Heinzer *et al.* 2015), which is higher than that reported by Young *et al.* (2002). However, authors believe that such results can be interpreted not only as an indication of changes in the health characteristics of the general population but also as a consequence resulting from the use of new criteria for diagnosing OSAS and the identification of respiratory sleep events that are more inclusive and better defined. Furthermore, the use of more advanced technologies for polysomnographic recordings that allow a more accurate identification and interpretation of respiratory events must be considered (Adams *et al.* 2016; Heinzer *et al.* 2016).

Although the clinical consequences of OSAS and the associated economic costs have been extensively reported, this pathology is markedly underdiagnosed worldwide. Epidemiological studies have demonstrated that 80% of men and approximately 90% of women with moderate-severe OSAS remain undiagnosed and are thus not treated correctly (Young *et al.* 1997). Therefore, interested dentists and experts in the field of respiratory disorders can help identify patients with suspected OSAS and collaborate in the appropriate multidisciplinary clinical and therapeutic management of such patients.

Snoring, the most frequently reported symptom in patients with suspected OSAS, is a very common phenomenon in approximately 30% of adults; therefore, it is essential to understand that patients with habitual snoring do not always develop OSAS but can present with an obstructive respiratory disorder of the upper airway, e.g., simple snoring or OSAS. These are two similar pathological conditions that involve very different clinical consequences. Patients with habitual snoring may also develop another respiratory sleep disorder presenting with incidental snoring or noisy breathing that manifests as snoring or is mistaken for snoring.

Therefore, a correct diagnostic classification system is the primary requirement for the adequate clinical and therapeutic management of patients with snoring.

International guidelines have confirmed that thorough sleep and clinical anamnesis are essential preliminary checkpoints for establishing a correct diagnosis of OSAS (Braghiroli *et al.* 2001; Collop *et al.* 2007; Epstein *et al.* 2009; Kapur *et al.* 2017).

However, several scientific studies have demonstrated that clinical anamnesis alone (even with the help of standardized questionnaires on various combinations of signs and symptoms) is not sensitive and specific enough to accurately diagnose OSAS (Hoffstein *et al.* 1993; Friedman *et al.* 1999), thus exposing patients with false-positive results to risks of inadequate treatment and those with false-negative results to risks of OSAS's complications not being treated.

Therefore, international guidelines state that it is fundamental to always combine clinical anamnesis with instrumental examinations, thus enabling the objective definition of the presence of a respiratory sleep disorder and its characteristics. Moreover, the evaluation of respiratory patterns during nocturnal sleep using polygraphic methods represents the gold standard to establish a diagnosis with certainty (Braghiroli *et al.* 2001; Collop *et al.* 2007; Epstein *et al.* 2009; Kapur *et al.* 2017).

The correct approach for patients with suspected OSAS includes the following:

- thorough **sleep anamnesis**, which investigates specific clinical signs and symptoms and allows the identification of possible diseases and the selection of the most suitable type of instrumental examination
- **internal medicine anamnesis** with an objective examination to identify predisposing factors and comorbidities
- **polysomnographic assessment** to distinguish simple snoring from OSAS, assess the severity of OSAS, or establish a differential diagnosis with other respiratory sleep disorders

A *correct diagnosis* and an *adequate evaluation of the severity of the disease* are the fundamental requirements for an effective therapeutic choice. Similarly, *evaluation of the anatomy of the upper airways*, a field pertaining to otolaryngologists, must also be considered.

Only by following this multistep and multispecialized approach can we possibly establish an individualized diagnostic and therapeutic approach for each patient, thus ensuring the best outcomes in terms of effectiveness and treatment adherence.

If not specified otherwise, in the following description of clinical signs and symptoms in patients with OSAS, we have referred the new International

Classification of Sleep Disorders [ICSD-3; American Academy of Sleep Medicine (AASM) 2014] and the manual "Principles and Practice of Sleep Medicine, 5th edition" (Kryger *et al.* 2011), which represent two reference texts in sleep medicine, whereas for the section above the instrumental diagnosis (whenever the bibliographic notes are not indicated in the text), we have referred the "Manual for Scoring Sleep and Associated Events" (Iber *et al.* 2012).

Sleep anamnesis

Table 2.1 summarizes the nocturnal and diurnal predictive symptoms of OSAS according to international diagnostic criteria, which will be discussed below.

2.1 Sleep anamnesis in patients with suspected OSAS.

	Nocturnal symptoms	Diurnal symptoms
Specific	Snoring Reported apnea Gasping or choking Nonrestorative sleep Insomnia	Sleepiness Tiredness
Nonspecific	Nocturia Xerostomia on awakening Diaphoresis Headache	**Cognitive disorders** **Depression** **Sexual dysfunction**
Other		Road accidents

Nocturnal symptoms

1. Snoring
2. Respiratory pauses or apnea during sleep, as reported by bed partners
3. Sudden awakenings with a gasping/choking sensation
4. Nonrestorative or fragmented sleep and insomnia

Other nonspecific symptoms based on the pathology include the following:

5. Nocturia and xerostomia or dry mouth on awakening or during arousals with a feeling of thirst, diaphoresis, and nocturnal headache on awakening

1. SNORING

The pivotal symptom in patients with suspected OSAS is **habitual snoring** (occurs at all or almost all nights) that is **persistent** for at least 6 months.

Snoring is characterized by an inspiratory noise caused by vibration of the oropharyngeal and hypopharyngeal soft tissues. Generally, it occurs every night and for the greater part of the sleep. It can be favored by the supine position, can occur only in the sleeping position or persist in all positions. Snoring often bothers the patients' bed partners who are sometimes forced to change their rooms; however, it can even be heard from another room in some cases.

Occasional snoring is less likely to indicate OSAS because it can be caused by temporary conditions such as consumption of alcohol, benzodiazepines, or myorelaxants, or it can be a result of irritative or intercurrent rhinopharyngeal inflammation factors.

The patients' bed partners or roommates are the primary reliable witnesses to describe how the patients breathe during the night, and it is always advisable to request their presence or provide indirect evidence (e.g., via telephone) during anamnesis.

Some patients with OSAS do not report snoring; this is more common in patients who sleep alone, such as women and elderly subjects.

Snoring can be clinically mistaken for other night respiratory noises such as nocturnal groaning and stridor.

- **Catathrenia** or *nocturnal groaning* is characterized by a considerably rare respiratory noise pattern that is very peculiar because it involves a protracted and noisy expiration, followed by deep inspiration (Vetrugno *et al.* 2001). It can occur for long or short durations during the night or even every night. Although the reported cases of nocturnal groaning in the literature are limited, this disorder is listed among respiratory sleep disorders in ICSD-3 (ICSD-3, page 114). This disorder does not have a clear clinical definition and does not require treatment, although in some cases wherein it occurs every night and disturbs both the patient and the bed partner, continuous positive airway pressure (CPAP) therapy has been proposed (Iriarte *et al.* 2007).
- **Nocturnal stridor** is characterized by an inspiratory sound caused by altered functionality of the vocal cords (reduced inspiratory space per paralysis in the abduction of one or both the vocal cords) occurring during sleep and in cases of some neurovegetative diseases (e.g., multiple system atrophy). It is also characterized by motor and vegetative disorders during wakefulness and by respiratory difficulties during sleep. The latter is dependent on a pathoetiological mechanism independent of OSAS (Vetrugno *et al.* 2007).

2. RESPIRATORY PAUSES OR APNEA DURING SLEEP, AS REPORTED BY BED PARTNERS

Respiratory pauses or sleep apnea have been reported by bed partners or roommates in 75% of patients with OSAS, and they are characterized by a specific respiratory pattern with snoring interrupted by considerably long silent pauses (apnea) that terminate with different noisy respiratory events (such as respiratory unblocking). After recovery of breathing at the termination of apnea, limb or overall body movements can be resumed (Hoffstein *et al.* 1995).

Because apnea occurs exclusively during sleep, patients are generally unaware about them, and similar to snoring, the only reliable witnesses are their bed partners or roommates who should always be investigated in this regard.

Patients who sleep alone can report apnea as awakening with a choking sensation, which could also be due to other causes (see below).

The incidence of apnea is higher in women with OSAS, as reported by their bed partners (Lin *et al.* 2008).

The reported cases of apnea do not necessarily indicate a pathology. Occasional sleep apnea can be normal; physiological events [e.g., rapid eye movement (REM)] that are usually sporadic may occur while falling asleep or dreaming. In such cases, patients can stop and restart breathing without any respiratory efforts (central apnea).

Furthermore, sleep apnea reported by bed partners can be different from obstructive apnea, particularly if they are not associated with snoring. In fact, there are other respiratory sleep disorders that appear as cyclical episodes of central apnea for protracted durations during the night (e.g., Cheyne-Stokes respiration in patients with cardiac diseases).

3. SUDDEN AWAKENINGS WITH A GASPING/CHOKING SENSATION

Some patients report sudden awakenings with a choking or gasping sensation that improves upon awakening or after a few seconds. This symptom has not been frequently reported in patients with OSAS (18%-31% of patients), but its presence is strongly correlated with the probability of the occurrence of the disease (Myers *et al.* 2013). Usually, patients return to sleep immediately when such awakenings occur rarely; however, generally anxious subjects and those patients in whom this symptom is frequent experience difficulties in falling back asleep and eventually have to consult a specialist.

Although they are very specific, sudden awakenings with a choking sensation may be caused by different factors (other than OSAS) such as nocturnal gastroesophageal reflux, paroxysmal nocturnal dyspnea, nocturnal asthma or bronchospasm, nocturnal hypoxemia, and nocturnal panic attacks. Sudden awakenings must be investigated, particularly if they are the only or the primary symptoms reported by the patients (For more detailed information on the different pathologies of OSAS that may cause awakenings with dyspnea or a choking sensation, including those listed below, please refer relevant text on internal medicine).

- *Nocturnal gastroesophageal reflux* is characterized by gastric secretions that flow from the esophagus to the larynx, particularly in the horizontal sleeping position, thus causing laryngospasm and eventual sudden awakenings with a choking sensation that generally persists for few breaths and is often associated with coughing. The symptom improves by consuming water or with repeated swallowing. These events appear more frequently in patients with a medical history or symptoms indicating gastroesophageal reflux disease (GERD), although subjects who do not present with other GERD symptoms may also be affected by these events because they are favored by increased negative intrathoracic pressures resulting from obstructive apnea as well as simple snoring.

- *Paroxysmal nocturnal dyspnea* is characterized by nocturnal awakenings associated with dyspnea or a choking sensation, which are typical of patients with cardiac failure diseases. Generally, it appears during phases of deficiency and is associated with semiorthopnea. Therefore, patients tend to sleep in the sitting position due to dyspnea while lying down. The clinical signs and symptoms of cardiac failure or cardiopathy must be investigated when evaluating such patients.
- *Nocturnal asthma attacks or bronchospasms* usually occur in subjects with an overt bronchial asthma diagnosis or with chronic obstructive pulmonary disease (COPD). These nocturnal dyspnea attacks are characteristically similar to daily attacks, which diminish with bronchodilator medication normally used by these patients.
- Episodes of *nocturnal hypoxemia*, which are independent of apnea and are characterized by a decrease in oxygenated blood levels during certain phases of sleep (especially during the REM phase), may occur with awakenings associated with dyspnea and a choking sensation. They are normally observed in subjects with secondary ventilatory failure with alterations in the pulmonary parenchyma (restrictive or obstructive lung diseases), thoracic cage (kyphoscoliosis), or the respiratory muscles (neuromyopathy) as well as in obese individuals with obesity hypoventilation syndrome. Even during wakefulness, these patients present with typical clinical signs and symptoms of the core disease (the arterial blood gas shows hypoxemia/hypercapnia), thus enabling a correct differential diagnosis with OSAS.
- *Anxiety disorder*, often disguised as somatic symptoms, may appear as anxiety or panic attacks only at night; they are characterized by sudden awakenings with a choking sensation or dyspnea. Its symptoms are generally associated with a sensation of anxiety that persists upon awakening and interferes with returning to sleep. It may recur several times during the night, thus disturbing the sleep. It appears in subjects with overt anxiety disorders or with nervous disposition.

4. NONRESTORATIVE OR FRAGMENTED SLEEP OR INSOMNIA

Patients with suspected OSAS often (50% of patients) report a scarcely restorative sleep with a **feeling of tiredness upon awakening** ("I feel like I did not sleep at all") even if the duration and quality of sleep are apparently satisfying. This feeling is justified by alterations in the sleep structure due to the respiratory disorder, which may appear as a modification in the sleep macrostructure (alterations in the sleep organization in phases) with a decrease particularly in the duration and quality of deep sleep as well as of REM sleep and fragmentation of the sleep microstructure [microawakenings (arousals) at the termination of each apnea].

In patients with apnea, bed partners often report restless sleep because of the patients' frequent limb or overall body movements and changes in sleeping positions that often occur at the termination of apnea (Maislin *et al.* 1995).

Some patients, particularly women, report real **insomnia** instead with *difficulty in maintaining the sleep because of repeated awakenings.* Some awakenings are caused by nocturia, whereas others do not have any apparent cause and are probably associated with respiratory events. The awakenings are often short and many in patients with apnea, whereas they are few, protracted (>30 minutes), and often occur in early mornings in patients with other forms of sleep-maintenance insomnia. In some patients, insomnia caused by other causes can be associated with OSAS, such as in menopausal women in whom both depression and OSAS represent risk factors (Shepertycky *et al.* 2005).

5. OTHER NOCTURNAL SYMPTOMS

Other frequent nocturnal symptoms that are **nonspecific** for the pathology (hence not included in the diagnostic criteria) in patients with OSAS are as follows:

- **Nocturia**, which is characterized by nocturnal awakenings with the need to urinate (2–7 awakenings per night). It is reported in 28% of patients with OSAS and is often attributed to urological complications when it is actually secondary to alterations in atrial natriuretic hormones due to changes in the intrathoracic pressure affecting the heart during obstructive apnea (Hajduk *et al.* 2003; Krieger *et al.* 1989).
- **Xerostomia or dry mouth upon awakening or intrasleep awakenings with a feeling of thirst**, which is reported in 74% of patients with OSAS, and nocturnal hypersalivation, which is reported in only 36% of patients. Both these symptoms indicate nocturnal mouth respiration.
- **Nocturnal diaphoresis** (excessive perspiration), particularly involving both the head and trunk, is possibly associated with respiratory efforts performed by patients during sleep.
- **Nocturnal headache or headache upon awakenings**, which normally has an oppressive characteristic (sensation of a heavy head) and often improves spontaneously a few hours after awakening. It often appears in noncephalalgic patients and can be an indication for increased levels of systemic arterial pressure during the night or upon awakening due to apneic episodes during sleep (Paiva *et al.* 1997).

Diurnal symptoms

1. Daytime sleepiness
2. Fatigue and fatigability

Other symptoms that are nonspecific to the pathology are as follows:
❸ Cognitive disorders, depression, and sexual dysfunction.

1. DAYTIME SLEEPINESS

Daytime sleepiness is the most important and complex symptom of OSAS.

- It appears in only 40%–60% of patients with OSAS [with apnea–hypopnea index (AHI) ≥ 5] and is possibly not associated with the severity of the syndrome; therefore, patients with severe OSAS do not present with sleepiness. However, sleepiness has been reported in 20% of patients with snoring with an AHI of <5 (Roure *et al.* 2008; Kapur *et al.* 2005).
- The cause of daytime sleepiness in patients with OSAS remains controversial because of lack of consistent observations. The presence of daytime sleepiness does not appear to be associated with the number of apneic/hypopneic events per hour of sleep. Its association with the level of compromised nocturnal oxygenation (index of SaO_2) is strong; however, it is not associated with an altered macrostructure of sleep but is associated with indices of the microfragmentation of sleep (although inconsistent). Furthermore, it appears to be associated with the presence of other sleep disorders or comorbidities (Roure *et al.* 2008; Kapur *et al.* 2005).
- The presence of daytime sleepiness in patients with OSAS influences therapeutic outcomes, particularly adherence to CPAP therapy, which is negligible in patients who do not present with sleepiness (Weaver *et al.* 2008).

Patients with OSAS demonstrate sleepiness by dozing in reduced stimulating conditions such as physical inactivity (sitting for long durations), boredom, repetitive activities, or relaxation, although it may also occur in increased stimulating conditions such as working or during social interactions (e.g., conversations). Generally, sleepiness can be prevented by body movements and stimulation activities (unlike a narcoleptic sleep attack).

The subjective perceptions of patients with OSAS about their sleepiness can considerably vary; it is often mistaken for tiredness, fatigue, boredom, or normal consequences of a tiring lifestyle. Furthermore, patients tend to adapt to their level of sleepiness and do not perceive it as a clinically significant problem.

Because of extreme variability in the subjective perceptions of patients with OSAS about sleepiness and the facts that sleepiness is not always observed in these patients and that its presence influences therapeutic choice, *daytime sleepiness must always be evaluated with standardized methods.*

Sleepiness assessment methods

Sleepiness assessment methods can be *subjective* (based on the perception and reports of the patients), *objective* (instrumental), *or indirect* (based on the consequences of sleepiness).

Subjective methods Sleepiness can be subjectively quantified on the basis of clinical criteria (simply by interviewing the patients about sleepiness when it occurs) and the descriptions presented below (American Academy of Sleep Medicine Task Force 1999):

Mild	Sleepiness occurs during activities that require minimal attention (i.e., watching television, reading, or traveling) with a mild impact on their quality of life
Moderate	Sleepiness occurs during activities that require a certain amount of attention (i.e., at meetings, concerts, theaters, and conferences) with a moderate impact on their quality of life
Severe	Sleepiness occurs during activities that require a maximum attention (i.e., during meals, conversations, and while driving) with significant impact on their quality of life

A rapid and more precise subjective method is the use of standardized self-administered questionnaires that can be given to patients while they are sitting in waiting rooms. The most frequently used questionnaire is the Epworth sleepiness scale (ESS) (Johns 1991), which measures daytime sleepiness by evaluating the tendency to doze in specific situations for a given duration of time (over the last month).

This makes it less susceptible to the influence of contingent and confounding factors (state-trait sleepiness). Therefore, ESS is the most universally used as well as the most recommended method for evaluating sleepiness. It has been translated and standardized in several languages, including Italian (Vignatelli *et al.* 2003) (📷 2.1).

A total ESS score of >10 indicates sleepiness and thus daytime sleepiness; when this score is >14, it usually represents markedly pathological sleepiness.

Although women with OSAS report daytime sleepiness equivalent to that reported by men, they often have lower ESS scores (Baldwin *et al.* 2004).

Other subjective methods are the Stanford sleepiness scale (SSS) and Karolinska sleepiness scale (KSS). These scales are based on "state," and therefore, they quantify sleepiness at specific moments in time and are more often used in research protocols and clinical practice (Hoddes *et al.* 1972; Kaida *et al.* 2006).

All subjective sleepiness assessment methods can be manipulated by patients according to their willingness to reveal or not to reveal the presence of daytime sleepiness, and this factor must always be considered when assessing the possible risk of sleepiness on driving.

Objective methods Objective methods are complex and costly and are not indicated at all in routine assessments of patients with OSAS. However, it is important to be aware of these methods because they can be necessary in spe-

EPWORTH SLEEPINESS SCALE (JOHNS 1991)

How likely are you to doze or fall asleep in the following situations in comparison with just feeling tired?

This refers to your recent routine activities.

Even if you have not performed some of these tasks recently, try to evaluate them based on how they would have affected you.

Use the following scale to select the most appropriate number corresponding to your answer for each situation:
0 = no chances of dozing or falling asleep
1 = slight chances of dozing or falling asleep
2 = moderate chances of dozing or falling asleep
3 = high chances of dozing or falling asleep

SITUATION	CHANCES OF DOZING (0–1)
1. Sitting and reading	_________
2. Watching television	_________
3. Sitting inactive at public places (e.g., at theaters or meetings)	_________
4. Traveling as a passenger in a car for an hour without any breaks	_________
5. Resting while lying down in the afternoon when circumstances permit	_________
6. Sitting and talking to someone	_________
7. Sitting quietly after lunch without consuming alcohol	_________
8. Sitting in a car stopped for a few minutes in the traffic	_________
Total	_________

This is a self-administered questionnaire, but it must be thoroughly explained to the patient to obtain correct answers

The patient must evaluate the chances of dozing or falling asleep in the abovementioned eight situations by assigning a score from 0 (no chances of dozing or falling asleep) to 3 (high chances of dozing or falling asleep) and referring to their routine activities over the past month.
The total score is determined by the sum of the single scores assigned to the different situations (0–24).

The cutoff for a normal score is 10
- Total score of ≤10: no daytime sleepiness
- Total score of 11–14: sleepiness
- Total score of >14: pathological sleepiness

The time for explaining and completing the questionnaire is <10 minutes.

2.1 Epworth sleepiness scale.

cific cases to precisely evaluate sleepiness, in comparison with that reported by the patients.

These methods employ polysomnographic procedures [electroencephalography (EEG) recordings] that enable the objective and accurate evaluations of sleepiness (time taken to fall asleep). They are usually performed at sleep laboratories with the assistance of specialized technologists. The test conditions are standardized, and the duration is 8 hours during which the patient has several opportunities to fall asleep (Littner *et al.* 2005).

There are two polysomnographic tests to assess alertness/wakefulness, and they evaluate two opposite aspects of sleepiness.

- **Multiple sleep latency test (MSLT)** evaluates the tendency to fall asleep in conditions of relaxation and lack of environmental stimuli (trying to sleep in the bed with the light off, in the sleep laboratory room). It is indicated for diagnosing idiopathic hypersomnia that is not associated with OSAS (e.g., narcolepsy). In four MSLT naps, an average sleep latency of <8 minutes is considered pathological sleepiness.
- **Maintenance wakefulness test (MWT)** evaluates the ability to stay awake and resist sleeping under conditions of extreme boredom and minimal stimulation (resisting falling asleep while sitting in a dimly lit sleep laboratory room). It is indicated for the evaluation of alertness/wakefulness in subjects exposed to potential risks of work-related accidents [e.g., commercial motor vehicle (CMV) drivers] or for demonstrating the effectiveness of therapy in patients with sleepiness (e.g., patients with OSAS receiving treatment). In four MWT naps of a maximum of 40 minutes, an average sleep latency of ≥30 minutes indicates a normal ability to resist sleep, that of <8 minutes indicates pathological sleepiness, and that between 8 and 30 minutes indicates borderline sleepiness, but its interpretation is controversial (Littner *et al.* 2005).

For further studies on modalities of the execution and interpretation of these tests, please refer to Littner *et al.* (2005).

The objective methods to assess sleepiness can also be partially manipulated by patients (in cases where they intentionally do not follow instructions), but to a lesser extent, this can be identified according to the performance tests.

Indirect methods These are performance tests that evaluate task execution. Errors in the execution of the given tasks indicate an indirect manifestation of sleepiness.

There are several tests to assess alertness/wakefulness; however, there is no standardized method. These tests comprise sessions evaluating the time of visual and motor responses (performance vigilance task). The Oxford sleep resistance test (OSLER) measures subjects' ability to maintain wakefulness and evaluates the capacity to respond to repeated visual stimuli (a light) with trials at different times of the day in a laboratory setting, which is similar to that in the MWT (Priest *et al.* 2001).

The more interesting and specialized tests are undoubtedly the driving simulation tests, which evaluate the driving performance of subjects in a laboratory setting using fairly complex simulators of a monotonous driving scenario for an extended duration of time (Contardi *et al.* 2004; Pizza *et al.* 2008; Philip *et al.* 2013). Although the results obtained in these tests reveal a high correlation among the polysomnographic alertness tests, they are not predictive of the risks of road accidents.

All performance tests, including the sleepiness evaluating tests, are strongly influenced by the patients' willingness to execute the test correctly, their capacity of paying attention and concentrating during the trial (age is an important factor), and learning.

The different subjective, objective, and indirect sleepiness assessment methods in patients with OSAS appear to demonstrate an unusual correlation between them and the risks of road accidents. This confirms that sleepiness is a complex problem in such patients, thus making it difficult to standardize a diagnostic method to evaluate sleepiness in patients with OSAS, particularly regarding their capability to drive.

When interviewing patients with snoring about their sleepiness, we must always be aware of the following fundamental physiological, behavioral, and clinical aspects of this phenomenon:

- a higher tendency to fall asleep and thus to sleepiness is physiologically normal in the early afternoon (13:00–16:00), independent of food consumption, and in the evening (after 21:00–22:00). Therefore, sleepiness reported at these times of the day could not be pathological
- the primary cause of excessive daytime sleepiness is chronic sleep deprivation, which is a common condition in the current society where sleep time is compromised to do "something else." To cause chronic sleep deprivation, it is sufficient to slightly reduce the duration of sleep (by 30 min) compared with the estimated sleep duration needed (average, 7 hours/day) every day for an extended duration of time
- daytime sleepiness can be caused by clinical problems that are different from OSAS, such as the following:
  - *Other sleep disturbances:* idiopathic hypersomnia (e.g., narcolepsy or idiopathic hypersomnia), motor dysfunctions that fragment the sleep (e.g., periodic limb movement disorder), parasomnia or other mood disorders during sleep, and sleep-wake disorders (ICSD-3)
  - *Neurological pathologies:* **such as Parkinson's disease, stroke, or forms of dementia**
  - *Depression*
  - *Obesity:* independent of the presence of associated OSAS
  - *Psychotropic drugs:* acting on the central nervous system and, to a lesser extent, other medications such as antihypertensive drugs (β-blockers) and antihistamines

All these clinical conditions may be associated with OSAS and may be responsible for a **failed improvement in daytime sleepiness** in the treated patients.

Therefore, during clinical anamnesis of patients with suspected OSAS, it is necessary to thoroughly investigate the duration and quality of sleep and verify the presence of other pathologies as well as analyze the medications they are taking.

Risks of road accidents

Excessive daytime sleepiness is commonly considered the cause of increased risks of road accidents in patients with OSAS. Although the most recent studies have demonstrated a weak and inconsistent correlation between the subjective and objective sleepiness assessment methods and the risks of road accidents, a study has also demonstrated a strong correlation between these assessment methods and the severity of OSAS (in terms of both respiratory events and SaO_2 indices) (Tregear *et al.* 2009).

All these studies have reported that the risk of road accidents is significantly increased in patients with OSAS compared with that in patients without OSAS (odds ratio of 1.22–4.89) both for car and CMV drivers even if the latter are more exposed to risk conditions (Tregear *et al.* 2009).

Therefore, it is always necessary to investigate patients with snoring about sleepiness while driving, accidents that were risked or that have occurred over the past years, and their profession. It is particularly important to determine whether patients are CMV drivers because the therapeutic choice for them must consider the need to reduce the risks of road accidents and eliminate sleepiness.

2. TIREDNESS

Tiredness is often reported by patients with OSAS. This symptom is frequently mistaken for sleepiness, which is the tendency to doze. Sometimes it is characterized by limited energy and easy fatigability due to nonrestorative sleep.

3. OTHER DIURNAL SYMPTOMS

Cognitive disorders and depression are other diurnal symptoms frequently associated with OSAS, but they are **nonspecific** for the pathology.

- **Cognitive disorders** are reported by a considerably high percentage (up to ca. 25%) of patients with OSAS. They are characterized by a deficit in executive functions, mainly presenting as a deterioration in information processing and decision-making capacity, a reduction in attention (on performance tests), and impaired memory in one or more domains (verbal, visual, and long- or short-term memory) (Kielb *et al.* 2012). Studies using functional magnetic resonance imaging (MRI) have highlighted that the affected brain areas in patients with OSAS were the prefrontal, frontal, and parietal cortices as well as the hippocampus. Neuronal damage is possibly attributed to different factors such as intermittent hypoxia, inflammatory processes associated with sleep-disordered breathing (SDB), altered sleep, and daytime sleepiness. The onset of cognitive disorders is considerably favored by concurrent conditions such as aging, male sex, a detrimental lifestyle (i.e., alcohol consumption and smoking), the presence of comorbidities (i.e., hypertension, diabetes mellitus, metabolic syndrome, and stroke), and a genetic predisposition to cognitive disorders (Lal *et al.* 2012).

- **Depression** is a mood disorder associated with OSAS and is present in 20% of the patients. When this symptom is secondary, it regresses with appropriate treatment of the respiratory disorder. Depression should be investigated when daytime sleepiness persists in patients with OSAS who are effectively treated. Similarly, the symptoms of OSAS should be investigated when patients with depression do not respond effectively to an antidepressant therapy (Schroder *et al.* 2005; Ejaz *et al.* 2011).
- Approximately one-third of patients with OSAS develop **sexual dysfunction**, particularly decreased libido and impotence. These disorders appear to be associated with the severity of nocturnal hypoxemia determined by apnea and can improve with therapy (Gonçalves *et al.* 2005).

Sex and sleep anamnesis in patients with OSAS

In the general population, the ratio of men:women with OSAS ranges from 3:1 to 8:1 among patients visiting sleep centers to be evaluated, indicating that women with OSAS are often not identified clinically because they report atypical symptoms or report symptoms in a different manner compared with men.

Notably, some scientific studies have demonstrated that women go to medical consultation alone and are not accompanied by their partners and that women report snoring as men, but their snoring is less intense and annoying. Apneic events witnessed by the patients' partners are more rarely reported, whereas women report more frequent awakenings with a choking sensation and palpitations. Regarding sleep disorders, they also complain of insomnia with difficulty in falling asleep, muscular pain, and migraines upon awakening. Diurnal symptoms include tiredness, limited energy, cognitive disorders, and depression (Lin *et al.* 2008).

The different clinical presentations in men and women may also depend on the fact that men develop more severe forms of OSAS more frequently.

As a result of the severity and atypicality of the presented symptoms, women are often erroneously diagnosed with a different pathology from OSAS, particularly in cases of depression, other sleep disorders, or internal medicine pathologies (e.g., fibromyalgia).

Clinical anamnesis and objective examinations

Performing a correct clinical analysis should be a part of general diagnostic work-ups when patients consult dentists, particularly those who are interested in respiratory sleep disorders; these dentists should:

- particularly focus on all the clinical conditions that are *predisposing factors* for OSAS and on the presence of pathologies that are strongly correlated with OSAS (*comorbidities*) to identify patients with suspected OSAS who are unaware of their pathology
- investigate the presence of comorbidities that influence individual therapeutic choices for patients already identified with snoring and suspected OSAS

Predisposing factors

The predisposing factors for OSAS include physiological, anatomical, and clinical conditions that are significantly associated with the pathology (■ 2.2).

Obesity. The association between respiratory sleep disorders and obesity has long been demonstrated. In fact, it was initially termed "Pickwickian syndrome" based on a character of Charles Dickens' "Pickwick Club,"—Joe, the fat boy "who is always asleep and who snores." Currently, ICSD-3 defines this term incorrect and unacceptable to identify OSAS because it may be confused for obesity hypoventilation syndrome, which has different pathophysiological characteristics (Bickelemann *et al.* 1956).

BMI (weight in kg/height in m2) is certainly the most used parameter to evaluate body weight. It distinguishes individuals according to normal weight (BMI 20.0–24.9 kg/m^2), overweight (BMI 25.0–29.9 kg/m^2), first-degree obesity (BMI 30.0–34.9 kg/m^2), second-degree obesity (BMI 35.0–39.9 kg/m^2), and third-degree obesity (BMI ≥ 40 kg/m^2).

■ **2.2** Predisposing factors for OSAS.

Body mass index	≥30 kg/m^2
Neck circumference	≥43 cm for men, ≥41 cm for women
Waist-to-hip ratio	>1.0 for men, >0.86 for women
Age	≤65 years
Sex	Male
	Female (women in menopause and pregnant women)
Heredity	Doubled risk in those whose relatives have developed the pathology
Anatomic factors	Craniofacial dysmorphism Skeletal conformation Syndromic patients
	Hypertrophy of the soft tissues in the oropharynx Tonsillar hypertrophy Mallampati Classes III and IV

Obesity is certainly the **primary predisposing factor for OSAS**. Epidemiological studies on the general population have demonstrated **a direct correlation between BMI and the prevalence of OSAS**. In the Sleep Heart Health Study, the prevalence of OSAS was 10% in subjects with a BMI of 16–24 kg/m^2, 13% in those with a BMI of 24–28 kg/m^2, 17% in those with a BMI of 28–32 kg/m^2, and 32% in those with a BMI of 32–59 kg/m^2 (Young *et al.* 2005).

Regarding patients with moderate or severe OSAS (AHI > 15), 58% of them are overweight or obese (Young *et al.* 2005), whereas the prevalence of OSAS was up to 80% in subjects with a BMI of ≥30 kg/m^2 and up to 98% in subjects with a BMI of ≥40 kg/m^2, as reported by studies on samples of obese individuals (Vgontzas *et al.* 1994; Valencia-Flores *et al.* 2000; Resta *et al.* 2001).

Generally, a BMI of ≥30 kg/m2 is an important risk factor for OSAS.

In particular, **central obesity**, i.e., fat distribution in androgen-dependent body areas (neck-torso-abdomen) is correlated with the development of OSAS.

A pathological **neck circumference** (2.2) of >43 cm in men and >41 cm in women is significantly correlated with the presence of OSAS and its severity, independent of visceral obesity, thus representing a predisposing factor for OSAS even in nonobese patients (Kawaguchi *et al.* 2011).

The **waist-to-hip ratio** (indicates pathology when this ratio is >1 in men and >0.86 in women) is another index of central obesity that is significantly correlated with the presence of a respiratory sleep disorder, which is independent of BMI. This ratio differs between patients with OSAS and healthy controls as well as those with simple snoring, particularly in men (Subramanian *et al.* 2012; Martinez-Rivera *et al.*, 2008).

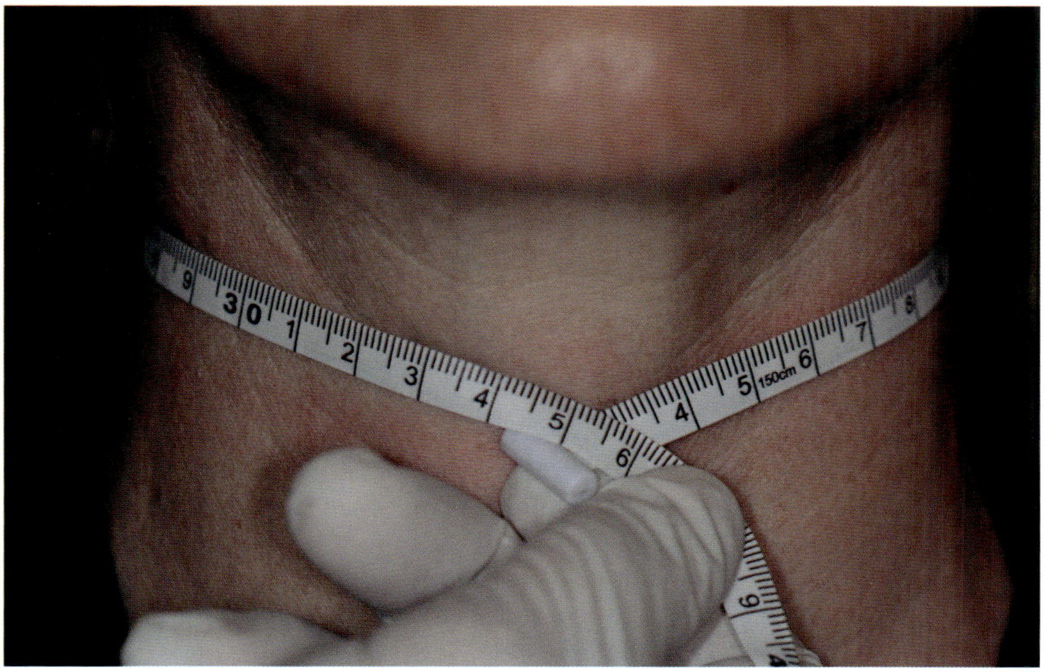

2.2 Measurement of the neck circumference.

Sex. Men are constitutionally more predisposed to develop snoring and OSAS than women, and in the general population, the ratio of men:women with OSAS ranges from 3:1 to 5:1. There are several possible causes for such differences, and factors related to anatomy (a longer and more collapsible oropharyngeal tract or a larger and retrodisplaced tongue) and functionality of the upper airways (men have less respiratory stability in response to stimuli and hormonal factors; estrogen and progesterone play a protective role, whereas testosterone plays a favoring role) must be investigated (Lin *et al.* 2008) The development of OSAS is also favored by the different deposition patterns of adipose tissue, which is visceral and deposits particularly in the neck and torso in men. Furthermore, weight gain worsens the severity of OSAS to a greater extent than that in women.

The prevalence of OSAS in women markedly increases after menopause, independent of age and BMI. Hormone replacement therapy appears to play a favorable role in the prevention and treatment of OSAS, although this is still controversial because of the risks associated with this therapy (Young *et al.* 2003; Bixler *et al.* 2001). Pregnancy, particularly during the last months, is a predisposing factor for OSAS, and it should always be investigated because it is significantly correlated with the risk of developing hypertension, glucose intolerance, and preeclampsia (Pien *et al.* 2013; Reutrakul *et al.* 2013).

Age. Epidemiological studies on subjects aged 30–70 years have demonstrated a linear correlation between age and the prevalence of OSAS (the proportion of patients with OSAS increases with aging according to all the different diagnostic criteria used). The increased risk of developing OSAS with age is more evident in women because it overlaps with changes that are correlated with menopause (Peppard *et al.* 2013). Studies on a population of a wider age range (Sleep Heart Health Study: 40–98 years) have highlighted that the risk of developing OSAS increases significantly between young and middle-aged subjects, whereas it stabilizes or even decreases in older subjects (aged >65 years), particularly becausE moderate-severe OSAS (≥15 apneic/hypopneic events per hour of sleep) is more significantly correlated with cardiovascular risks (Young *et al.* 2002).

Furthermore, the presence of OSAS is weakly correlated with obesity as well as with clinical symptoms that are indicative of the pathology (strong and persistent snoring, reported apnea and sleepiness) in subjects aged >65 years. Moreover, some studies have also reported this weak correlation with the presence of cardiovascular complications. Therefore, OSAS should be thoroughly investigated in older subjects, independently of the presence of predictive factors, to decide whether there is an indication for appropriate treatment (Young *et al.* 2002).

The risk of fatal complications of OSAS is also correlated with age in men; considering all the causes, men with moderate-severe OSAS present a mortality risk that is higher if they are younger than 50 years old (Lavie *et al.* 2005). In conclusion, patients with a higher risk are those aged between 30 and 65 years, whereas the risk for fatal complications of moderate-severe OSAS is higher in young men aged <50 years than in older men (Lavie *et al.* 2005).

Ethnicity. OSAS has been indicated in all races. Compared with Caucasians, OSAS is more frequent in African Americans, Hispanics, and inhabitants of the Pacific Islands and Eastern Asia (particularly Chinese). Despite their slim build, the latter present craniofacial characteristics as predisposing factors for OSAS (O'Connor *et al.* 2003).

Heredity. Individuals whose relatives have developed OSAS are twice as likely to develop OSAS depending on the hereditariness of craniofacial conformation and ventilatory control.

Predisposing anatomical conditions. These represent important predisposing factors for OSAS, particularly in slim patients. These factors can be more accurately evaluated by specific and specialized examinations (e.g., endoscopy, radiology, and telecephalometry). A simple objective evaluation of patient enables the overall identification of favoring conditions that might require further investigation.

The presence of craniofacial dysmorphism due to even minor skeletal alterations in the facial bones (e.g., a retropositioned and vertically oriented mandible, narrow and arched palate, occlusal alterations, and bimaxillary retroposition) must always be evaluated, and dentists usually have the required equipment and tools to perform such evaluations.

Furthermore, the so-called syndromic patients are affected by complex syndromes and craniofacial dysmorphism that predispose them to OSAS. In such cases, the symptoms of the disease are often undervalued, whereas they should always be investigated (Down syndrome, acromegaly, achondroplasia, mucopolysaccharidosis, Marfan syndrome, Apert syndrome, Pierre Robin sequence, and Treacher Collins syndrome) (Villa *et al.* 2005).

Hypertrophy of the oropharyngeal soft tissues and its role in the collapse of the upper airways can only be properly evaluated via an endoscopy during wakefulness or sleep; moreover, approximate objective evaluations enable the identification of conditions that highly predispose individuals to OSAS. These include the following:

- adenotonsillar hypertrophy (the primary cause of OSAS in children and adolescents) or only tonsillar hypertrophy in adults, which can be precisely evaluated using the tonsillar hypertrophy grading scale (Friedman *et al.* 2002)
- macroglossia, which is better evaluated with the modified Mallampati classification (Mallampati *et al.* 1985)
- uvula and soft palate hypertrophy

After being examined by dentists, patients with suspected OSAS who present clear craniofacial dysmorphism or hypertrophy of the oropharyngeal soft tissue must always be investigated by a competent specialists (facial maxillary surgeon and/or otolaryngologist) for proper therapeutic planning.

Pathological conditions associated with OSAS (comorbidities)

Several internal medicine pathologies are significantly correlated with OSAS. With fairly strong evidence, OSAS has been identified as an independent risk factor (from other confounding factors, i.e., obesity) in some pathologies, whereas OSAS can be an aggravating or advancing factor in other pathologies (■ 2.3 e 2.4).

These pathologies must always be investigated in clinical anamnesis for two reasons. First, because their presence suggests an association with OSAS that needs to be subsequently investigated with sleep anamnesis. Second, because the presence of physical comorbidities influences the choice of the most appropriate therapy in patients with OSAS (Epstein *et al.* 2009).

The primary internal medicine pathologies for which OSAS represents a proven or possible significant **risk factor** are:

- arterial hypertension, particularly diastolic and not treated with drugs (proved as independent risk factors for OSAS)
- type 2diabetes mellitus (possible independent risk factors for OSAS)
- previous ischemic stroke or recurrent transient ischemic attacks (possible independent risk factor of OSAS)
- atrial fibrillation or nocturnal cardiac arrhythmia (possible independent risk factor OSAS)
- coronary diseases (possible independent risk factor for OSAS).

■ **2.3** Primary comorbidities for which OSAS is a significant risk factor.

Arterial hypertension	Particularly diastolic and if it is not treated with drugs OSAS sicuro fattore di rischio indipendente
Type 2 diabetes mellitus	Proven independent risk factor for OSAS
Previous ischemic stroke or recurrent transient ischemic attacks	Probable independent risk factor of OSAS
Atrial fibrillation or nocturnal cardiac arrhythmia	Possible independent risk factor for OSAS
Coronary disease	Possible independent risk factor for OSAS

■ **2.4** Primary comorbidities for which OSAS is an aggravating or advancing factor.

Congestive cardiac failure	Aggravating or advancing factor for OSAS in comorbidities with other cardiac pathologies
Pulmonary hypertension	Aggravating or precipitating factor of OSAS in comorbidities with other cardiac or pulmonary pathologies
Gastroesophageal reflux disease	Negative endothoracic pressure due to apnea favor reflux, particularly in patients with hiatal hernia

The primary internal medicine pathologies for which OSAS is an aggravating or advancing factor are:

- congestive cardiac failure (aggravating or advancing factor for OSAS in comorbidities with other cardiac pathologies);
- pulmonary hypertension (aggravating or precipitating factor of OSAS in comorbidities with other cardiac or pulmonary pathologies);
- gastroesophageal reflux disease (negative endothoracic pressure due to apnea favor reflux, particularly in patients with hiatal hernia).

Instrumental examination (polysomnography)

Over the years, several studies have demonstrated and confirmed that there is neither a clinical model comprising a combination of objective signs and symptoms nor a standardized subjective questionnaire (the Berlin and STOP-Bang questionnaires are the most studied and used ones) that can reliably predict the presence and severity of OSAS. However, clinical signs and symptoms are fundamental for evaluating the risk of OSAS, which is based on selecting the modality of the instrumental examination (there are several methods of polysomnographic recording) and determining how urgent it is to establish the patients' diagnosis and proceed with treatment (according to the clinical risks associated with OSAS) (Fleetman *et al.* 2011; Epstein *et al.* 2009; Kapur *et al.* 2017).

Therefore, international guidelines affirm that to achieve a correct diagnosis of OSAS, it is always necessary to perform an instrumental examination to objectively evaluate the respiratory pattern during sleep. This examination is generically known as **polysomnography**, and it allows the continuous and simultaneous recording of different physiological parameters during spontaneous sleep at night, thus enabling the precise identification of respiratory events and their consequences (Braghiroli *et al.* 2001; Epstein *et al.* 2009; Kapur *et al.* 2017).

The data from the medical literature on the variability in respiratory patterns across different nights indicate that one night of instrumental recording with at least 4 hours of sleep (recorded or estimated) is sufficient to establish a diagnosis of OSAS. Furthermore, it is recommended that patients must spend at least 10% of their time in the supine position (ca. 20–30 minutes) to evaluate its effect on respiratory sleep patterns and to correctly identify patients with positional OSAS (POSA) (Epstein *et al.* 2009; Braghiroli *et al.* 2017).

Different types of polysomnography

The modalities of polysomnographic recordings differ according to the setting in which the examination is performed (at a sleep laboratory or at the patient's home) and the number of recorded parameters.

An attended examination is performed at a sleep laboratory; it requires the continuous presence of a specialized healthcare team (sleep technician, nurse, or respiratory physiotherapist) assisting the patients and monitoring the quality of the recording track throughout the examination. This allows us to correct any technical problems that may have occurred during the night, which would otherwise affect the interpretation of the examination; obtain precise information about the patients during the examination, and intervene in cases if necessary.

An unattended examination is performed at the patient's home; it only requires the presence of specialized personnel at its initiation and completion (to place and remove the sensors for recording), without monitoring the patient or the recording.

It is obvious that the attended examination is always reliable and correctly interpretable. However, it is very costly because of the continuous presence of the specialized healthcare team for 8–9 hours/day. Conversely, the unattended examination is less costly because it does not require a clinical setting, and the personnel are only present for a limited time. The risk of obtaining recordings that cannot be correctly interpreted in the case of technical problems occurring during the night, which compromise the quality of the signals or polysomnographic patterns because the behavior of the patient at that precise moment of the recording is unknown. Several clinical trials comparing the two methods have demonstrated that approximately 10% of patients who were evaluated using a sleep testing device at home had to be re-evaluated at a sleep laboratory to ensure their appropriate management. This partly reduces the real economic advantage of the unattended method (El Shayeb *et al.* 2014).

AASM identifies four levels of instrumental recordings that can be used for diagnosing OSAS according to decreasing complexity and costs (Ferber *et al.* 1994; Kushida *et al.* 2005) (■ 2.5).

- **Full-night polysomnography at a sleep laboratory or standard polysomnography (Level I)**. This enables the recording of sleep, respiratory parameters, SaO_2, cardiac activity, inferior limb movement, body position, and any other parameter that is considered necessary for the clinical diagnosis (>7 parameters). A video recording of the patients throughout the night can be used (video polysomnography). The examination is continuously attended.
- **Full-night unattended polysomnography, ambulatory testing (Level II)**. This enables the recording of the same parameters (>7 parameters), but it is unattended.
- **Respiratory monitoring (Level III)**. This does not record the sleep but records all the other parameters, i.e., airflow, respiratory effort, SaO_2, cardiac frequency [electrocardiography (ECG)], body position and if necessary the movement of the inferior limbs (>4 parameters). It is usually unattended.

2.5 Instrumental examination methods for diagnosing OSAS according to AASM.

	Level I Night polysomnography in a sleep laboratory	Level II Full-night ambulatory polysomnography	Level III Cardiorespiratory monitoring/ polygraphy	Level IV Nocturnal oximetry
Minimum parameters	>7 EEG EOG Submental EMG Airflow Respiratory effort (from thoracoabdominal movements) SaO_2 ECG	>7 EEG EOG Submental EMG Airflow Respiratory effort (from thoracoabdominal movements) SaO_2 ECG	>4 Airflow Respiratory effort (from thoracoabdominal movements) SaO_2 ECG or cardiac frequency	<4 SaO_2 Cardiac frequency + airflow or respiratory effort
Lower limb movements EMG lower limbs	Recommended	Recommended	Possible	Not possible
Body position	It can be documented by a video recording or can be objectively evaluated	It must be objectively evaluated	It must be objectively evaluated	Not measured
Noise of snoring	Desirable but optional	Desirable but optional	Desirable but optional	Not recorded
Personnel	Constantly present	Not present	Not present	Not present
Intervention during examination	Possible	Not possible	Not possible	Not possible

Instrumental evaluation methods according to AASM

EEG: measurement of electrical brain activity for the interpretation of wake-sleep monitored by surface electrodes placed on the scalp. The recommended derivations are: F4/M1 + C4/M1 + O2/M1 (*).

EOG: measurement of ocular movements for the interpretation of wake-sleep (REM sleep) detected by surface electrodes placed at the side of the eyes. The recommended derivations are: E1/M2 (right eye) + E2/M2 (left eye) (*).

EMG: muscular activity measured by surface electrodes placed in the middle of the muscle. The recommended muscles are submentalis for detecting muscle atonia in REM sleep and tibialis anterior for detecting nocturnal myoclonus in the lower limbs. It is possible to use any other muscle according to the clinical needs of the patient (*).

EEG + EOG + SUBMENTAL EMG: essential parameters for sleep evaluation

AIRFLOW: passage of air through the upper airways (nasopharynx) measured with a nasal cannula and/or oronasal thermistor. Recommended: nasal cannula to identify hypopnea (*) and oronasal thermistor to identify apnea. When it is not possible to apply both the devices and only once can be used, the nasal cannula is recommended. In cases of malfunctioning of the previously mentioned sensors, the flow can be indirectly derived from the thoracoabdominal dynamics (X-flow) (*).

RESPIRATORY EFFORT: the characteristics of the respiratory activity are detected through the chest and abdomen movements. Recommended: torso movements detected by a plethysmography belt placed around the ribcage; abdomen movements detected via a plethysmography belt placed in the periumbilical area (*).

ECG: detection of electrical heart activity using surface electrodes placed on the torso. The placement of a single derivation II on the torso (one electrode on the right clavicle and the reference electrode on the left midaxillary line) is recommended.

SaO_2: Arterial oxygen saturation detected with a pulse oximeter, usually applied to a finger (sampling >3 v/s). This sensor also detects the cardiac frequency.

Legend:

Upper frame: characteristics of different instrumental evaluation methods accepted by AASM for diagnosing OSAS

Lower frame: definitions and recommendations relative to the recordable parameters

(*): Further clarification about which sensors to employ and their correct placement can be found in AASM Manual for Scoring Sleep and Associated Events, 2nd Ed., Westchester, 2012.

Sources: Ferber *et al.* 1994; Kushida *et al.* 2005; Collop et al. 2007; Iber *et al.* 2012

- **Monitoring 1–3 bioparameters (Level IV).** This records a limited number of cardiorespiratory parameters (<4 parameters) usually through pulse oximeter sensor measuring SaO_2 and cardiac frequency. Airflow and respiratory efforts can also be investigated. It is always unattended.

Due to the increasing availability and widespread use of ambulatory recording systems in the diagnosis of OSAS, AASM has recently dismissed the distinction among ambulatory methods (Levels II–IV) by defining them as out-of-center (sleep) testing and proposing a new and more complex classification system labeled with the acronym SCOPER (Sleep, Cardiac, Oximetry, Position, Effort, and Respiration) (Collop *et al.* 2011). The SCOPER score can be calculated for every recording system available in the market. It allows the precise identification of the technical characteristics of the system (type of sensors used) and an evaluation of the complexity of the instrumental recording that was previously classified according to different levels (with sleep recording, without sleep recording but with recording of all respiratory parameters, and with recording of only some of the respiratory parameters).

Considering the technological advancements and the growing complexity of the ambulatory methods, this scoring system has mainly been established with the aim to simplify and make AASM certification more efficient for the facilities provided in the US, such as instrumental services outside sleep medicine centers (corresponding with our service of providing sleep medicine at the patient's home). However, this classification system has not yet been used in guidelines or scientific studies, which extensively use the Level I–IV classification system to date. Therefore, we have also used the Level I–IV classification system in this chapter. Moreover, we aimed to maintain consistency with other similar classification systems used by other international and national scientific societies (see below).

The **European Sleep Research Society** (ESRS) acknowledges three instrumental procedures used for diagnosing sleep disorders (Fischer *et al.* 2012) (■ 2.6).

- **Full-night polysomnography**, which records the sleep and all other physiological parameters required for diagnosis (same as Level I and II examinations). It can be performed at a sleep laboratory (same as Level I polysonography) or unattended (same as Level II polysonography)
- **Polygraphy**, which does not record sleep but records all the cardiorespiratory parameters (level III respiratory monitoring)
- **Reduced/limited monitoring**, which records only a limited number of cardiorespiratory parameters (equivalent to Level IV monitoring)

Italian guidelines. The Italian Association of Sleep Medicine (AIMS)-*Associazione Italiana Pneumologi Ospedalieri* (AIPO; Italian Association of Hospital Pulmonologists) procedures to diagnose OSAS in adults identify four modalities of instrumental recording that coincide with the four AASM levels (Braghiroli *et al.* 2001).

- **Full-night polysomnography at a sleep laboratory**, which records the sleep and all other parameters required (same as Level I).

2.6 Instrumental evaluation methods according to ESRS.

	Full-night polysomnography (attended or unattended)	Polygraphy	*Limited monitoring*
Minimum parameters	>7 EEG EOG Submental EMG Airflow Respiratory effort (from thoracoabdominal movements) SaO_2 ECG	>4 Airflow Respiratory effort (from thoracoabdominal movements) SaO_2 ECG or cardiac frequency	<4 SaO_2 cardiac frequency + airflow or respiratory effort
Lower limbs movement EMG of lower limbs	Recommended	Possible	Not possible
Body Position	It can be documented by a video recording or can be objectively measured	It must be objectively measured	Not measured
Noise of snoring	Desirable but optional	Desirable but optional	Not recorded
Personnel	Present in the attended procedure	Not present	Not present
Intervention during the examination	Possible	Not possible	Not possible

EEG: electroencephalography, EOG, electrooculography; EMG, electromyography

- **Full-night ambulatory polysomnography at the patient's home**, which records the sleep and all other parameters required (same as Level II).
- **Full-night cardiorespiratory monitoring at the patient's home**, which records all the cardiorespiratory parameters but not sleep (same as Level III).
- **Reduced/limited cardiorespiratory monitoring**, which records a limited number of cardiorespiratory parameters (e.g., SaO_2, cardiac frequency, airflow, and body position) (same as Level IV).

It is important to identify the correct names for the several methods of instrumental recording used for diagnosing OSAS because this allows the most adequate type of examination that can be requested of each patient and an understanding of the characteristics of the performed examination in patients who have already been analyzed. Table 2.7 summarizes the comparison between the recording procedures used by the AASM, ESRS, and AIMS-AIPO guidelines.

2.7 Comparison of the instrumental evaluation methods according to the AASM, ESRS, and AIMS-AIPO guidelines.

AIMS-AIPO	Full-night polysomnography at a sleep laboratory	Full-night ambulatory polysomnography	Full-night cardiorespiratory monitoring	Limited cardiorespiratory monitoring
AASM	Level I	Level II	Level III	Level IV
ESRS	Full-night polysomnography		Polygraphy	Limited monitoring

Which instrumental method can be used for diagnosing OSAS?

All international and national guidelines consider full-night polysomnography at a sleep laboratory the gold standard because it evaluates sleep and all cardiorespiratory parameters while continuously monitoring the patient and the recording. Therefore, it has an accuracy of 100% for OSAS diagnosis, disease severity staging, and differential diagnosis with other respiratory sleep disorders (Kushida *et al.* 2005; Collop *et al.* 2007; Kapur *et al.* 2017). However, this examination can only be performed at a sleep laboratory, and it involves high costs that significantly limit its diagnostic accessibility.

Home sleep apnea testing (HSAT) ambulatory recording methods, particularly cardiorespiratory monitoring systems or Level III polygraphy, are currently used by major international scientific societies for diagnosing OSAS because comparative studies have revealed that these methods provide good diagnostic accuracy and good capacity to correctly direct the patients to a therapy (Collop *et al.* 2007; Phurroug *et al.* 2009; Fleetham *et al.* 2011). However, their use must be limited in some cases, which must be fundamentally identified and considered in daily clinical practice (Collop *et al.* 2007; Gay *et al.* 2010, Kuna 2010; Kapur *et al.* 2017).

The latest AASM guidelines on the diagnosis of OSAS in adult patients specify that (Kapur *et al.* 2017):

- HSAT is acceptable to establish a diagnosis of OSAS *only* if associated with a thorough clinical anamnesis of the patients
- HSAT is acceptable to establish a diagnosis of OSAS *in uncomplicated adult patients with an increased risk of moderate or severe OSAS*
- *uncomplicated patients* are those who do not present with clinical conditions that favor the presence of respiratory disorders of a central type (cardiopathy, neurological pathologies, or the use of opiates) or other sleep disorders that may interfere with the reliability of HSAT (e.g., insomnia, motor disorders or behavioral sleep disorders, or other forms of hypersomnia)
- *indicative signs and symptoms of an increased risk of OSAS* are excessive daytime sleepiness and at least two of the following three symptoms or comorbidities: loud habitual snoring, reported respiratory pauses during sleep, awakening with a choking sensation, and a diagnosis of arterial hypertension
- recording with cardiorespiratory monitoring/polygraphy (HSAT) must be technically appropriate, i.e., it must include the *minimum number of parameters* (airflow, thoracoabdominal movements with inductive plethysmography, and SaO_2) recorded with the *recommended modalities and sensors* (AASM Manual for the Scoring of Sleep and Associated Events [Berry *et al.* 2012]), which can be correctly interpreted for at least 4 hours (at least airflow + SaO_2) during the time of habitual sleep (therefore, daytime recordings are not acceptable)

- HSAT must be performed under the *supervision of a certified sleep specialist* or a certified supplier who can guarantee a manual analysis of the recording and its correct interpretation
- HSAT is *highly discouraged* in patients with suspected OSAS who present with significant comorbidities, such as cardiac failure with an ejection fraction of <40%, recent stroke, neuromuscular pathologies, hypoventilation in wakefulness and sleep, moderate-severe COPD, and the chronic use of opiates. For such patients, *full-night polysomnography* is preferred
- when the results of a patient with a pretest high probability of developing OSAS (presenting daytime and night symptoms and/or predisposing factors) are negative with a cardiorespiratory monitoring system, it is necessary to perform a re-evaluation with a more complex instrumental method (full-night polysomnography)

Unlike the Level III monitoring systems, the level IV/portable monitoring systems (e.g., nocturnal blood oxygen saturation) are not acceptable for diagnosing OSAS in several guidelines (AASM and ESRS), whereas other scientific societies (e.g., the Canadian Thoracic Society and the American Medicare Service) specify that portable monitoring systems measuring at least three parameters (oximetry + one respiratory sensor) show an acceptable diagnostic capability only if they are performed by an experienced sleep clinician on patients with a high probability of moderate-severe OSAS. The clinician should be thoroughly familiar with the clinical situation of the patient. If needed, the possibility of performing full-night polysomnography must be available (Collop *et al.* 2007; Fisher *et al.* 2012; Fleetham *et al.* 2011).

Although they are antecedents, the *Italian guidelines for diagnosing* OSAS are aligned with the more recent international guidelines. In particular, they affirm that the most appropriate instrumental examination must be selected for diagnosing OSAS according to the clinical situation of the patient:

- based on the reported clinical symptoms and the presence of predisposing factors; the higher the probability of a patient developing OSAS, the simpler the recording method can be (cardiorespiratory monitoring or portable/reduced monitoring)
- if the patient's clinical situation is highly complex (sleepiness not associated with a sleep disorder, comorbidities with other sleep disorders, or cardiological or ventilatory pathology), the method of recording should also be more complex (full-night polysomnography at home or at a sleep laboratory) (Braghiroli *et al.* 2001)

Respiratory events

The instrumental recording of the patient with suspected OSAS enables us to:

- identify the presence of respiratory events, namely, alterations in the respiratory pattern that are typical of the disease (obstructive apnea/hypo-

pnea) with *easily identifiable beginning and end* phases and a duration between ≥10 and <180 seconds
- calculate the indices by determining the frequency of the respiratory events over time, which allows an evaluation of the severity of the disease
- distinguish the typical obstructive events of OSAS from other types of events and thus make a differential diagnosis with other respiratory sleep disorders

The AASM "Manual for the Scoring of Sleep and Associated Events" (Iber *et al.* 2012; Berry *et al.* 2012) reports the criteria for a correct and reproducible identification of such events (Table 3). The primary criteria to identify these events can be found in the manual of AIPO (the Italian Association of Hospital Pulmonologists guidelines), which also lists the primary recommendations for diagnosing and treating respiratory sleep disorders (AIPO 2011).

PRINCIPAL RESPIRATORY SLEEP EVENTS

La Table 2.8 summarizes the characteristics of the primary respiratory sleep events: apnea, hypopnea, and reduced airflow.

Apnea and hypopnea

Apnea

1. Absence of or ≥90% decrease in the airflow (passage of air at the oronasal site)
2. Duration of ≥10 seconds.
3. They can be associated with the following:
   - decreased SaO_2 (desaturation) of any entity
   - arousal from sleep

Apnea can be classified into **three types** according to the correlation between the absence of airflow and the thoracoabdominal dynamics.

Obstructive apnea (📷 2.3): absence of airflow due to upper airway narrowing with persistent respiratory efforts characterized by the presence of thoracoabdominal movements (the central respiratory drive is present, but the upper airways are obstructed). Usually, respiratory efforts are increased during obstructive apnea because the patient increases the thoracoabdominal bellows to overcome the upper airway obstruction. This can determine the onset of paradoxical breathing characterized by thoracoabdominal movements in a reverse pattern during the obstructed respiratory events (the thorax expands and the abdomen contracts). When the airways are open, normal breathing recovers and the respiratory movements return to the normal pattern (the thorax and abdomen expand in a synchronous manner).

2.8 Respiratory events.

Respiratory event	Description	Duration	Characteristics
Apnea	Absence of or ≥90% decrease in the airflow (passage of air at the oronasal site)	≥10 seconds	*It is associated with:* 1) It could be associated with decreased SaO_2 (desaturation) of any entity 2) arousal from sleep
Hypopnea	≥30% decrease in the airflow (passage of air at the oronasal site)	≥10 seconds	*It is associated with:* 1) desaturation of ≥3% (AASM criterion, 2012) or ≥4% (AIPO criterion) and/or 2) arousal from sleep (2.6)*
Respiratory effort-related arousal (RERA)	Series of respiratory events with progressive respiratory efforts and/or airflow decrease (<30%), with a flattening of the airflow curve (identified by the nasal cannula), which ends abruptly with an arousal** (2.7)	≥10 seconds	Without desaturation
Flow limitation arousal (FL arousal)	Series of respiratory events with flattening of the airflow curve during inspiration (identified by the nasal cannula), manifestation of a partial obstruction of the upper airways (<30%), it abruptly returns to normal in association with an arousal**	≥10 seconds	Without desaturation
Events of flow limitation associated with AA	Series of respiratory events with flattening of the airflow curve during inspiration (identified by the nasal cannula), manifestation of a partial obstruction of upper airways (<30%), it abruptly returns to normal in association with an AA***	≥10 seconds	It is associated with AA identified by: 1) Vasoconstriction identified on the plethysmographic waveform from the pulse oximeter 2) Increase in cardiac frequency of 6 beats/minute for 2 consecutive minutes
Desaturation event	Rapid and phasic decrease in SaO_2 (≥3% or ≥4%) with rapid recovery	≥10 seconds	Usually associated with apnea or hypopnea

*In cases of ambulatory recording systems that do not record sleep, hypopnea is only identified when it is associated with a desaturation of 3% because there is no EEG recording and the arousal cannot be highlighted.

**They are only correctly identifiable with full-night polysomnography because they require a sleep recording with EEG to identify the arousal associated with them.

***The electroencephalographic arousal is usually associated with an increase in vegetative sympathetic activity (increase in cardiac frequency + peripheral vasoconstriction), which is identified by the so-called autonomic arousal (AA) characterized by a sudden increase in cardiac frequency and a reduction in the plethysmographic waveform recorded with the pulse oximeter. Therefore, the AA can be recognized without EEG recording (Johnson PL et al. 2005; AIPO 2011).

Central Apnea (2.4): Absence of airflow due to the absence of respiratory efforts, characterized by the absence of thoracoabdominal movements but with open upper airways (there is no respiratory drive; therefore, the air does not flow despite the upper airways being open).

Mixed apnea (2.5): Absence of airflow due to the absence of respiratory efforts (central component) in the first part of the event and then due to narrowing of the upper airways when the thoracoabdominal movement resumes (obstructive component).

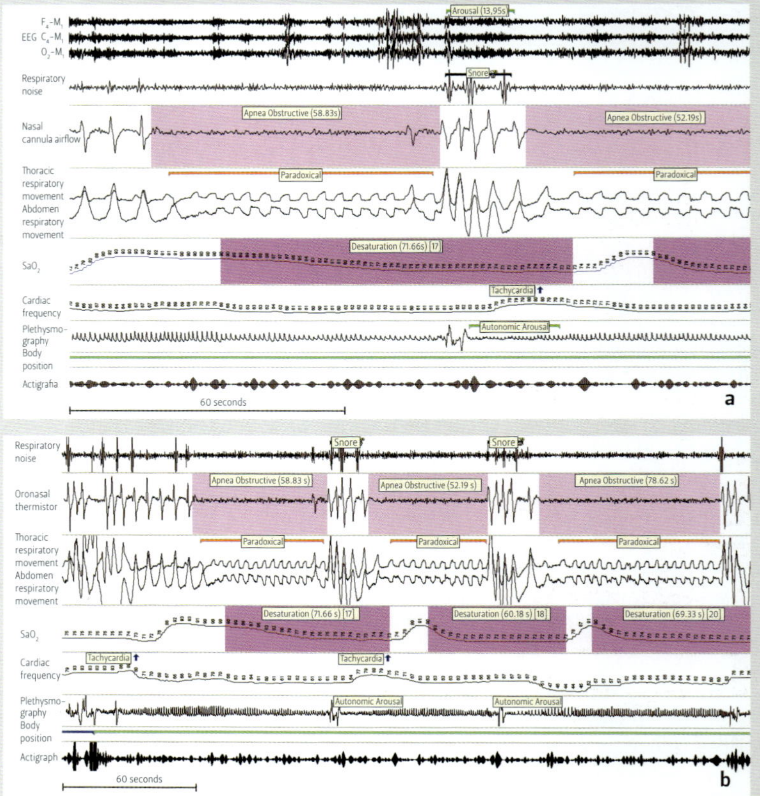

2.3 a. **Obstructive apnea:** absence of airflow, manifestation of a complete obstruction of the upper airways (obstructive apnea on nasal cannula airflow), persistence of thoracoabdominal movements with respiratory efforts and paradoxical breathing (paradoxical on thoracoabdominal respiratory movements), desaturation: rapid decrease in SaO_2 secondary to the event with rapid recovery (SaO_2 desaturation), arousal with resumed breathing: rapid modification in frequency on EEG (arousal on EEG), rapid snoring resuming at the end of apnea (snoring on respiratory noise), tachycardia at the end of apnea (cardiac frequency), vasoconstriction at the end of apnea as a manifestation of autonomic arousal on oximeter plethysmography corresponding with EEG arousal.
b. Sequence of obstructive apnea.

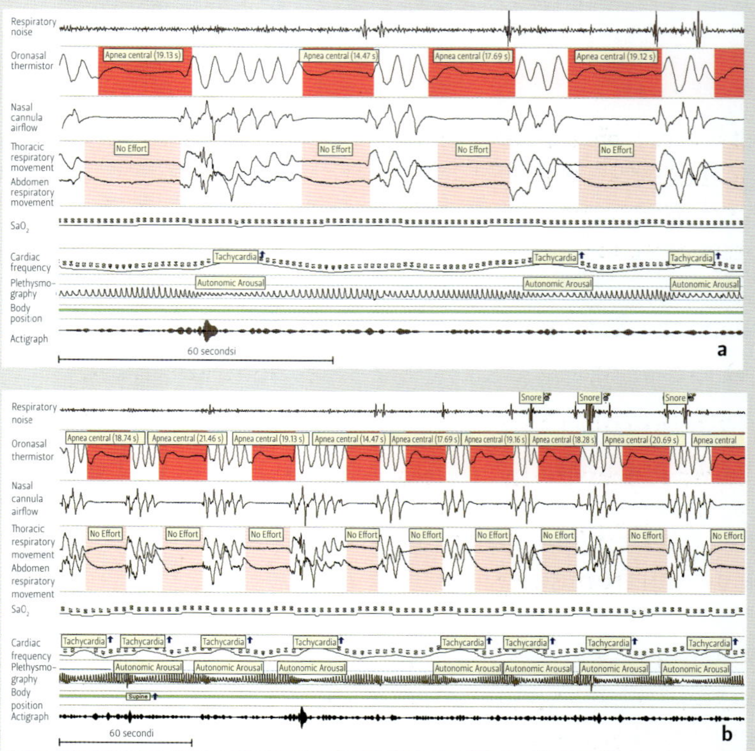

2.4 a. **Central apnea**: absence of airflow (central apnea on nasal cannula airflow), absence of thoracoabdominal movements and respiratory efforts (no effort of thoracoabdominal respiratory movements), no desaturation in this case (rapid decrease in SaO_2 secondary to the event with rapid recovery) but can be present (SaO_2), absence of snoring when breathing resumes (respiratory noise), tachycardia at the end of apnea (cardiac frequency), vasoconstriction at the end of apnea as a manifestation of autonomic arousal on oximeter plethysmography.
b. Sequence of central apnea

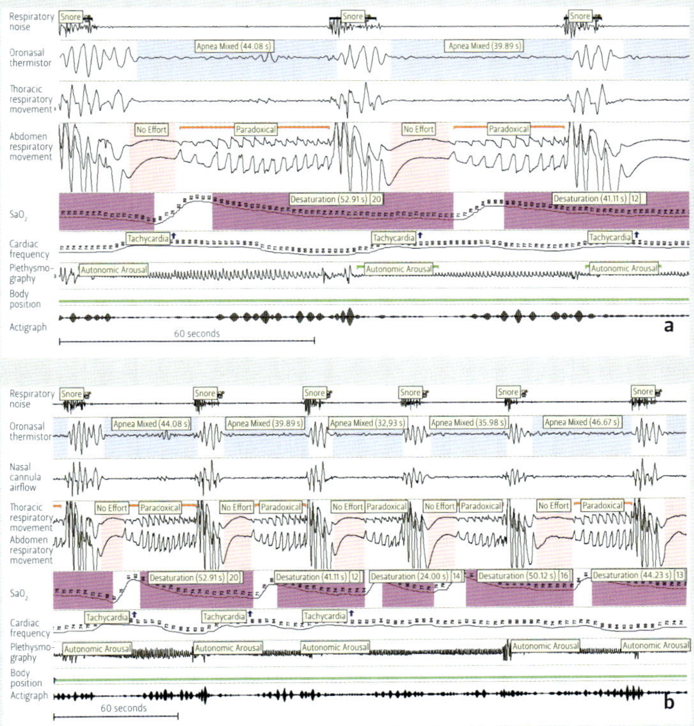

2.5 a. Mixed apnea: absence of airflow (mixed apnea on nasal cannula airflow), absence of thoracoabdominal movements in the initial phase of apnea and subsequent resumption of movements with respiratory efforts and paradoxical breathing (no effort of thoracoabdominal respiratory movements and then paradoxical on thoracoabdominal respiratory movements), desaturation: rapid increase in SaO_2 secondary to the event with rapid recovery (SaO_2 desaturation), rapid snoring resuming at the end of apnea (snoring on respiratory noise), tachycardia at the end of apnea (tachycardia on cardiac frequency), vasoconstriction at the end of apnea. **b.** Sequence of mixed apnea.

Obstructive and mixed apnea are typical of OSAS, whereas central apnea are typical of other nonOSAS respiratory sleep disorders [central sleep apnea syndrome (CSAS) and Cheyne-Stokes breathing], although a certain number of central apnea can also be identified in patients with OSAS.

Hypopnea (2.6)

1. Decrease of ≥30% in the airflow (passage of the air at oronasal site).
2. Duration of ≥10 seconds.
3. It must necessarily be associated with the following:
   - desaturation of ≥3% (AASM 2012 criterion) or ≥4% (AIPO criterion) and/or
   - arousal from sleep

In cases of ambulatory recording systems that do not record sleep, hypopnea is identified only when it is associated with a desaturation of 3% (or 4% according to AIPO criteria) because there is no EEG recording and the arousal cannot be identified (Iber *et al.* 2012).

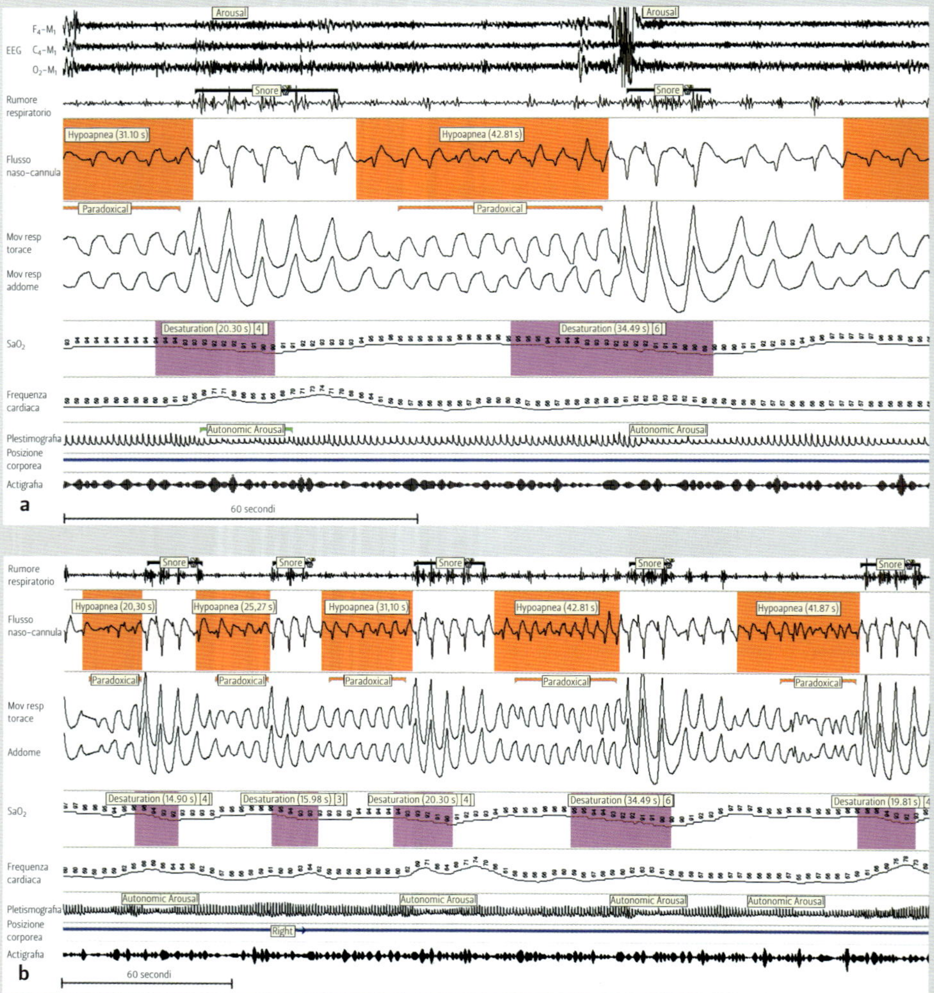

2.6 **a. Obstructive hypopnea:** reduction of ≥30% in airflow, manifestation of a partial obstruction of the upper airways (hypopnea on nasal cannula flow), persistence of thoracoabdominal movements with respiratory efforts and paradoxical breathing (paradoxical on thoracoabdominal respiratory movements), desaturation: rapid decrease in SaO_2 secondary to the event with rapid recovery (SaO_2 desaturation), arousal with resumption of breathing: rapid modification in the frequency on EEG (arousal on EEG), abrupt snoring resumes at the end of apnea (snoring on respiratory noise), tachycardia at the end of apnea (cardiac frequency), vasoconstriction at the end of apnea as a manifestation of autonomic arousal on oximeter plethysmography corresponding with EEG arousal . **b.** Sequence of obstructive hypopnea.

There are **two types of hypopnea.**

Obstructive hypopnea: when the airflow is reduced and the airflow curve is flattened, there is a manifestation of an obstruction to the passage of air, and the thoracoabdominal movements are in reverse phase or increased, similar to major respiratory efforts.

Central hypopnea: when both the airflow and the respiratory efforts are reduced but with regular and coordinated movements.

In clinical practice, it is essential to distinguish the different types of hypopnea while analyzing a polysomnographic recording because this influences the final diagnosis (OSAS, nonOSAS respiratory disorders, and OSAS + other respiratory disorder), whereas the distinction between the two types of

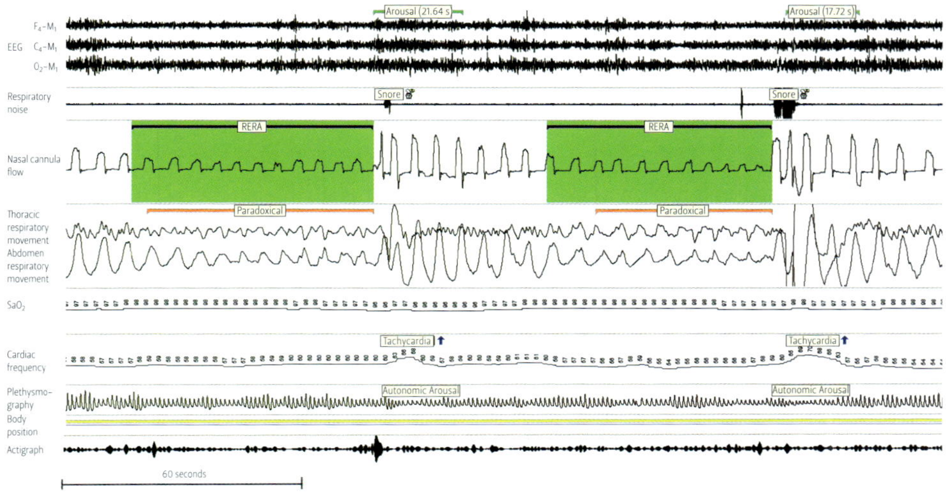

2.7 Respiratory effort-related arousal (RERA): sequence of respiratory events with airflow reduction (<30%), flattening of the airflow curve, manifestation of a partial obstruction of the upper airways (RERA on nasal cannula flow), persistence of thoracoabdominal movements with respiratory efforts and paradoxical breathing (paradoxical on thoracoabdominal respiratory movements), absence of modification in SaO_2, arousal with the resumption of breathing: rapid modification in the frequency on EEG (arousal on EEG), tachycardia at the end of the event (tachycardia on cardiac frequency), vasoconstriction at the end of the event as a manifestation of autonomic arousal on oximeter plethysmography corresponding with EEG arousal.

hypopnea is optional and recommended only in particular clinical situations wherein the percentage of central hypopnea is significant (e.g., an association between OSAS and periodic breathing) in a majority of the cases. However, only the generic number of hypopnea is calculated in the majority of cases (Berry *et al.* 2012; Iber *et al.* 2012).

Other *obstructive respiratory sleep events do not satisfy the criteria for apnea or hypopnea* despite having the same pathophysiological mechanisms. These are phasic events characterized by a partial obstruction of the upper airways, which are minor events in comparison with apnea and hypopnea (airflow reduction of <30%), and increased respiratory effort without affecting oxygen saturation but affecting the quality of sleep because they are associated with an arousal (a rapid and short sleep reduction).

Respiratory Effort-Related Arousal o RERA (2.7))

- Series of respiratory events with a progressive increase in respiratory efforts and/or reduction in airflow (<30%) and flattening of the airflow curve (identified by a nasal cannula) terminating abruptly with an arousal
- Without desaturation.
- Duration of ≥10 seconds (Iber *et al.* 2012)

Flow Limitation Arousal o FL-Arousal

- Series of respiratory events with flattening of the airflow curve in the inspiratory phase (identified by a nasal cannula) that normalizes abruptly in association with an arousal
- Without desaturation
- Duration of ≥10 seconds

Clinical definitions of these two events *overlap*. They can *only be correctly identified with full-night polysomnography* because they require a sleep recording with EEG to evaluate the arousal associated with them (Ayappa *et al.* 2000).

EEG arousal is usually associated with an increase in vegetative sympathetic activity (increase in cardiac frequency + peripheral vasoconstriction), which is identified by the so-called AA characterized by an abrupt increase in cardiac frequency (6 beats/minute for 2 consecutive beats) and a reduction in the amplitude of the plethysmographic waveform recorded with the pulse oximeter. Thus, AA can also be identified without EEG recording (Johnson *et al.* 2005; AIPO 2011).

Consequently, RERA/FL arousal can also be identified at an acceptable approximation using systems that do not record sleep by investigating the events of flow limitation that determine AA.

Thus, in the Level III instrumental recordings (cardiorespiratory monitoring or polygraphy), where it is not possible to evaluate EEG arousal, it is possible to identify the events of flow limitation associated with AA (2.8):

- series of respiratory events with flattening of the airflow curve in the inspiratory phase (identified by a nasal cannula) and the manifestation of partial obstruction of the upper airways (<30%) that normalizes abruptly in association with AA (identified with oximeter/EEG parameters)
- without desaturation
- duration of ≥10 seconds

The AASM manual classifies RERAs specifying that they cannot be identified in the Level III recordings because they do not include the flow limitation event associated with the AA; moreover, to the best of our knowledge, no validating studies have been performed using standard polysomnography. In contrast, the AIPO manual recommends the identification of RERAs.

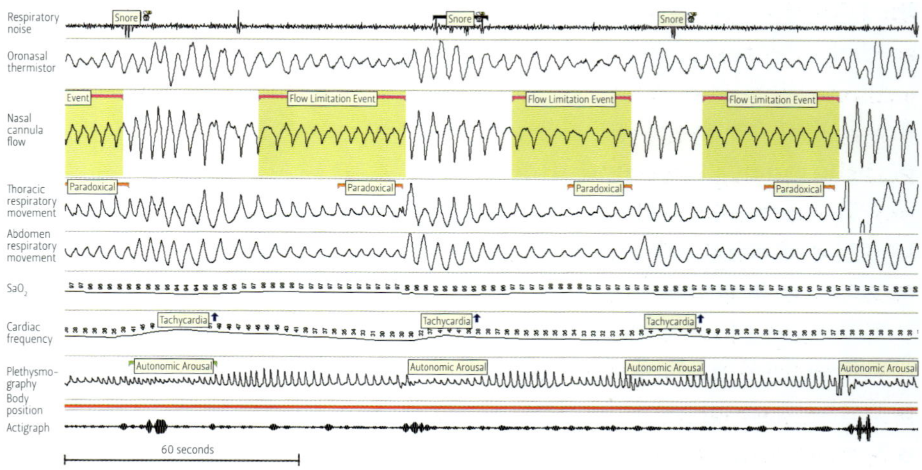

2.8 Event of airflow limitation associated with AA: sequence of breaths with a reduction in airflow (>30%) and flattening of the airflow curve, manifestation of a partial obstruction of the upper airways (flow limitation event on nasal cannula flow), persistence of thoracoabdominal movements with an increase in respiratory efforts and paradoxical breathing (paradoxical on thorax and abdomen respiratory movements), absence of SaO_2 modifications (SaO_2) and abrupt resumption of snoring at the end of the event (snoring on respiratory noise), tachycardia at the end of the event (tachycardia on cardiac frequency), vasoconstriction at the end of the event as a manifestation autonomic arousal on oximeter plethysmography.

These minor obstructive events are not characteristic of patients with typical OSAS. Their identification on polysomnographic recording is more difficult, particularly without an EEG recording. Usually, automatic analysis does not identify them correctly; therefore, the identification and scoring of such events are considered optional (recommended only in particular clinical situations) in the standard interpretation of an instrumental examination performed on patients with suspected OSAS (Iber *et al.* 2012). However, these events must be identified and included in the scoring of the respiratory disorder index (RDI) in cases of patients with sleepiness presenting an atypical clinical situation that is scarcely indicative of OSAS or if the sleepiness persists on verifying the efficacy of the therapy.

Apnea and hypopnea usually cause a phasic decrease of varying amounts in SaO_2 (3%–20%), according to the characteristics of the respiratory event (presence of respiratory efforts), its duration, and the clinical (especially cardiovascular) condition of the patient. Desaturation reaches its minimum slightly after the end of the respiratory event. Subsequently, SaO_2 resumes rapidly, returning to the baseline values in the majority of cases. However, in some severe forms of OSAS or in comorbid patients, SaO_2 cannot return to the baseline values even after breathing has resumed.

A **desaturation event** has the following characteristics:

- phasic and rapid decrease in SaO_2 (≥3% or ≥4%) with abrupt recovery
- duration of ≥10 seconds
- usually associated with apnea or hypopnea (📷 2.3).

Other respiratory patterns

There are other respiratory patterns that are not characteristics of patients with OSAS but can appear in periods associated with obstructive events, particularly in patients with cardiocerebral comorbidities. The most characteristic respiratory pattern is **Cheyne-Stokes respiration**, a periodic modification (for at least three cycles) in breath amplitude with a typical crescendo-decrescendo pattern (identical duration of the two phases confers a diamond shape to the respiratory signal). Often, central apneic events are interposed between breathing oscillations. The duration of central apnea and the resumption of breathing are almost constant, conferring a pattern of marked periodicity (📷 2.9). It is considered clinically significant when it is associated with at least five central apneic events per hour of sleep or when it lasts for at least 10 consecutive minutes (Iber *et al.* 2012).

This respiratory alteration is typical in patients with cardiac failure and recent stroke (OSAS is often associated with both these conditions). Additionally, it can also be found in patients with OSAS and stable cardiological or neurological comorbidities.

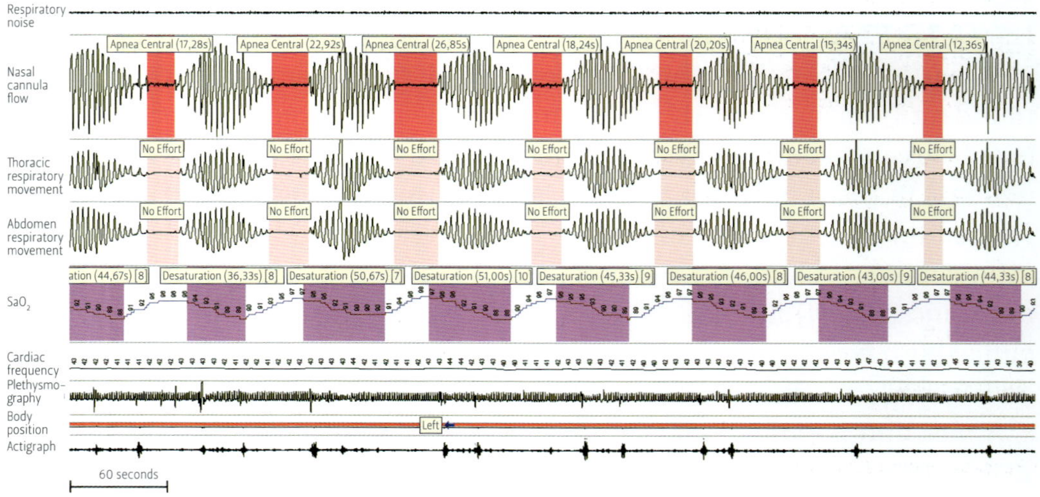

2.9 Cheyne–Stokes respiration: periodic modification in breath amplitude with a typical crescendo-decrescendo and diamond-shaped pattern. Synchronous oscillation on all the respiratory tracks (nasal cannula flow and thoracoabdominal respiratory movements), interposed central apnea (central apnea on nasal cannula flow and no efforts on thoracoabdominal respiratory movements), desaturation: rapid decrease in SaO_2 secondary to the event with a cup-shaped trend (decrease phase of equal duration to the recovery phase) (SaO_2 desaturation). Generally, the duration of central apnea and the resumptive phase of breathing are constant, conferring marked periodicity to such a pattern.

Respiratory indices

The identification of respiratory events enables the calculation of different indices of respiratory sleep disorders, i.e., the number of respiratory events per hour of sleep (total number of respiratory events/total sleep duration × 60), which are the main measures of disease severity in OSAS.

In polysomnographic recording, the calculation is performed using **time of sleep as measured on EEG.**

Sleep is not recorded in cardiorespiratory monitoring/polygraphy; therefore, the index can be calculated based on the following:

- *monitoring time* or estimated time of sleep, namely, the total recording time minus the periods in which it is assumed that the patients are awake, according to what is reported by the patients in their sleep diary completed on the night of the recording or because they are in the standing position or significant motor activity or a very irregular respiratory pattern is present
- *total time of recording*, which is not recommended because the index may be underestimated if the recording system is activated before going to bed or the patient stays awake for durations of time during the night
- *total time in the supine position* (patient in bed), which may result in an underestimated index if the patient remains awake in bed

Monitoring time (TM) is recommended by international criteria. It should always be used because it allows the calculation of indices that are closer to the time of polysomnography (Iber *et al.* 2012).

TM evaluates the indices of respiratory sleep disorder to estimate the severity of OSAS. Therefore, it is important to determine if these indices have been calculated based on electroencephalographic sleep (Level I and II systems), estimated sleep, or recording time (Level III and IV systems). This data should always be specified in the instrumental examination report.

2.9 Respiratory indices.

Respiratory index	Description	Characteristics
Apnea–hypopnea index (AHI)	Number of apneic + hypopneic events per hour of sleep	If not specified otherwise, this index comprises all types of apnea
Central apnea index	Number of central apneic events per hour of sleep	When the apneic events have only been distinguished as obstructive, mixed, or central
Obstructive apnea index	Number of obstructive apneic events per hour of sleep	
AHIC	Central apneic + central hypopneic events per hour of sleep	These indices are obtained when all hypopneic events have been distinguished as central or obstructive in the analysis of the recording track
AHIo	Obstructive and mixed apneic + obstructive hypopneic events per hour of sleep	
AHI SUPINE	Apnee + ipopnee per ora di sonno in posizione supina	Some patients with OSAS present with apnea/hypopnea mainly or exclusively in the supine position during the recorded night. For these patients, it is important to distinguish AHI per position
AHI NONSUPINE	Apnea + hypopnea in the nonsupine sleeping position	
Respiratory disorder index (RDI)	Number of apnea + hypopnea + RERA/FL arousal per hour of sleep	Besides apnea and hypopnea (already considered in AHI), this index also includes minor obstructive events that affect sleep structure but not nocturnal oxygen saturation. Thus, it is the most detailed method to grade the severity of OSAS.
Respiratory event index	Number of apneic + hypopneic events per hour of estimated sleep (monitoring time) during evaluation with an ambulatory recording system (ICSD-3 2014)	In the criteria for diagnosing OSAS, the new ICSD-3 guidelines suggests the use of this index when diagnosis is performed with an ambulatory system (HSAT) to distinguish it from AHI or RDI, which are obtained with a polysomnographic recording
Oxygen desaturation index (ODI)	Number of desaturation events per hour of sleep	This index almost always overlaps with AHI, although there are certain patients with apnea that do not cause a desaturation (in such cases, AHI will be higher than ODI), whereas other patients present desaturation events that can be correlated with small modifications in respiratory patterns, and they cannot be classified as respiratory events (in these cases, ODI will be higher than AHI). By definition, ODI is lower than RDI, which contains all the minor obstructive respiratory events that do not modify SaO_2

Table 2.9 summarizes the most commonly used respiratory indices, which are described below.

1. AHI = number of apneic + hypopneic events per hour of sleep. If not specified otherwise, this index comprises all types of apnea. Generally, patients with OSAS present a major portion of respiratory events as the obstructive or mixed type, whereas central apnea represents the smallest percentage and thus does not affect the overall value of the index. In contrast, when central apneic events appear in a significant number, it is important to distinguish central apnea from obstructive and mixed types by calculating the following:

   - **cAI (central apnea index)** = number of central apneic events per hour of sleep;
   - **oAI (obstructive apnea index)** = number of obstructive + mixed apneic events per hour of sleep

In analyzing the recording track, if hypopnea has also been distinguished as central and obstructive events, we can obtain more precise indices such as the following:

- **cAHI** = central apneic + central hypopneic events per hour of sleep;
- **oAHI**= obstructive and mixed apneic + obstructive hypopneic events per hour of sleep.

Whenever a high number of central respiratory events occur, the presence of other pathologies associated with OSAS (especially cardiological or neurological pathologies) or a respiratory disorder other than OSAS must always be considered. A cardiorespiratory monitoring system may be insufficient to diagnose both these conditions, which may require a closer examination with polysomnography. Some patients with OSAS present with apnea/hypopnea mainly or exclusively in the supine position. Thus, their total AHI depends on the amount of sleeping time spent in such position during the recorded night. For these patients, it is important to differentiate AHI per position as follows:

- **Supine AHI** = apneic + hypopneic events per hour of sleep in the supine position;
- **Nonsupine AHI** = apneic + hypopneic events in a position other than supine (on their side or prone).

The presence of respiratory events occurring mainly in the supine position may significantly influence therapeutic choice, especially in mild or moderately severe cases (for more detailed explanation, see the paragraph about POSA).

❷ **Respiratory disorder index (respiratory disorder/disturbance index, RDI)** = number of apnea + hypopnea + RERA/FL arousal per hour of sleep. Besides apnea/hypopnea (already considered in AHI), this index also includes minor obstructive events that affect the sleep structure but not the nocturnal oxygen saturation. Thus, this is a more detailed method of grading the severity of OSAS. For a correct calculation, it is necessary to perform polysomnography with the sleep evaluation to identify RERA or FL arousal. However, it can also be calculated to a reasonable approximation with cardiorespiratory monitoring by identifying the events of flow limitation associated with AA (see above). AHI and RDI are often wrongly considered equivalent. In fact, the second index also includes the minor obstructive events. Therefore, in patients with OSAS presenting only obstructive and mixed apnea/hypopnea (the majority), the two indices will correspond, whereas for those with several RERA/FL arousals, AHI underestimates the severity of the disorder, and RDI is the more correct index that should be calculated, especially if the patient presents daytime sleepiness. When the report of an instrumental examination on a patient with suspected OSAS shows RDI, it is essential to understand how it has been calculated and which respiratory events have been considered.

3. **Respiratory event index (REI)** = number of apneic + hypopneic events per hour of monitoring time (ICSD-3 2014). The AASM Manual for the Scoring of Sleep and Associated Events suggests that REI be used with an ambulatory system (HSAT) that does not record sleep, to distinguish it quickly and clearly from AHI or RDI, which are calculated on the actual sleeping time recorded by polysomnography (Iber *et al.* 2012).
4. **Oxygen desaturation index (ODI)** = number of desaturation events per hour of sleep. This index almost always overlaps with AHI. However, there are certain patients with apnea in whom desaturation events are not observed (in such cases, AHI will be higher than ODI), whereas other patients present desaturation events that can be correlated with small modifications in respiratory pattern; therefore, they cannot be classified as respiratory events (in these cases, ODI will be higher than AHI). By definition, ODI is lower than RDI, which includes all the minor obstructive respiratory events that do not modify SaO_2.

In the recordings performed with ambulatory systems, a significant discrepancy between AHI and ODI (with ODI > AHI) may sometimes suggest that the analyses of the recording track have been automatically performed without manual correction. In fact, automatic correction for desaturation events can be simple and precise, but it is more complex for apnea/hypopnea and can therefore be significantly incorrect.

Thus, when evaluating the index of respiratory sleep disorders to grade the severity of OSAS, it is important to determine if they have been calculated in encephalographic sleep (Level I and II systems), estimated sleep, or the recording period (Level III and IV systems). This data should always be specified in the instrumental examination report.

Other values of SaO_2 during sleep

AHI or RDI is sufficient to establish a diagnosis of OSAS; however, it is necessary to consider other indices of the sleep disorder to correctly assess its severity. In particular, the different values of SaO_2 during sleep are essential. The more commonly calculated values by the recording systems are as follows (2.10):

- **Mean SaO_2** = the average of all SaO_2 values during sleep. It is affected by basal SaO_2 in the periods without respiratory events, the amount of desaturation with apnea/hypopnea, and the recovery of SaO_2 at the end of apnea/hypopnea;
- **Minimum SaO_2** = the minimum value of SaO_2 during sleep;
- **Mean SaO_2 desaturation** = the average of the desaturation values associat-

2.10 Values of SaO_2 during sleep.

Respiratory Index	Description	Characteristics
Mean SaO_2	Average of all SaO_2 values during sleep	It is influenced by basal SaO_2 in the respiratory events, the amount of desaturation with apnea/hypopnea, and the recovery of SaO_2 at the end of apnea/hypopnea
Minimum SaO_2	Minimum value of SaO_2 reached during sleep	
Mean desaturation (SaO_2)	Average of the desaturation values associated with respiratory events (amount of phasic decrease in SaO_2 associated with the respiratory events)	It can be influenced by basal SaO_2 in patients with ventilatory pathologies
Mean SaO_2 of minimum peaks	Average of the minimum SaO_2 values reached with desaturation events	It can be influenced by basal SaO_2 in patients with ventilatory pathologies
Sleeping time with SaO_2 < 90% (cumulative time, CT 90%)	% of sleeping time spent with SaO_2 < 90%	
Sleeping time with SaO_2 < 80% (CT 80%)	% of sleeping time spent with SaO_2 < 80%	

ed with the respiratory events (amount of the phasic decrease in SaO_2 associated with the respiratory events). It can be influenced by basal SaO_2 in patients affected by ventilatory pathologies.

- **Mean SaO_2 of minimum peaks** = the average value of SaO_2 reached with desaturation events. It can be influenced by basal SaO_2 in patients affected by ventilatory pathologies.
- **Sleeping time with SaO_2 < 90% (cumulative time, CT 90%)** = the percentage of sleeping time spent with SaO_2 < 90%;
- **Sleeping time with SaO_2 < 80% (CT 80%)** = the percentage of sleeping time spent with SaO_2 < 80%.

Currently, all the digital polysomnographic recording systems (from Level I to IV) are provided with software that automatically analyzes data collected from the patient during the night (raw data) and performs an automatic analysis of the recording track. This analysis is performed according to the preset software criteria, which must correspond with international diagnostic criteria for identifying sleep and associated events. Automatic analysis provides sleep interpretation, an identification of the respiratory events and the counts of indices, the evaluation of oxygen saturation indices, and an analysis of the plethysmography waveform, the ECG, and the movements of lower limbs in some cases. It is important to highlight that this type of recording track analysis is never completely reliable, especially in unattended ambulatory recordings where the quality of signals for analysis may worsen during the night.

Therefore, all the guidelines agree that the presence of a clinician who is experienced in sleep disorders and who will always perform a manual analysis before writing the report is necessary to obtain a correct diagnosis of OSAS (Collop *et al.* 2007; Braghiroli *et al.* 2001).

The use of automatic analysis of the recording track alone poses significant risks in the patients is associated with a risk of receiving inappropriate treatment, whereas the clinician is associated with a legal risk of inappropriate behavior.

Criteria for diagnosing OSAS

Diagnosis of OSAS

According to AASM's ICSD-3, it is necessary to examine the following factor to establish a diagnosis of OSAS for an adult patient:

1. A combination of the following clinical and instrumental criteria (A + B):

   A. The presence of at least one of the following symptoms or criteria:

   - excessive daytime sleepiness, nonrestorative sleep, daytime tiredness, or insomnia
   - awakenings with a choking sensation
   - loud snoring and/or respiratory pauses during sleep, as reported by the bed partner
   - diagnosis of arterial hypertension, mood disorder, cognitive deficit, coronary artery disease, stroke, cardiac failure, atrial fibrillation, or type 2 diabetes mellitus

   B. Five or more respiratory events that are mainly obstructive per hour of sleep, as recorded on polysomnography or an ambulatory system (HSAT). It is recommended that RDI must be used in cases of obstructive and mixed apnea + hypopnea + RERA for polysomnographic recordings and REI in cases of obstructive and mixed apnea + hypopnea for HSAT recordings.

Or

2. The instrument only criterion in the absence of clinical symptoms or criteria (C):

   C. Fifteen or more respiratory events that are mainly obstructive per hour of sleep and recorded with polysomnography or an ambulatory system (HSAT). It is recommended that RDI must be used in cases of obstructive and mixed apnea + hypopnea + RERA for polysomnographic recordings and REI for cases of obstructive and mixed hypopnea for HSAT recordings.

   D. In both diagnostic conditions, the disorder cannot be explained by other neurological or medical pathologies.

To establish a correct diagnosis of OSAS, it is essential to apply international diagnostic criteria, which are the fundamental requirements for appropriate therapeutic choices.

Despite the ICSD-3 recommendations, AHI is frequently used rather than the obstructive RDI to diagnose OSAS in clinical practice. This is acceptable except in the following cases:

- when central apnea appears at a considerable number (cAI ≥ 5). In these cases, it is recommended that oAHI (obstructive) rather than overall AHI be evaluated
- when there is a significant number of RERA/FL arousals that must be quantified and added to the index

The diagnostic criteria for OSAS proposed by AASM in ICSD-3 are completed agreed to and accepted by all other scientific societies.

Severity of OSAS

According to all international guidelines, the severity of OSAS is the key element for consideration when choosing the most appropriate treatment to propose to the patient.

The primary important element to assess the severity of OSAS is the number of respiratory events per hour of sleep, namely, AHI (or RDI if RERA/FL arousals are included). Based on AHI, the severity of OSAS is stratified as indicated in Tabella 2.11 (American Academy of Sleep Medicine Task Force 1999).

The epidemiological data on cardio- and cerebrovascular risks in patients with OSAS are based on this severity classification.

However, if we consider the severity of the respiratory disorder from the viewpoint of a therapeutic strategy (i.e., searching for the best therapy for each patient), it is crucial to consider the following aspects:

- *AHI per position* is the presence of POSA, particularly if AHI for the nonsupine sleeping position is <5 and if there are no important comorbidities that require therapies other than CPAP
- *impaired SaO_2* during sleep (evaluated by saturation indices), which is significant when it presents hypoxemia during sleep for extended duration of time (CT for >90% is ≥20%–30%). It preferably directs toward therapies with positive pressure (CPAP or bilevel positive airway pressure)
- *presence of daytime sleepiness*, which may represent a risk of road and work-related accidents, particularly when the patient has a risky profession, particularly driving a mode of transportation. This makes it necessary to choose a therapy based on the scientific data of its efficacy on the risk of accidents

2.11 Classification of the severity of OSAS.

Mild	AHI (or RDI) ≥ 5 and < 15
Moderate	AHI (or RDI) ≥ 15 and < 30
Severe	AHI (or RDI) ≥ 30

- *presence of significant comorbidities* of cardiological, neurological, or ventilatory types, which makes it necessary to choose a therapy with proven efficacy in reducing cardiocerebrovascular risks and improving ventilation (CPAP)

When discussing therapeutic choices, it is essential to consider the role of the anatomy of the upper airways. This is evaluated with instrumental methods by an otorhinolaryngologist who plays a key role in selecting surgical techniques, which in turn influences the efficacy of nonsurgical therapies (The factors required for a correct therapeutic and differentiated choice are thoroughly described in Chapter 4).

Clinical and pathophysiological subtypes of OSAS

Remaining within the framework of the abovementioned international diagnostic criteria, some patients with OSAS present with peculiar clinical and polysomnographic aspects, which may influence therapeutic choice in some cases.

POSITIONAL OSAS

Although the importance of the supine sleeping position in ascertaining OSAS and snoring has always been known, its clinical recognition has remained scarce in the therapeutic and diagnostic guidelines (Robin 1948).

Respiratory physiology studies have shown that the supine position determines a modification in the morphology and dimension of the airway geometry at the pharynx level (also due to gravity) and an increase in collapsibility, a reduction of the lung volumes, and a major instability of ventilatory control (Issa *et al.* 1984; Pevernagie *et al.* 1995; Joosten *et al.* 2014). All these elements explain why the supine position can significantly aggravate OSAS.

Polysomnographic studies on patients with OSAS have highlighted that obstructive respiratory events are more frequent and last longer in the supine position, particularly during REM sleep, which results in a higher desaturation, and that the presence of a certain body position (respiratory events are predominant in the supine position) is the main cause of underestimating the severity of OSAS (in 20%–40% of patients) based on AHI of a single recorded night (Oksenberg *et al.* 2010; Eiseman *et al.* 2010) (2.10 e 2.11).

The diagnosis of POSA was arbitrarily classified by Cartwright in the 1980s with the following definition: number of apneic/hypopneic events per hour of sleep in the nonsupine position (nonsupine AHI) (Cartwright 1984; Cartwright *et al.* 1991).

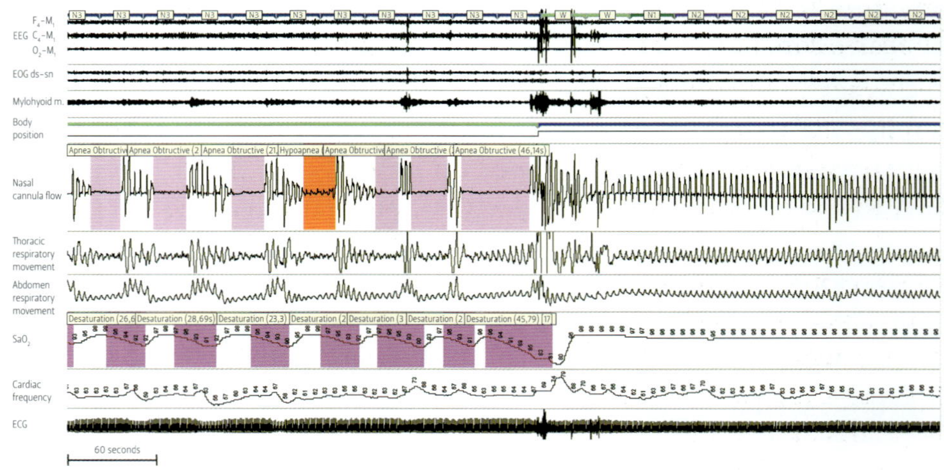

2.10 Obstructive apnea correlated with the supine position In the first part of the image, the patient was evaluated in the supine position (identified by the green line on the body position signal) with a sequence of obstructive apnea associated with desaturation; in the center, corresponding with an awakening [on EEG passage from N3 (deep sleep) to W (wakefulness)], the patient changes body position. In the second part of the image, the patient was evaluated in the lateral posture (identified by the blue line on the body position signal), the respiratory pattern became regular, and the fre-

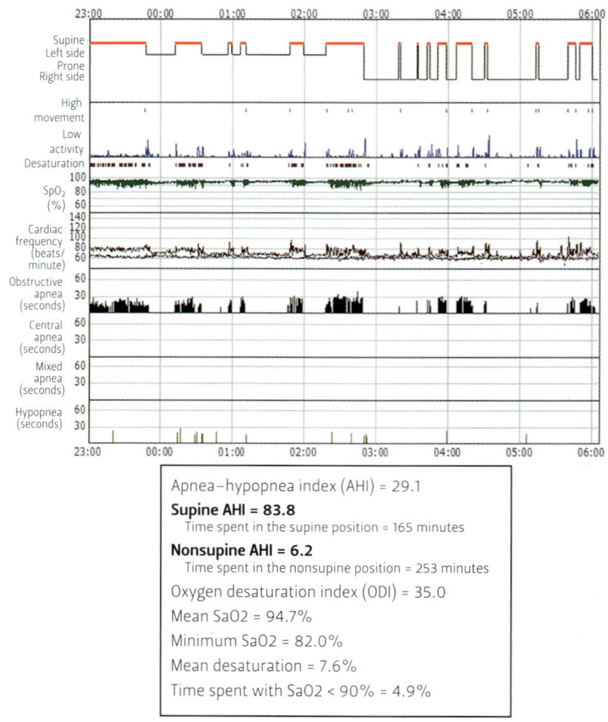

2.11 Cardiorespiratory monitoring of a patient with positional OSAS. Obstructive apnea/hypopnea and the associated desaturation events show a clear correlation with the body position (red bars on the body position signal). The positional OSAS is highlighted by AHI calculated with the patient's estimated sleeping time and differentiated by position (supine AHI, nonsupine AHI).

Since then, this diagnostic criterion has been used worldwide; however, several subsequent studies have restrictively adapted this criterion by setting a maximum limit for the nonsupine AHI (<5, <10, or <15) until the most restrictive criterion, namely, the supine AHI, which should be at least double compared with the nonsupine AHI + nonsupine AHI of <5 (Mador *et al.* 2005; Ravesloot *et al.* 2013).

Recently, it has been proposed that two forms of positional OSAS be distinguished (Joosten *et al.* 2014).

1. **Supine-predominant OSAS** (OSAS with a positional component) with a supine AHI that is twice as high or higher than the nonsupine AHI without

any limit to the nonsupine AHI; namely, patients with respiratory events appearing mainly in the supine position and to a lesser extent when assuming the nonsupine position;

2. **Supine-isolated OSAS** (isolated POSA) with a supine AHI that is twice as high or higher than the nonsupine AHI + nonsupine AHI of <5; namely, patients with respiratory events appearing only in the supine position.

More recently, Frank *et al.* have proposed a new classification system (Amsterdam Positional OSAS Classification, APOC) to optimize the indications for treatment with positional therapy. It distinguishes patients with OSAS into three categories: APOC I, II, and III (For more detailed explanation, see Chapter 5) (Frank *et al.* 2015).

To establish a diagnosis of POSA, it is crucial that patients spend *sufficient time in the supine* and *nonsupine positions during the recorded night*. However, there is no common indication establishing a minimum necessary time. The majority of studies set this limit between 20 and 60 minutes (as exclusion/inclusion criterion for the study) (Chung *et al.* 2010; Bignold *et al.* 2011; Joosten *et al.* 2014). More recently, the authors who have proposed the APOC classification system (whose aimed to standardize the identification criteria for POSA) suggested a minimum time for both the worst (supine) and the best (nonsupine) sleeping position of at least 10% of the sleeping time (Frank *et al.* 2015).

All the studies agreed that 50%–60% of patients with OSAS present a *positional disorder*, whereas patients presenting with a positional disorder only (supine-isolated OSAS) represent 25%–30% of patients with OSAS who are Caucasians. Recent studies on Asian populations have highlighted a higher percentage at 70%–75% (nonsupine AHI < 5), which is probably correlated with the different facial morphologies of these populations (Oksenberg *et al.* 1997; Richard *et al.* 2006; Mo *et al.* 2011; Joosten *et al.* 2014).

The percentage of positional patients is higher among patients with mild-moderate OSAS (84%–87%), and it decreases significantly among patients with severe OSAS (44%).

Positional patients are younger and slimmer than nonpositional ones, which has been confirmed by all literature reviews. Furthermore, some studies suggest that positional patients are the least drowsy, have a better quality of night sleep, and present lower values of both diastolic and systolic arterial pressures (these last characteristics are correlated with a milder respiratory sleep disorder) (Oksenberg *et al.* 1997; Mo *et al.* 2011; Joosten *et al.* 2014).

Changes in body weight can significantly influence the positionality of patients with OSAS: a significant weight gain can worsen the respiratory disorders by significantly increasing the nonsupine AHI so that it progresses into nonpositional AHI, whereas weight loss can reduce the respiratory events in the nonsupine position, thus revealing a positionality (Oksenberg *et al.* 2012).

In patients with POSA, AHI may vary considerably according to each night owing to the time spent in the supine position, which may influence the diagnosis of the disease (AHI ≥ 5) in approximately 40% of patients who are not diagnosed with OSAS. Moreover, this can lead to underestimation of the severity (approximately 39% of patients with mild-moderate OSAS would be diagnosed with severe OSAS if they slept the entire night in the supine position [Sunnergreen *et al.* 2013]).

Thus, it is crucial to always monitor the sleeping position during polysomnography or a polygraph recording as well as calculate AHI distinguished by position.

Unfortunately, there is a lack of precise indications of how to monitor sleeping positions and about the accuracy of body position sensors. Even the AASM's Manual for Scoring of Sleep and Associated Events does not provide specific indications on where to place the sensors and which ones should be used (whereas it is indicated for other polysomnographic parameters). To the best of our knowledge, only one study has specified that it is recommended to record body positions during sleep (it must always be evaluated) (Iber *et al.* 2012).

The commonly used body position sensors are those placed on the thorax, which detect the torso position. However, recent studies have demonstrated that the position of the head (detected with a sensor placed on the center of the forehead) during sleep may play a crucial role. In fact, a double sensor (the head and torso) enables a better identification of patients with POSA (Schwab 2011; Van Kesteren *et al.* 2011). Currently, the use of a double sensor (head and torso) is not recommended by international guidelines, although it may have important implications in the future, particularly in evaluating therapeutic response in patients treated with an oral device and/or positional therapy.

It has been speculated that the prone position could also affect OSAS. In fact, some studies have reported worsening of the respiratory pattern in such position, whereas others have reported an improvement. However, a recent review and metaanalysis has established that it is not possible to affirm that the prone position plays a role in determining obstructive respiratory events (Menon *et al.* 2013).

In conclusion, because patients with POSA are mainly young, slim, and present with respiratory sleep disorders of mild-moderate severity with peculiar characteristics (respiratory events appearing only in the supine position), it is clear how identification of the positionality can have important consequences on the management of such patients and their treatment. In general, because of the limited severity of this type of OSAS, these patients tend to be less adherent to CPAP therapy, whereas they respond more effectively to therapy with mandibular advancement devices (positionality is one of the criteria for selecting this therapy) and are only partially adherent to surgery of the soft tissues of the upper airways (which significantly reduces nonsupine AHI). These patients can benefit from positional therapy (see Chapter 5).

REM-RELATED OSAS

In normal sleep, the *REM phase* (dreaming sleep) occurs on an average of 3–5 times per night (corresponding with the nonrapid eye movement [NREM]-REM sleep cycles). The majority of REM sleep occurs in the second half of the night when REM sleep cycles are longer and higher in activity (REM and myoclonus).

From a neurological viewpoint, REM sleep is characterized by a condition of pre- and postsynaptic inhibition both at the sensory and motor levels with a subsequently increased arousal threshold (awakening) and considerable muscular hypotonia.

From a respiratory viewpoint, REM sleep is physiologically characterized by an irregular respiratory pattern (irregular respiratory events in frequency and amplitude), increased resistance and collapsibility of the upper airways, reduced lung volumes (both secondary to the hypotonia of the pharynx dilator muscles and intercostal muscles), decreased ventilatory response to both hypoxia and hypercapnia (capacity to increase ventilation in response to a chemical stimulus), and increased arousal threshold triggered by the hypoxic stimulus (brain aptitude to remain awake in response to stimuli) (Kryger *et al.* 2011).

During REM sleep, these physiological respiratory changes favor the onset of hypoventilation in patients who have already developed ventilatory pathologies during wakefulness (COPD, neuromuscular pathologies, kyphoscoliosis, and obesity hypoventilation syndrome) and the appearance or aggravation of a respiratory sleep disorder with obstructive apnea/hypopnea.

The data from the literature show that obstructive respiratory events are longer and cause a higher desaturation during REM sleep even if they are not more frequent during NREM sleep. In fact, AHI-NREM is usually higher or equal to AHI-REM (the number of apneic + hypopneic events per hour of REM Sleep) in patients with severe OSAS (AHI ≥ 30) (Muraki *et al.* 2008; Loadsman *et al.* 2000).

REM-related OSAS refers to a subgroup of patients with OSAS who present with obstructive respiratory events predominantly or exclusively during REM sleep.

The most commonly used diagnostic criterion is the number of apneic + hypopneic events per hour of REM Sleep (AHI-REM), which must be at least double compared with the number of apneic + hypopneic events per hour of NREM sleep (AHI-NREM) (AHI-REM/AHI-NREM ≥ 2) (Haba-Rubio *et al.* 2015) (Figure 2.12).

Several authors are engaged in this topic and have proposed additional criteria, such as the concurrent presence of AHI-NREM < 15 or < 10 (adding the time spent in the REM phase for at least 10 minutes) until the most restrictive criteri-

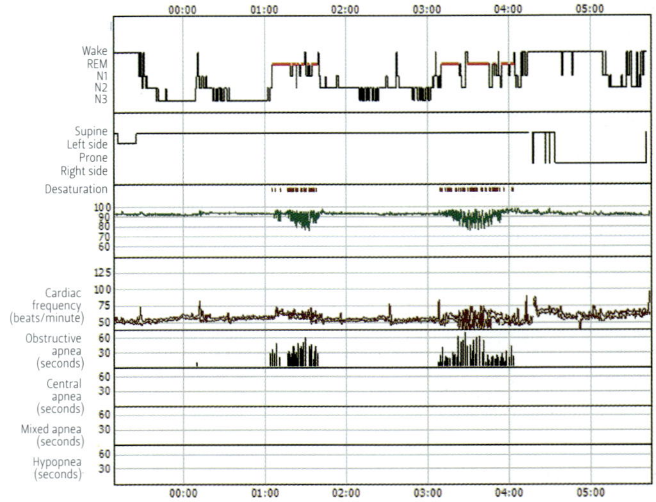

Apnea-hypopnea index (AHI) = 16.5
AHI-REM = 47.1
AHI-NREM = 6.1
Oxygen desaturation index (ODI) = 47.1
Mean SaO_2 = 93.2%
Minimum SaO_2 = 82.0%
Mean desaturation = 7.2%
Time spent with SaO_2 < 90% = 9.4 %

2.12 Full-night polysomnography of patients with REM-related OSAS. Apnea/hypopnea only appear in sequences during the REM sleep phases (red bars correspond with REM on the sleep recording track), whereas there is no direct correlation with the supine position. AHI is calculated based on the sleeping time estimated by the patient and distinguished per REM-NREM. It highlights REM-related OSAS.

on of AHI-NREM < 5/hour + AHI-REM ≥ 5/hour with at least 30 minutes of recording spent in the REM phase, which is currently recommended to correctly identify this subgroup of patients (Conwell *et al.* 2012; Mokhesi *et al.* 2012).

According to the different diagnostic criteria employed, the prevalence of REM-related OSAS ranges between 10% (restrictive criteria) and 36% (AHI-REM/AHI-NREM ≥ 2) (Conwell *et al.* 2012; Mokhesi 2012).

To date, studies have failed to clearly standardize this subgroup of patients with OSAS according to the clinical symptoms, outcome, and therapy. Some authors attribute this to the diagnostic criteria employed, which are quite variable in range (Mokhesi *et al.* 2012; Mokhesi 2012).

All studies agree that patients with REM-related OSAS are young individuals (aged <55 years) who are predominantly women (24% women vs. 8% men) presenting with mild-moderate OSAS (Koo *et al.* 2008).

Although the initial studies associated REM-related OSAS with increased daytime sleepiness, wide-ranging epidemiological studies have not confirmed such a hypothesis (Chami *et al.* 2010).

A recent Asian study on a wide range of patients with OSAS wherein the REM-related OSAS subgroup was identified (without recruiting with restrictive criteria) has demonstrated that patients with REM-related OSAS do not differ from other patients in terms of sleepiness (measured with ESS) and quality of life (assessed with standardized questionnaires), whereas they report a significantly minor prevalence of depression and cardiovascular diseases (Su *et al.* 2012).

Furthermore, the therapeutic consequences do not differ among patients with REM-related OSAS: the efficacy and adherence to CPAP treatment overlaps in patients with OSAS and REM-related OSAS even if slightly inferior pressures are more effective for the latter (Su *et al.* 2012).

In conclusion, because of the lack of evidence of a real difference in terms of clinical presentation, outcome, and therapeutic choice between patients with REM-related OSAS and patients with OSAS, there are insufficient factors to consider REM-related OSAS a distinct clinical or pathophysiologic subtype (ICSD-3, 2014; Mokhesi *et al.* 2012; Mokhesi 2012).

UPPER AIRWAY RESISTANCE SYNDROME (UARS)

UARS has been observed in patients with shoring, tiredness, and nonrestorative night sleep who presented with normal AHI (<5) but a high number of minor obstructive events (later identified with RERA) that affected the quality of sleep but not the nocturnal oxygenation at the polysomnographic recording.

Patients with UARS may present with the typical symptoms of OSAS, although they mainly report atypical symptoms such as insomnia characterized by difficulty in falling asleep and maintaining the sleep with considerable tiredness and asthenia rather than daytime sleepiness (ESS is often within the limits), pain, and muscular fatigability. Moreover, they tend to be hypotensive rather than hypertensive individuals and are young and slim; it is more common in women than in men (Guilleminault *et al.* 2000; Guilleminault *et al.* 2001).

Owing to these atypical characteristics, the underlying respiratory sleep disorder is often unidentified, and rheumatologic diseases or depression are diagnosed with subsequent prescription of antidepressant, sleeping, and stimulant drugs (Guilleminault *et al.* 2000).

A 5-year follow-up of untreated patients with UARS highlighted that the respiratory disorder remained unchanged, whereas insomnia and depression had worsened. In patients who had gained weight, UARS progressed into OSAS but cardiovascular complications were not reported (Guilleminault *et al.* 2006).

The effective therapy for this subgroup of patients is the same as that proposed for OSAS, and it causes a regression of atypical symptoms. More often, therapeutic choice is directed toward therapies other than CPAP (Guilleminault *et al.* 2000).

Because of its clinical differences, UARS was previously identified as a nosological entity autonomous from OSAS. Subsequently, the common pathophysiological mechanisms (obstruction of the upper airways) and overlapping therapeutic indications (subobstruction of the upper airways) were considered. The International Classification of Sleep Disorders (2005) proposed UARS as part of OSAS by replacing AHI (ICSD-2, 2005) with RERA in RDI, which is required to establish a diagnosis.

Even the new ICSD-3 (2014) has included UARS in the OSAS description as follows: "Data suggest that this condition is a variant of OSAS where the obstructive events determine arousals and minimally affect oxygenation [...]. The prevalence of this group is unknown [...]. By using correct sensors and standardized criteria to identify respiratory events, the majority of the patients satisfy the diagnostic criteria of OSAS (calculating RDI = apnea + hypopnea + RERA per hour of sleep)." In conclusion, there is no evidence to distinguish patients with UARS from patients with OSAS, albeit they present with peculiar clinical characteristics, because the underlying pathophysiological mechanisms and therapeutic possibilities and responses overlap.

Elements of differential diagnosis

In cases of patients with habitual snoring or those reporting respiratory sleep disorders who do not satisfy the diagnostic criteria for OSAS after investigation, it is important to be able to hypothesize an alternative diagnosis to suggest an appropriate diagnostic-therapeutic course. Thus, it is necessary to determine the primary elements of differential diagnosis for OSAS and other respiratory sleep disorders.

For a more detailed and thorough explanation of isolated snoring and all the other nonOSAS respiratory sleep disorders, please refer to ICSD-3.

Isolated snoring

ICSD-3 includes isolated snoring under the subchapter heading "Isolated Symptoms and Normal Variants" in the chapter about sleep-related breathing disorders (ICSD-3, 2014, pages 136–140) to highlight the nonpathological paraphysiological significance of this condition.

Isolated snoring is clinically characterized as a condition where patients report loud and habitual snoring that may bother their bed partners or roommates. It does not cause a change in the quality of sleep (continuous and restful sleep), daytime sleepiness, or other consequences, and AHI or RDI is <5 with an instrumental diagnostic recording (polysomnography or polygraph).

The presence of habitual snoring in patients with other metabolic or cardiovascular pathologies should always suggest the presence of OSAS, which must be thoroughly investigated even in the absence of other symptoms or signs that are indicative of OSAS.

Isolated snoring does not appear to be associated with high cardiocerebrovascular risks. Some previous epidemiological studies have indicated an increased risk for such pathologies (hypertensive stroke, coronary heart disease, or heart attack), whereas a recent observational study with polysomnographic methods has demonstrated that patients with habitual snoring without apnea do not present with increased risks of death or cardiovascular morbidities (Rich *et al.* 2011).

To establish a diagnosis of isolated snoring and exclude OSAS in patients with habitual snoring, the following steps are essential:

1. always perform instrumental recordings (polysomnography or polygraphy) that are appropriate in terms of the sensors used and the correctness of the analysis of the recording tracks;
2. always evaluate AHI or RDI in different sleeping positions because patients can be affected by POSA or have slept in the supine position for a very little time or not at all;
3. verify that patients have sufficiently slept during the recorded night (>4 h) and that AHI or RDI has been appropriately calculated (in cases of a cardiorespiratory monitoring system, and if REI is calculated rather than AHI or RDI, ensure that the recording time does not differ from the estimated sleeping time; in such cases, it is recommended to calculate AHI or RDI based on the estimated sleeping time).

Isolated snoring has a pathophysiologic mechanism similar to that of OSAS (subobstruction of the upper airways appearing during sleep), but by definition it does not cause clinical consequences or represent a risk factor for other pathologies. Therefore, no treatment is indicated unless the patients request it because their conditions have become a social problem (a nuisance for their bed partner).

Other nonOSAS respiratory sleep disorders

SDB must be considered in patients with snoring or when patients report a respiratory sleep disorder and the recording detects a pattern that is mainly characterized by nonobstructive respiratory events or breathing irregularities that cause changes in SaO_2 over an extended period of time.

NonOSAS SDB:

- epidemiologically less frequent than OSAS
- usually presents in patients with other (cardiac, neurologic, medical, or ventilatory) comorbidities at an elderly age
- must be investigated with more complex instrumental methods (polysomnography Levels I and II) and evaluated by a clinician who is experienced in sleep medicine
- can be associated with OSAS

As specified previously, ICSD-3 is used as the reference text for a correct and detailed nonOSAS SDB classification; here we will summarize and illustrate the main categories and the most important characteristics of nonOSAS SDB.

CENTRAL SLEEP APNEA SYNDROME

CSAS is clinically characterized by awakenings with a choking sensation, fragmented and nonrestorative nocturnal sleep, or insomnia and daytime sleepiness. Snoring can also be present.

Central apnea and hypopnea are exclusively or predominantly present (≥50% of the events are central) with cAI ≥ 5; desaturation is determined by such respiratory events and is variable but generally with a minor difference compared with that after an obstructive event.

It can be associated with Cheyne-Stokes periodic breathing, with the typical crescendo-decrescendo pattern mixed with central apnea (standard characteristics described in the respiratory events) for extended periods during the night.

ICSD-3 identifies idiopathic CSAS as not associated with other pathologies, which is not clearly defined from an epidemiologic viewpoint (rare event), and whose physiopatogenetic mechanisms appear to be correlated with low levels of CO2 in the blood (generally, these patients present a low CO2 in wakefulness, <40 mmHg). The course and outcome of CSAS are not fully known.

CSAS can be associated with other common clinical or pathophysiologic conditions; it has been observed in the following:

- patients with *cardiac diseases*, particularly but not exclusively in cardiac failure phases. Its presence increases the risk of mortality (Cheyne-Stokes breathing-CSAS) (Lanfranchi *et al.* 1999)
- patients with *neurologic diseases*, particularly those involving the brainstem, where the respiratory center is located (e.g., stroke, demyelinating diseases, degenerative diseases, and Chiari malformation). In these cases, Cheyne-Stokes-breathing is not present (CSAS due to medical causes without Cheyne-Stokes breathing)
- patients taking opiates or after taking medication that suppresses respiratory center activity (for instance, after general anesthesia) (medication-induced CSAS)
- patients traveling to and sleeping at high altitudes (≥2500 m and even >1500 m in some patients) (high-altitude CSAS)
- some patients with OSAS treated with CPAP who present with very frequent central apneic events (so-called complex SAS) (CPAP-induced CSAS)

SLEEP-RELATED HYPOVENTILATION/HYPOXEMIC SYNDROMES

These are characterized by alterations in respiratory sleep pattern associated with decreased basal SaO_2 (hypoxemia) for an extended period during the night and possibly with hypercapnia (when measured). Sometimes, both central and obstructive apnea can also be associated, although they do not represent the prevalent respiratory pattern, whereas they associate more often with hypoxemia and hypercapnia during wakefulness. They are detectable with an arterial blood gas analysis.

Primary or idiopathic forms of these syndromes are very rare; they can be congenital or acquired and are defined as a congenital central hypoventilation syndrome (also known as Ondine's syndrome).

The secondary forms are normally associated with other pathologies that cause an alteration in ventilatory function. The most well-known pathology among them is obesity hypoventilation syndrome, which appears in very obese patients and can be comorbid with OSAS and hypoventilation associated with medical causes, such as obstructive ventilatory pathologies (COPD), parenchymal lung disease (pulmonary fibrosis), ribcage pathologies (kyphoscoliosis), or neuromuscular diseases.

When these secondary hypoventilation syndromes are associated with OSAS, the medical case is defined as overlap syndrome.

REFERENCES

Adams R, Appleton S, Taylor A, McEvoy D, Wittert G. Are the ICSD-3 criteria for sleep apnoea syndrome too inclusive? *Lancet Respir Med.* 2016;4(5):e19-e20.

AIPO Associazione Italiana Pneumologi Ospedalieri. *Raccomandazioni per la Diagnosi e Cura dei Disturbi respiratori nel Sonno (DRS).* Milano: AIPO Ricerche; 2011.

American Academy of Sleep Medicine Task Force. Sleep-related breathing disorders in adults: recommendations for syndrome definition and measurement techniques in clinical research. *Sleep.* 1999;22(5):667-689.

American Academy of Sleep Medicine. *International Classification of Sleep Disorders.* 3rd ed. (ICSD-3). 2014, pp. 53-62.

Ayappa I, Norman RG, Krieger AC, Rosen A, O'Malley RL, Rapoport DM. Non-Invasive detection of respiratory effort-related arousals (RERAs) by a nasal cannula/pressure transducer system. *Sleep.* 2000 Sep 15;23(6):763-767.

Baldwin CR, Kapur WK, Holberg CJ, Rosen C, Nieto FJ. Association between gender and measures of daytime somnolence in the Sleep Heart Health Study. *Sleep.* 2004;27:305-311.

Berry RB, Budhiraja R, Gottlieb DJ, et al. Rules for scoring respiratory events in sleep: update of the 2007 AASM Manual for the Scoring of Sleep and Associated Events. Deliberations of the Sleep Apnea Definitions Task Force of the American Academy of Sleep Medicine. *J Clin Sleep Med.* 2012;8(5):597-619.

Bickelmann AG, Burwell CS, Robin ED, et al. Extreme obesity associated with alveolar hypoventilation: a Pickwickian syndrome. *Am J Med.* 1956;21(5):811-818.

Bignold JJ, Mercer JD, Antic NA, McEvoy RD, Catcheside PG. Accurate position monitoring and improved supine-dependent obstructive sleep apnea with a new position recording and supine avoidance device. *J Clin Sleep Med.* 2011;7(4):376-383.

Bixler E, Vgontzas A, Lin H, et al. Prevalence of sleep-disordered breathing in women. *Am J Respir Crit Care Med.* 2001;167(3pt1):608-613.

Braghiroli A, Marrone O, Sanna A, et al. Linee guida di procedura diagnostica nella sindrome delle apnee ostruttive nel sonno nell'adulto. Commissione paritetica Associazione Italiana Medicina del Sonno (AIMS) e Associazione Italiana Pneumologi Ospedalieri (AIPO). *Rassegna di Patologia dell'Apparato Respiratorio.* 2001;16:278-280.

Cartwright RD, Diaz F, Lloyd S. The effects of sleep posture and sleep stage on apnea frequency. *Sleep.* 1991;14(4):351-353.

Cartwright RD. Effect of sleep position on sleep apnea severity. *Sleep.* 1984;7(2):110-114.

Chami HA, Baldwin CM, Silverman A, et al. Sleepiness, quality of life, and sleep maintenance in REM versus non-REM sleep-disordered breathing. *Am J Respir Crit Care Med.* 2010;181(9):997-1002.

Chung JW, Enciso R, Levendowski DJ, Westbrook PR, Clark GT. Patients with positional versus nonpositional obstructive sleep apnea: a retrospective study of risk factors associated with apnea-hypopnea severity. *Oral Surg Oral Med Oral Pathol Oral Radiol Endod.* 2010;110(5):605-10.

Collop N, Anderson W, Boehlecke B, et al. Clinical guidelines for the use of unattended portable monitors in the diagnosis of obstructive sleep apnea in adult patients. Portable Monitoring Task Force of the American Academy of Sleep Medicine. *J Clin Sleep Med.* 2007;3(7):737-747.

Collop NA, Tracy SL, Kapur V, et al. Obstructive Sleep apnea Devices for Out-Of-Center (OOC) testing: technology Evaluation. *J Clin Sleep Med.* 2011;7(5):531-548.

Contardi S, Pizza F, Sancisi E, Mondini S, Cirignotta F. Reliability of a driving simulation task for evaluation of sleepiness. *Brain Res Bull.* 2004;63(5):427-431.

Conwell W, Patel B, Doeing D, et al. Prevalence, clinical features, and CPAP adherence in REM-related sleep-disordered breathing: a cross-sectional analysis of a large clinical population. *Sleep Breath.* 2012;16(2):519-526.

Eiseman NA, Westover MB, Ellembogen JM; Bianchi MT. The Impact of body posture and sleep stages on sleep apnea severità. *J Clin Sleep Med.* 2012;8(6):655-666.

Ejaz SM, Khawaja IS, Bhatia S, Hurwitz TD. Obstructive sleep apnea and depression: a review. *Innov Clin Neurosci.* 2011;8(8):17-25.

El Shayeb M, Topfer LA, Stafinski T, Pawluk L, Menon D. Diagnostic accuracy of level 3 portable sleep tests versus level 1 polysomnography for sleep-disordered breathing: a systematic review and meta-analysis. *CMAJ.* 2014;186(1):E25-E51.

Epstein L, Kristo D, Strollo PJ, et al. Clinical guideline for the evaluation, management and long-term care of obstructive sleep apnea in adults. *J Clin Sleep Med.* 2009;5(3):263-276.

Ferber R, Millman R, Coppola M, et al. Portable recording in the assessment of obstructive sleep apnea. ASDA standards of practice. *Sleep.* 1994;17(4):378-392.

Fischer J, Dogas Z, Bassetti CL, et al. Standard procedures for adults in accredited Sleep Medicine Centres in Europe. *J Sleep Res.* 2012;21(4):357-368.

Fleetham J, Ayas N, Bradley D, et al. Canadian Thoracic Society Sleep Disordered Breathing Committee. Canadian Thoracic Society 2011 guideline update: diagnosis and treatment of sleep disordered breathing. *Can Respir J.* 2011;18(1):25-47.

Frank MH, Ravesloot MJ, van Maanen JP, Verhagen E, de Lange J, de Vries N. Positional OSA part 1: Towards a clinical classification system for position-dependent obstructive sleep apnoea. *Sleep Breath.* 2015;19(2):473-480.

Friedman M, Ibrahim H, Bass L. Clinical staging for sleep-disordered breathing. *Otolaryngol Head Neck Surg.* 2002;127(1):13-21.

Friedman M, Tanyeri H, La Rosa M, et al. Clinical predictors of obstructive sleep apnea. *Laryngoscope.* 1999;109(12):1901-1907.

Gay PC, Selecky PA. Are Sleep Studies appropriately done in the home? *Respir Care.* 2010;55(1):66-73.

Gonçalves MA, Guilleminault C, Ramos E, Palha A, Paiva T. Erectile dysfunction, obstructive sleep apnea syndrome and nasal CPAP treatment. *Sleep Med.* 2005;6(4):333-339.

Guilleminault C, Black J, Palombini L, Ohayon M. Clinical investigation of obstructive sleep apnea syndrome and upper airway resistance syndrome patients. *Sleep Med.* 2000;1:51-56.

Guilleminault C, Kim YD, Chowdhuri S, Horita M, Ohayon M, Kushida C. Sleep and daytime sleepiness in upper airway resistance syndrome compared to obstructive sleep apnea syndrome. *Eur Respir J.* 2001;17:838-847.

Guilleminault C, Kim YD, Palombini L, Li K, Powell N. Upper airway resistance syndrome and its treatment. *Sleep.* 2000;23 Suppl 4:S197-S200.

Guilleminault C, Kirisoglu C, Poyares D, et al. Upper airway resistance syndrome: a long-term outcome study. *J Psychiatr Res.* 2006;40(3):273-279.

Haba-Rubio J, Janssens JP, Rochat T, Sforza E. Rapid eye movement-related disordered breathing: clinical and polysomnographic features. *Chest.* 2005;128(5):3350-3357.

Hajduk IA, Strollo PJ Jr, Jasani RR, et al. Prevalence and prediction of nocturia in obstructive sleep apnea-hypopnea syndrome—a retrospective study. *Sleep.* 2003;26:61-64.

Heinzer R, Marti-Soler H, Haba-Rubio J. Prevalence of sleep apnoea syndrome in the middle to old age general population. *Lancet Respir Med.* 2016;4(2):e5-e6.

Heinzer R, Vat S, Marques-Vidal P, Marti-Soler H, Andries D, Tobback N, et al. Prevalence of sleep-disordered breathing in the general population: the HypnoLaus study. *Lancet Respir Med.* 2015;3(4):310-318.

Hoddes E, Dement W, Zarcone V. The development and use of Stanford Sleepiness Scale (SSS). *Psychophysiology.* 1972;9:150.

Hoffstein V, Mateika S, Hanly P. Snoring and arousals: a retrospective analysis. *Sleep.* 1995;18(10):866-872.

Hoffstein V, Szalai JP. Predictive value of clinical features in diagnosing obstructive sleep apnea. *Sleep.* 1993;16(2):118-122.

Iber C, Ancoli-Israel S, Quan SF (for the American Academy of Sleep Medicine). *The AASM manual for the scoring of sleep and associated events: rules, terminology, and technical specifications.* 2nd ed. Westchester, Il: American Academy of Sleep Medicine; 2012.

Iriarte J, Alegre M, Urrestarazu E, Viteri C, Arcocha J, Artieda J. Continuous positive airway pressure as treatment for catathrenia (nocturnal groaning). *Neurology.* 2006;66(4):609-610.

Issa FG, Sullivan CE. Upper airway closing pressures in obstructive sleep apnea. *J Appl Physiol.* 1984;57(2):520-527.

Johns MW. A new method for measuring daytime sleepiness: the Epworth Sleepiness Scale. *Sleep.* 1991;14(6):540-545.

Johnson PL, Edwards N, Burgess K, Sullivan C. Detection of increased upper airway resistence during overnight polysomnography. *Sleep.* 2005;28(1):85-90.

Joosten SA, O'Driscoll DM, Berger PJ, Hamilton GS. Supine position related obstructive sleep apnea in adults: pathogenesis and treatment. *Sleep Med Rev.* 2014;18(1):7-17.

Kaida K, Takahashi M, Akerstedt T, Nakata A. Validation of the Karolinska sleepiness scale against performance and EEG variables. *Clin Neurophysiol.* 2006;117(7):1574-1581.

Kapur VK, Auckley DH, Chowdhuri S, Kuhlmann DC, Mehra R, Ramar K, Harrod CG. Clinical practice guideline for diagnostic testing for adult obstructive sleep apnea: an American Academy of Sleep Medicine clinical practice guideline. *J Clin Sleep Med.* 2017;13(3):479-504.

Kapur VK, Baldwin RN, Resnick HE, Gottlieb DJ, Nieto J. Sleepiness in patients with moderate to severe Sleep Disordered Breathing. *Sleep.* 2005;28(4):472-477.

Kawaguchi Y, Fukumoto S, Inaba M, et al. Different impacts of neck circumference and visceral obesity on the severity of obstructive sleep apnea syndrome. *Obesity.* 2011;19(2):276-282.

Kielb SA, Ancoli-Israel S, Rebok GW, Spira AP. *Cognition in obstructive sleep apnea-hypopnea syndrome (OSAS): current clinical knowledge and the impact of treatment. Neuromolecular Med.* 2012;14(3):180-193.

Koo BB, Dostal J, Ioachimescu O, Budur K. The effects of gender and age on REM-related sleep-disordered breathing. *Sleep Breath.* 2008;12(3):259-264.

Krieger J, Laks L, Wilcox I, et al. Atrial natriuretic peptide release during sleep in patients with obstructive sleep apnoea before and during treatment with nasal continuous positive airway pressure. *Clin Sci.* 1989;77:407-411.

Kryger MH, Roth T, Dement WC. *Principle and practice of sleep medicine*, 5th ed. Elsevier, 2011.

Kuna TS. Portable-Monitor Testing: An Alternative for Managing Patients with Obstructive Sleep Apnea Syndrome. *Respir Care.* 2010;55(9):1196-1212.

Kushida CA, Littner MR, Morgenthaler T, et al. Practice parameters for the indications for polysomnography and related procedures: an update for 2005. *Sleep.* 2005;28(4):499-521.

Lal C, Strange C, Bachman D. Neurocognitive impairment in obstructive sleep apnea. *Chest.* 2012;141(6):1601-1610.

Lanfranchi PA, Braghiroli A, Bosimini E, et al. Prognostic value of nocturnal Cheyne-Stokes respiration in chronic heart failure. *Circulation.* 1999;99(11):1435-1440.

Lavie P, Lavie L, Herer P. All-cause mortality in males with sleep apnoea syndrome: declining mortality rates with age. Eur *Respir J.* 2005;25(3):514-520.

Lin CM, Davidson, TM, Ancoli-Israel S. Gender differences in Obstructive Sleep Apnea and treatment implications. *Sleep Med Rev.* 2008;12(6):481-496.

Littner MR, Kushida C, Wise M, et al. Practice parameters for clinical use of the multiple sleep latency test and manteinance of wakefulness test. *Sleep.* 2005; 28(1):113-121.

Loadsman JA, Wilcox I. Is obstructive sleep apnoea a rapid eye movement-predominant phenomenon? *Br J Anaesth.* 2000;85(3):354-358.

Mador MJ, Kufel TJ, Magalang UJ et al. Prevalence of positional sleep apnea in patients undergoing polysomnography. *Chest.* 2005;128(4):2130-2137.

Maislin G, Pack AI, Kribbs NB, et al. A survey screen for prediction of apnea. *Sleep.* 1995(18):158-166.

Mallampati SR, Gatt SP, Gugino LD, et al. A clinical sign to predict difficult tracheal intubation: a prospective study. *Can Anaesth Soc J.* 1985;32(4):429-434.

Martinez-Rivera C, Abad J, Fiz JA, Rios J, Morera J. Usefulness of truncal obesity indices as predictive factors for obstructive sleep apnea syndrome. *Obesity.* 2008;16(1):113-118.

Menon A, Kumar M. Influence of body position on severity of obstructive sleep apnea: a sistematic review. *ISRN Otolaryngol.* 2013;2013:670381.

Mo JH, Lee CH, Rhee CS, Yoon IY, Kim JW. Positional dependency in Asian patients with obstructive sleep apnea and its implication for hypertension. *Arch Otolaryngol Head Neck Surg.* 2011;137(8):786-790.

Mokhlesi B, Punjabi NM. "REM-related" obstructive sleep apnea: an epiphenomenon or a clinically important entity? *Sleep.* 2012;35(1):5-7.

Mokhlesi B. REM-related obstructive sleep apnea: to treat or not to treat? *J Clin Sleep Med.* 2012;8(3):249-250.

Muraki M, Kitaguchi S, Ichihashi I, et al. Apnoea-hypopnea index during rapid eye movement and non-rapid eye movement sleep in obstructive sleep apnoea. *J Int Med Res.* 2008;36(5):906-913.

Myers KA, Mrkobrada M, Simel DL. Does this patient have obstructive sleep apnea? The Rational Clinical Examination systematic review. *JAMA.* 2013;310(7):731-741.

O'Connor G, Lind B, Lee E, et al. Variation in symptoms of sleep-disordered breathing with race and etnicity: the Sleep Heart Health Study. *Sleep.* 2003;26(1):74-79.

Oksenberg A, Arons E, Nasser K, Vander T, Radwan H. REM-related obstructive sleep apnea: the effect of body position. *J Clin Sleep Med.* 2010;6(4):343-348.

Oksenberg A, Dynia A, Nasser K, Gadoth N. Obstructive sleep apnea in adults: body postures and weight changes interactions. *J Sleep Res.* 2012;21(4):402-409.

Oksenberg A, Silverberg DS, Arons E, et al. Positional vs non positional obstructive sleep apnea patients: anthropomorphic, nocturnal polysomnographic, and multiple sleep latency test data. *Chest.* 1997;112(3):629-639.

Paiva T, Farinha A, Martins A, Guilleminault C. Chronic headaches and sleep disorders. *Arch Intern Med.* 1997;157:1701-1705.

Park JG, Morgenthaler TM, Gay PC. Novel and emerging nonpositive airway pressure therapies for sleep apnea. *Chest.* 2013;144(6):1946-1952.

Peppard PE, Young T, Barnet JH, Palta M, Hagen EW, Hla KM. Increased prevalence of sleep-disordered breathing in adults. *Am J Epidemiol.* 2013;177(9):1006-1014.

Pevernagie DA, Stanson AW, Sheedy PF 2nd, Daniels BK, Shepard JW Jr. Effects of body position on the upper airway of patients with obstructive sleep apnea. *Am J Respir Crit Care Med.* 1995;152(1):179-185.

Philip P, Chaufton C, Taillard J, et al. Maintenance of Wakefulness Test scores and driving performance in sleep disorder patients and controls. *Int J Psychophysiol.* 2013;89(2):195-202.

Phurroug S, Jacques L, Strille J, Brechner R. *Coverage Decision Memorandum for sleep testing for obstructive Sleep Apnea (OSA)(CAG00405N).* Baltimore Centers for Medicare and Medicaid; 2009.

Pien GW, Pack AI, Jackson N, Maislin G, Macones GA, Schwab RJ. Risk factors for sleep-disordered breathing in pregnancy. *Thorax.* 2013 doi:10.1136/thoraxjnl-2012-202718.

Pizza, F, Contardi S, Ferlisi M, Mondini S, Cirignotta F. Daytime driving simulation performance and sleepiness in obstructive sleep apnoea patients. *Accid Anal Prev.* 2008;40(2):602-609.

Priest B, Brichard C, Aubert G, Liistro G, Rodenstein D. Microsleep during a simplified maintenance of wakefulness test. A validation study of the OSLER test. *Am J Respir Crit Care Med.* 2001;163(7):1619-1625.

Ravesloot MJL, van Maanen JP, Dun L, de Vries N. The undervalued potential of positional therapy in position-dependent snoring and obstructive sleep apnea — a review of the literature. *Sleep Breath.* 2013;17(1):39-49.

Resta O, Foschino-Barbaro MP, Legari G, et al. Sleep-related breathing disorders, loud snoring and execessive daytime sleepiness in obese subjects. *Int J Obes Relat Metab Disord.* 2001;25(5):669-675.

Reutrakul S, Zaidi N, Wroblewski K, et al. Interactions between pregnancy, obstructive sleep apnea, and gestational diabetes mellitus. *J Clin Endocrinol Metab.* 2013;98(10):4195-4202.

Rich J, Raviv A, Raviv N, Brietzke SE. An epidemiologic study of snoring and all-cause mortality. *Otolaryngol Head Neck Surg.* 2011;145:341-344.

Richard W, Kox D, den Herder C, Laman M, van Tinteren H, de Vries N. The role of sleep position in obstructive sleep apnea syndrome. *Eur Arch Otorhinolaryngol.* 2006:263(10):946-950.

Robin IG. Snoring. *Proc R Soc Med.* 1948;41(3):151-153.

Roure N, Gomez S, Mediano O, et al. Daytime sleepiness and polysomnography in obstructive sleep apnea patients. *Sleep Med.* 2008;9(7):727-731.

Schröder CM, O'Hara R. Depression and obstructive sleep apnea (OSA). *Ann Gen Psychiatry.* 2005;4:13.

Schwab RJ. A quantum advance in PSG recordings: the importance of head position in mediating the AHI. *Sleep.* 2011;34(8):985-986.

Shepertycky MR, Banno K, Kryger MH. Differences between men and women in the clinical presentation of patients diagnosed with obstructive sleep apnea syndrome. *Sleep.* 2005 Mar;28(3):309-14.

Su CS, Liu KT, Panjapornpon K, Andrews N, Foldvary-Schaefer N. Functional outcomes in patients with REM-related obstructive sleep apnea treated with positive airway pressure therapy. *J Clin Sleep Med.* 2012;8(3):243-247.

Subramanian S, Jayaraman G, Majid H, Aguilar R, Surani S. Influence of gender and anthropometric measures on severity of obstructive sleep apnea. *Sleep Breath.* 2012;16(4):1091-1095.

Sunnergren O, Broström A, Svanborg E. Positional sensitivity as a confounder in diagnosis of severity of obstructive sleep apnea. *Sleep Breath.* 2013;17(1):173-179.

Tregear S, Reston J, Schoelles K, Phillips B. Obstructive sleep apnea and risk of motor vehicle crash: systematic review and meta-analysis. *J Clin Sleep Med.* 2009;5(6):573-581.

Valencia-Flores M, Orea A, et al. Prevalence of sleep apnea and electrocardiographic disturbances in morbidly obese patients. *Obesity Research.* 2000;8(3):262-269.

Van Kesteren ER, van Maanen JP, Hilgevoord AA, Laman DM, de Vries N. Quantitative effects of trunk and head position on the apnea hypopnea index in obstructive sleep apnea. *Sleep.* 2011;34(8):1075-1081.

Vetrugno R, Liguori R, Cortelli P, et al. Sleep-related stridor due to dystonic vocal cord motion and neurogenic tachypnea/tachycardia in multiple system atrophy. *Mov Disord.* 2007 Apr 15;22(5):673-678.

Vetrugno R, Provini F, Plazzi G, Vignatelli L, Lugaresi E, Montagna P. Catathrenia (nocturnal groaning): a new type of parasomnia. *Neurology.* 2001;56(5):681-683.

Vgontzas A, Tan T, Bixler E, Martin L, Shubert D, Kales A. Sleep apnea and sleep disruption in obese patients. *Arch Intern Med.* 1994;154(15):1705-1711.

Vignatelli L, Plazzi G, Barbato A, et al. Italian version of the Epworth sleepiness scale: external validity. *Neurol Sci.* 2003;23(6):295-300.

Villa MP, Pagani J, Miano S, Parisi P. Sindrome delle apnee ostruttive nel sonno in età pedatrica. *Area Pediatrica.* 2005; Dossier - Anno 6, nr. 7.

Weaver TE, Grunstein RR. Adherence to continuous positive airway pressure therapy: the challenge to effective treatment. *Proc Am Thorac Soc.* 2008 Feb 15;5(2):173-178.

Young T, Evans L, Finn L, Palta M. Estimation of the clinically diagnosed proportion of sleep apnea syndrome in middle-aged men and women. *Sleep.* 1997;20(9):705-706.

Young T, Finn L, Austin D, Peterson A. Menopausal status and Sleep-Disordered breathing in the Wisconsin Sleep Cohort Study. *Am J Respir Crit Care Med.* 2003;167(9):1181-1185.

Young T, Palta M, Dempsey J, Skatrud J, Weber S, Badr S. The occurrence of sleep-disordered breathing among middle-aged adults. *N Engl J Med.* 1993;328(17):1230-1235.

Young T, Peppard P, Gottlieb D. Epidemiology of obstructive sleep apnea: a population health perspective. *Am J Respir Crit Care Med.* 2002;165(9):1217-1239.

Young T, Peppard P, Taheri S. Excess weight and sleep-disordered breathing. *J Appl Physiol.* 2005;99(4):1592-1599.

Young T, Shahar E, Nieto F, et al. Predictors of sleep-disordered breathing in community-dwelling adults: the Sleep Heart Health Study. *Arch Intern Med.* 2002;162(8):893-900.

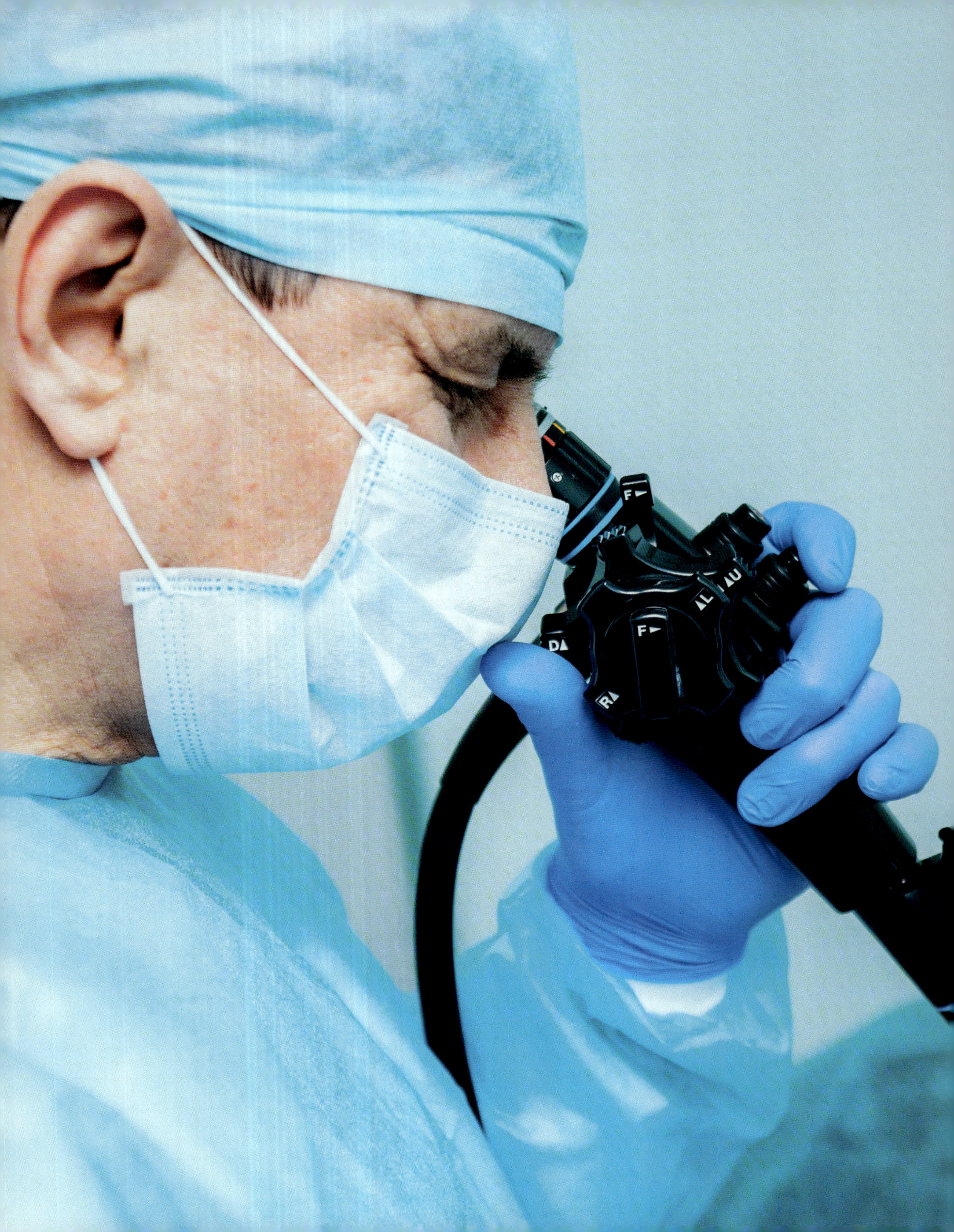
F
U
L
F
D
R

Clinical and instrumental diagnosis of obstructive sites

Giovanni Sorrenti ▪
Irene Pelligra ▪ Ottavio Piccin ▪
Riccardo Albertini ▪ Giuseppe Caccamo

Objectives

- Learning the ear, nose, and throat (ENT) diagnostic work-up of patients with obstructive sleep apnea syndrome (OSAS)
- Understanding the operative indications, limitations, and modalities of advanced drug-induced sleep endoscopy (DISE)
- Learning to identify the main obstructive sites and the related therapeutic choices

Introduction

One of the main factors responsible for the onset of snoring and OSAS is the presence of morphological alterations reducing the lumen of the upper airways, particularly in nonobese individuals. Accordingly, we can deduce the importance of an accurate evaluation of the caliber and collapsibility of the first segments of the upper airways as an essential tool to identify the site where the obstruction occurs and its pattern and formulate an adequate non-continuous positive airway pressure (non-CPAP) therapeutic approach.

Owing to the expertise required in this field, specialized otolaryngologists play a key role in the diagnostic work-up of patients with OSAS. This requires a clinical and instrumental protocol articulated in different steps, in which the complexity is due to the multifactorial origin of OSAS and the complex (not yet clarified) pathophysiological relationship between anatomic and functional factors. There are no morphological anomalies specific to patients with OSAS nor is there a direct relationship between the presence of such anomalies and the severity of the nocturnal respiratory disorder.

Furthermore, examinations performed on awake patients do not provide definite information about the possible sites of pharyngeal obstruction during sleep.

The introduction of DISE has significantly contributed to understanding the obstructive mechanisms during sleep despite the limitations inherent to this method, which will be discussed in the relevant paragraphs. Currently, this examination is the most advanced and reliable diagnostic tool for evaluating the site, grading, and pattern of obstruction in patients with OSAS who are candidates for receiving a non-CPAP therapy.

Clinical evaluation

The epidemiological impact, cardiovascular complication risks, and poor quality of life resulting from daytime sleepiness give OSAS the characteristics of a social pathology that needs to be identified and treated accordingly. A thorough evaluation of the diurnal and nocturnal symptoms is certainly the initial component required to direct the diagnosis, acquire predictive information about the presence and severity of the nocturnal respiratory disorder, and identify patients who require further examinations (polygraphic recordings) based on a priority criterion of a suspected severity.

After classifying patients who require further examination by evaluating the diurnal and nocturnal symptoms of the general clinical conditions, nonessential habits, and medication therapies, the presence of symptoms belonging to the ENT sphere must be investigated.

The association between OSAS and gastroesophageal reflux is very frequent, such that the negative endoluminal pressure generated by apneic events favors the aspiration of the gastric content into the pharynx, and the acidic pH of the gastric flow aggravates the laryngopharyngeal mucosa with consequent chronic inflammation and edema of the tissues, which in turn aggravates the obstructive site in a vicious circle. These symptoms are characterized by awakenings with a gasping sensation associated with the reflux episodes and by characteristic choking sounds.

Similarly, it is important to evaluate the presence of a nasal respiratory insufficiency due to functional or anatomic causes (nonallergic and allergic rhinitis and craniofacial traumas with altered anatomy of the facial skeleton), which can aggravate the nocturnal obstructive symptoms and invalidate the compliance and/or therapeutic efficacy of other treatments, as described later in this chapter.

Objective examinations

The diagnostic outcomes of the ENT objective examinations are described in Table 3.1. The evaluated anatomic sites and the necessary examinations are presented in Table 3.2.

3.1 Diagnostic outcomes of the ENT objective examinations.

Identifying anatomic anomalies that are potentially associated with OSAS
Detecting predictive factors of the presence and severity of the nocturnal respiratory disorder, with an aim to identify and assess patients who require further examinations (nocturnal recordings) based on a priority criterion of the suspected severity
Diagnosing possible pathologies in the ENT sphere (particularly neoformations in the nasal cavity or pharyngolaryngeal tract) that need to be independently treated from OSAS
Defining the anatomic factors of the upper airways for determining the therapeutic plan

3.2 Stages of the ENT objective examinations.

Anatomic site	Diagnostic method	Semeiotics
Nose	Rhinoscopy	Nasal patency Aspects of the nasal mucosa Morphology of middle and inferior turbinates Presence of deviations in the septum and bone spurs Presence of polyps or neoformations
Oral cavity and orohypopharynx	Orohypopharyngoscopy	Morphology and aspects of the soft palate and uvula Ratio between the tongue and soft palate (modified Mallampati score) Tonsillar hypertrophy grading

Rhinoscopy

Objective nasal examinations are crucial to evaluate patients with OSAS for the following reasons:

- An increase in nasal resistance can cause an increase in the negative pressure at the beginning of the upper airway, contributing to pharyngeal collapse;

- Oral breathing occurs at the base of a malposition of the tongue, which tends to fall back, thus aggravating both the retropalatal and pharyngeal obstruction;
- In patients who need a non-CPAP therapy, their compliance regarding the device (a MAD, tongue retaining device, or another sort of OSA treatment) may be reduced because of the increased pressure that must be applied in the case of nasal respiratory stenosis. Similarly, in patients treated with mandibular advancement devices (MAD), the presence of a nasal respiratory obstruction may reduce the tolerability and efficacy of MAD.

From a practical viewpoint, the nasal cavity, the middle and inferior meatus, and the nasopharynx are investigated, followed by evaluations of the nasal mucosa (presence of edema, hyperemia, or pathological secretions); the morphology of the middle and inferior turbinates; the presence of deviations in the nasal cavity, nasal septal crests, or spurs; the presence of polyps, adenoids, or other neoformations; and conditions that can alter the nasal airflow and increase nasal resistance.

In cases of suspected sinusitis, computed tomography (CT) of the nose and paranasal sinuses must be performed to verify a possible obstruction of the sinus ostium associated with anatomic anomalies.

Orohypopharyngoscopy

The pharynx plays a crucial role in respiratory obstruction during sleep. Therefore, evaluation of the oral cavity of the orohypopharynx is primarily important in patients with OSAS.

The evaluation is initiated by investigating the soft palate and uvula and identifying possible anomalies, such as elongation and/or hypertrophy of the uvula, overabundant palatal mucosa, and faucial pillars, which are characteristics of patients with OSAS. This is followed by determining the ratios between the soft palate and the tongue using the Mallampati score modified according to Friedman, which allows an immediate assessment of the tongue impediment encumbrance. This score is calculated by determining the plane of the posterior portion of the tongue and the profile of the soft palate with an open mouth; the tongue remains inside the mouth. This scoring is performed according to four degrees of severity, as reported in Table 3.3.

The Mallampati score can also be a useful index of hypopharyngeal obstruction. In fact, a close correlation among hypopharyngeal obstruction, Mallampati scoring, and OSAS severity has been demonstrated.

The degree of tonsillar hypertrophy is also an important predictive factor for OSAS and its severity. Tonsillar hypertrophy can be classified into four degrees according to its severity, as described in Table 3.4. A high tonsillar grade is considered a positive predictive factor for successful pharyngeal surgery.

3.3 Mallampati scores modified according to Friedman.

Grade I	Tonsils, faucial pillars, and soft palate are clearly visible
Grade II	Uvula, pillars, and superior tonsillar pole are visible
Grade III	Only part of the soft palate is visible
Grade IV	Soft palate is not visible; only the hard palate is visible

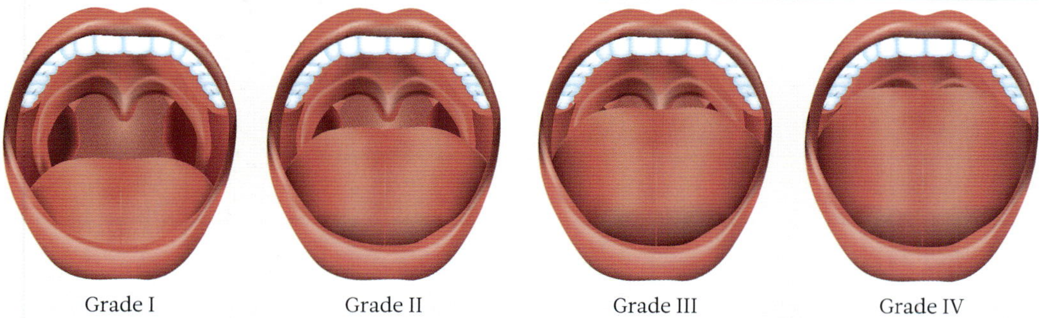

3.4 Tonsillar hypertrophy grading.

Grade I	Surgically removed tonsils
Grade II	Atrophic intravelic tonsils
Grade III	Tonsils are barely visible and are slightly out of the anterior pillar
Grade IV	Hypertrophic tonsils occupy three-quarters of the midline region

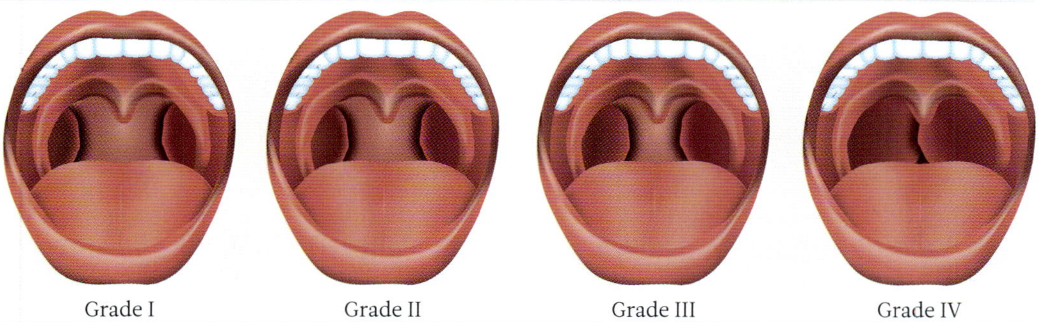

Fibroendoscopy with Müller's maneuver

Fibroendoscopy is performed at the end of the general objective examination. This examination enables a more thorough visualization of the upper aerodigestive tract. In particular, it allows the following:

- to evaluate the presence of deviations in the nasal septum, hypertrophy of the turbinates, polyps or edema of the nasal mucosa, and rhinopharyngeal obstruction with more accuracy than a standard rhinoscopy;
- to define the length of the soft palate and uvula, the tonsillar encumbrance, the characteristics of the tongue base, the sections of the aerodigestive tract at different sites, the presence of edema in the mucosa (expression of chronic traumatism associated with snoring), and the possible presence of a neoformation in the pharyngolaryngeal tract;

3.5 Lingual tonsil hypertrophy grading.

Grade I	Complete view of the glossoepiglottic and epiglottic valleculas
Grade II	Lingual tonsil occupying less than 50% of the vallecula
Grade III	Lingual tonsil occupying more than 50% of the vallecula
Grade IV	Glossoepiglottic and epiglottic valleculas are not visible

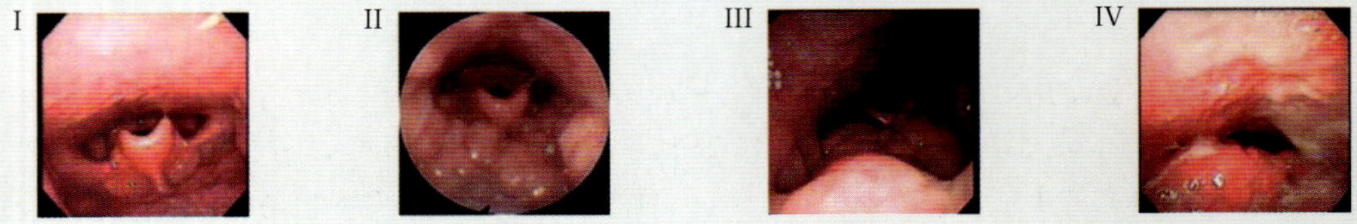

Source: Friedman 2015

- to detect the grade of hypertrophy of the lingual tonsils. This can be particularly obvious in patients who have undergone adenotonsillectomy, obese individuals, subjects presenting with gastroesophageal reflux, or those receiving specific medications such as phenytoin. Hypertrophy of the lingual tonsils is classified into grades I–IV according to the visibility of the epiglottic vallecula (3.5);
- to observe the morphology of the epiglottis, which can be small and omega-shaped, flaccid, or retrodisplaced, thus suspecting its role in the obstruction;
- to evaluate the glottic plane. Although it is rarely involved in the obstruction, it may present with anatomic or functional alterations (neoformations or uni- or bilateral vocal cord paralysis), which may have clinical impacts during sleep.

The endoscopic examination is completed with the Müller's maneuver, which comprises forced inspiration with a closed mouth and pinched nose to generate negative pressure inside the airway. By simulating what happens during an apneic event, this depression favors pharyngeal collapse and allows the dynamic evaluation of the degree of the pharyngeal collapse at the retropalatal and retrolingual levels.

DESCRIPTION OF THE TECHNIQUE

Endoscopy is performed on awake patients using a diagnostic fiberscope (3.5 mm caliber, 30 cm in length, and angular adjustment of 105°) under conditions of oral breathing, nasal breathing, and snoring simulation to better identify the possible vibration sites. At first, patients are examined in a sitting position and later in a supine position.

After evaluating the nasal cavity accurately, the nasopharynx, which is a possible site for an airflow obstruction due to the presence of hypertrophic adenoid tissues or neoformations, is examined. Then, the soft palate and uvula (particularly their length, thickness, and distance from the posterior wall) are

3.6 Percentage of obstruction determined by Müller's maneuver.

Score	Percentage of reduction in the airway diameter
1 +	Percentage of reduction in the airway diameter
2 ++	Minimum reduction in the airway area (<25%)
3 +++	Reduction in the airway area by ca. 50%
4 ++++	Reduction in the airway area by ca. 75%

examined and evaluated for possible hypertrophy and vertical orientation of the tongue base. The investigation ends with an examination of the hypopharyngolaryngeal tract to determine the presence of hypertrophy of the tongue base, a malformed or flaccid epiglottis, vocal cord paralysis, or masses that obstruct the laryngeal lumen.

The percentage of obstruction detected by Müller's maneuver is determined according to the classification proposed by Sher in 1985 Table 3.6. It is necessary to determine the pattern of collapse, which can be circular or concentric and lateral or anteroposterior.

In summary, fibroendoscopy with Müller's maneuver is a useful tool for diagnostic work-ups of patients with OSAS because it is minimally invasive and it allows the static and dynamic evaluation of the airway in a simple, rapid, and cost-effective manner. Its limitations are that it is performed on awake patients and it requires the cooperation of patients. Furthermore, the interpretation of the obtained data is strictly dependent on the operator. Over the past years, the reliability of the data obtained with sleep endoscopy has been questioned, particularly regarding obstruction at the tongue base and the epiglottis. Fernandez-Julian *et al.* (2014) have reported changes in the surgical plan for patients who had mainly been subjected to basic clinical evaluations, endoscopy with Müller's maneuver, and cephalometry in 40% of patients after sleep endoscopy. Such changes could be mainly attributed to a missed detection of the hypopharyngeal obstruction (tongue-epiglottis) on general objective examinations and to endoscopy performed on awake patients.

Diagnosis by imaging

Lateral teleradiography

Skeletal anomalies cannot be neglected when determining the pathology of OSAS. It has been extensively documented that patients with a maxillar-mandibular retrusion (or skeletal class II malocclusion) have a higher risk of OSAS than those without skeletal abnormalities, considering that, ultimately, this results from a disproportion between the volume of the container (facial skeleton) and the volume of the soft tissues. In clinical practice, it is possible to deduce useful information on the impact of such anomalies based on the lateral teleradiography of the head.

Cephalometric analysis with lateral teleradiography was introduced in sleep surgery approximately 25 years ago, and it still represents a rapid and cost-effective tool to evaluate the whole upper airway in patients with OSAS. This analysis comprises linear and angular measurements detected on lateral teleradiography of the skull obtained with strictly defined geometric conditions (a head unit holds patients immobile in the Frankfurt plane, and the distance from the radiation source to the fixed plate is 1.5 m). This analysis offers a panoramic view to evaluate the relationships between skeletal structures and soft tissues.

Sleep surgery has widely adopted the analysis proposed by Stanford's group in 1983; this analysis considers only some fundamental parameters: skeletal class malocclusion, the distance from the hyoid bone to the mandibular plane, the length of the soft palate, and the width of the posterior airway space.

These morphological data are evaluated with other essential indicators [apnea-hypopnea index (AHI), body mass index (BMI), Mallampati score, tonsillar hypertrophy grading, and endoscopic staging], and they may play an important role in identifying the obstructive sites and thus enabling to choose a more adequate treatment: surgery (intervening the bony or soft-tissue parts) or dentistry.

The advantages of lateral teleradiography are easy accessibility, noninvasiveness, reproducibility, and cost-effectiveness. The disadvantages are represented by its bidimensionality, with the impossibility of providing volumetric data and demonstrating the structures laterally delimiting the pharynx (tonsils, palatine arches, and the lateral pharyngeal wall), as well as by the fact that this examination is performed on patients in an erect position and a wakefulness state.

Cephalometric tracing will be described later in this chapter. From a surgical view point, the presence of mandibular retrusion, a reduced pharyngeal airway space (PAS < 10 mm), and a caudal dislocation of the hyoid bone [medial pterygoid (MP)-hyoid bone (Hy) > 15 mm] are clinically significant data, which are indicative factors for retrolingual obstruction. Such data reveal limited therapeutic outcomes achieved only by pharyngeal surgery and the need to correct the retrolingual obstruction.

CT

CT is useful in evaluating the morphology of cranial-cervical regions in patients with apnea. Conventional CT allows us to identify anatomical bone anomalies, evaluate morphological alterations in different sites of the upper airways, and gain a panoramic view of the pharyngolaryngeal tract components. Furthermore, CT enables us to analyze the cross-sectional regions of the air lumen at the different sites and evaluate the thickness of the pharyngeal walls. Sagittal reconstructions, particularly those detected on spiral CT, allow us to determine the length of the soft palate correctly and guarantee a complete view of the lingual components, particularly the relationship of the soft palate with its base and the mandibular plane. The 3D reconstruction of the craniofacial structures is also useful to evaluate airway modifications in patients subjected to oropharyngeal surgery or bimaxillary advancement. Owing to the costs and radiation exposure, this procedure is used in the field of snoring surgery research instead of clinical practice.

Magnetic resonance

Similar observations regarding CT can be applied to magnetic resonance (MR). MR works very well in cervicofacial region examinations because this region is rich in soft-tissue parts, which results in a better range of contrast. It provides images of different cross-sections that are highly detailed for airway cavities as well as their delimiting soft-tissue parts. In a sagittal projection, it is possible to execute a precise analysis of the morphology of the tongue, the floor of the mouth, and their relationship with the bone frame. This analysis is important, particularly in view of a surgical intervention directly on the hyoid lingual complex because it allows us to identify and determine the pharyngeal obstruction due to volume anomalies and the position of the tongue. Besides evaluating the caliber of the airway, the axial projection is also useful for determining through magnetic resonance the concentration of the adipose tissue in the pharyngeal wall and parapharyngeal spaces.

Unlike CT, MR does not expose patients to ionizing radiation; however, the examination duration, high cost, and applicability limitations for obese individuals restrict the use of MR in the research field.

The advantages and disadvantages of the three methods discussed above are listed in Table 3.7.

3.7 Medical imaging.

Methods	Indications	Advantages	Disadvantages
Lateral teleradiography	Evaluation of the relationship between the skeletal and soft tissues	Easy accessibility Noninvasive Reproducible Cost-effective	Bidimensional Insufficient identification of significant anatomic anomalies Erect position Wakefulness state
Computed tomography	Evaluation of the morphology of the cranial-cervical region Analysis of the cross-sectional region of the air lumen at different sites	Tridimensional Volumetric reconstructions Reproducible Evaluation of the thickness of the lateral wall	High cost Radiation exposure Wakefulness state
Magnetic resonance	Evaluation of the airway cavities, particularly the delimiting soft tissues Analysis of the tongue morphology, the floor of the mouth, and their relationship with the bone frame	Tridimensional Noninvasive Volumetric reconstructions Reproducible Evaluation of the thickness of the lateral wall	Duration of the examination High cost Applicability limitations in obese individuals Wakefulness state

Sleep endoscopy

To date, we have presented the diagnostic work-ups of patients with OSAS; these diagnostic work-ups comprise multiple steps, and none of them alone is sufficient to establish a topographic diagnosis of the obstruction.

The discussed diagnostic tools are useful and commonly used in clinical practice. However, they have disadvantages of being performed in a wakefulness state and not considering the dynamic aspects of the obstruction, which are as important (if not more) as the purely morphological aspects.

Sleep endoscopy involves the evaluation of the airway of patients with OSAS under conditions that are at least coinciding (if not the same) with those of physiological sleep. This has enabled us to shift the attention to evaluating the dynamic morphology of the pharynx, thus discovering the predominant role of lateral pharyngeal collapse in identifying the obstruction and, in turn, supporting its interpretation. Several studies and the experience of our authors with more than 600 patients have confirmed that lateral pharyngeal collapse is the most frequent obstructive modality. Accumulation of such data is the basis of a profound change in the surgical approach for patients with OSAS, particularly regarding the pharyngeal surgical techniques. After the introduction of sleep endoscopy, obstruction removal-based techniques [uvulopalatopharyngoplasty (UPPP) and laser-assisted uvula palatoplasty (LAUP)] have been gradually abandoned in favor of functional surgical techniques [expansion sphincter pharyngoplasty (ESP), functional expansion pharyngoplasty (FEP), and their related variants] whose targets is not the removal of excessive soft tissue but rather stabilization of the pharyngeal walls. This resulted in an increase in the percentage of successful outcomes from 40%-60% using the conventional techniques to 80%-85% using the current techniques.

Furthermore, sleep endoscopy has allowed us to improve our understanding on how the tongue and epiglottis participate in the genesis of the obstruction. Their role is often underestimated during examinations performed in a wakefulness state.

Despite the limitations owing to the action of drugs, the reproducibility of a sleep that is as close as possible to a physiological sleep and the subjectivity of the interpretation of the obtained data make sleep endoscopy the currently most reliable diagnostic method for evaluating the site, percentage, and pattern of obstruction in patients with OSAS who are candidates for a non-CPAP therapy.

Sleep endoscopy was introduced by Pringle in 1981, and since then, it has undergone several modifications. In 2013, the European Position Paper defined its minimum requirements as reported below.

DESCRIPTION OF THE TECHNIQUE

Sleep endoscopy must be performed in a surgical or endoscopic room equipped with a standard system to monitor the patients. The minimum equipment set comprises the following:

- a flexible fiberscope with optical fibers, preferably connected to a video-recording system for offline visualization of the examination;
- mechanical pump or target-controlled infusion (TCI) for administering the sleep-inducing drug (propofol);
- equipment for pulse oximetric and electrocardiographic monitoring during sedation;
- equipment for electroencephalographic monitoring (bispectral index, BIS®) (optional)

Sleep endoscopy is performed on patients in the supine position on the operating table in a dimmed and silent surgery room. This analysis is initiated by infusing a sleep-inducing drug, preferably propofol (2,6-diisopropylphenol), which is considered the most adequate because of its rapid onset (less than 1 minute), duration of action (3–10 minutes), short half-life, and minimum adverse effects. The drug can be administered using the bolus technique and a mechanical or TCI pump. The latter allows for a more standardized sedation because the amount of drug infused is calculated using an algorithm that considers the pharmacodynamic and pharmacokinetic characteristics of the drug and the characteristics (weight and height) of the patients; therefore, the drug is able to guarantee a constant concentration of the infuse drug at the obstructive site. The level of sedation can be controlled using a continuous electroencephalographic monitoring system (BIS®), which is indicated as optional by the European Position Paper but considered as a part of the standard setting for sleep endoscopy by our authors. This enables us to monitor the level of sedation in almost real time; moreover, along with the TCI pump, it allows optimal and constant maintenance of the specific drug used for sedation during the procedure. This is a key requirement to reproduce snoring without inducing respiratory depression, central-type apneic episodes, or sudden awakenings. PO2 levels maintained between a mean saturation and nadir saturation level are indicative of induced sleep overlapping with physiological sleep and are displayed on the polysomnographic equipment. Regarding BIS®, it has been recommended that these levels should be maintained between 70 and 50.

Once drug sedation has been initiated, a flexible fiberscope is inserted in the patients' airways by positioning its tip on the nasopharynx, while awaiting the onset of snoring or apneic episodes. The evaluation is performed at retropalatal, retrolingual, and supraglottic laryngeal levels. To simulate the action and evaluate the possible benefits of MAD, a mandibular pull-up maneuver, which comprises the manual advancements of the mandible, is performed. The examination duration is approximately 20–25 minutes. Generally, patient awakenings do not present a problem, as experienced and documented in the literature by our authors.

At the end of the procedure, the obtained data are described according to one of the several proposed classifications; the most commonly used clas-

3.8 VOTE classification.

Structure	Degree of obstruction*	Pattern		
		Anteroposterior	Lateral	Concentric
Velum (palatine velum)				
Oropharynx				
Tongue base				
Epiglottis				

*Degree of obstruction: 0, absence of obstruction; 1, partial obstruction (vibration); 2, complete obstruction; 3, nonvisualized site.

Source: Kezirian et al. 2011.

3.9 OHL classification.

Site	Nose (static obstruction)	Oropharynx	Hypopharynx	Larynx a: supraglottic b: glottic
Obstruction grade value %	0%–25%: 1	0%–25%: 1	0%–25%: 1	Positive or negative collapse/obstruction
	25%–50%: 2	25%–50%: 2	25%–50%: 2	
	50%–75%: 3	50%–75%: 3	50%–75%: 3	
	75%–100%: 4	75%–100%: 4	75%–100%: 4	

Source: Vicini et al. 2012

sifications are the velum oropharynx tongue base epiglottis (VOTE) and the nose oropharynx hypopharynx and larynx (NOHL) (Table 3.8 and 3.9).

Sleep endoscopy has been performed as a routine practice since 2006 at the hospital unit where our authors perform operations, and since 2012, it has been performed in an advanced setting (advanced sleep endoscopy).

Besides sleep-inducing drug infusion with a TCI pump and BIS® monitoring, this setting requires the following:

- **online cardiorespiratory monitoring** to control the action of the drug on respiratory events (identifying and excluding any central apneas, which recur more frequently in the first 10 minutes after sedation, from observations) and to verify the good technical quality of the procedure based on the real-time comparison between the intraDISE polygraphic data and diagnostic recording data. Furthermore, the simultaneous recordings of endoscopic and polygraphic data enable us to associate each respiratory event with its corresponding obstructive pattern. In clinical practice, sensors are placed on the patients before sleep induction. These are the same sensors that are used for home monitoring (nasal cannula, thermistor, pulse oximeter, and microphone to record snoring), and they transmit the relative data to a control panel via a wireless router provided with a specific software that is placed inside the surgery room;

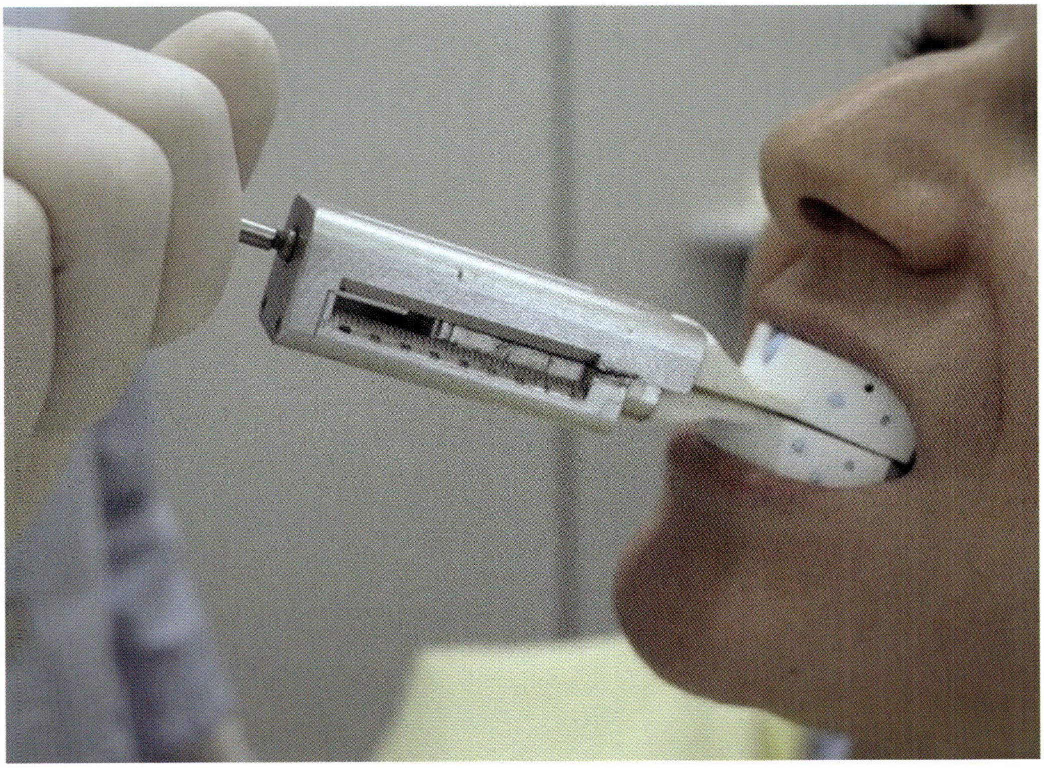

3.1 Positioning of the MAD simulator.

- **simulation of the mandibular advancement using the George Gauge device (*custom*-made).** This aims to compensate for the main limitations of a mandibular advancement simulated with a pull-up maneuver, which sets an arbitrary and nonrepeatable advancement without considering the vertical disruption obtained with MAD and whose effects on airway collapse are not negligible. In clinical practice, our authors perform this maneuver using a silicon putty with the George Gauge Bite device (5 mm vertical opening), whose advancement corresponds to the most comfortable and protruded position achieved by the patients (3.1). The simulator is placed in the oral cavity when the patients are awake. After adequate time (10–15 minutes), the simulator is removed and the evaluation is completed under basal conditions. The MAD simulator has allowed us to improve our understanding of the airway dynamics of mandibular advancement and to evaluate its therapeutic potential more accurately not only for retrolingual obstruction (as described previously) but also for retropalatal obstruction;
- **transoral DISE (TO-DISE)** to evaluate the position of the tongue and its possible role in oropharyngeal obstruction;
- **lateral rotation of the head** to evaluate the role of the position on the obstruction.

Figure 3.2. illustrates the advanced sleep endoscopy setting.

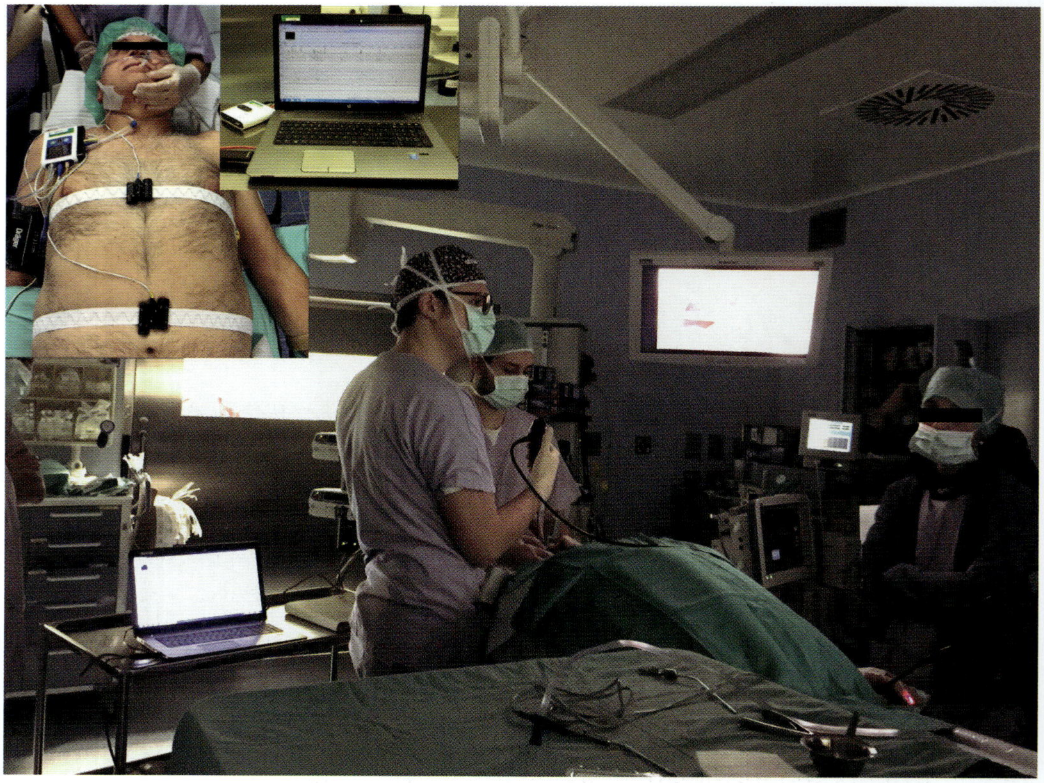

3.2 Advanced sleep endoscopy setting.

Our authors believe that such implementations offer multiple advantages, mainly the possibility to control the bias that is inherent to the method (an essential process to obtain reliable information from the procedure and to formulate individualized therapeutic proposals for treatments), thereby responding to the need for an individualized therapy, whose requirement has been increasingly stated in the modern literature.

Furthermore, advanced sleep endoscopy provides reliable information on the obstructive site, grade, and pattern that can be useful for the morphological and functional phenotyping of patients with OSAS, namely, classifying the patients based on the type of prevalent obstruction, with the ultimate aim of providing a decisional algorithm for the therapeutic approach.

Indications and limitations

The main indication for sleep endoscopy is investigating a nonventilatory therapeutic option for patients with OSAS who refuse or are intolerant to CPAP therapy. It is also indicated before therapeutic re-planning for patients in whom the first surgical procedure has failed and for patients who do not respond adequately to a ventilatory therapy.

The main limitations are represented by the depressant action of hypnotic drugs on the muscular tone, with a possible overestimation of the obstruction, and by the impossibility of reproducing a regular sleep architecture, particularly a rapid eye movement (REM) sleep. Therefore, patients with REM-related OSAS are not eligible for sleep endoscopy. Moreover, the nonnegligible costs, which can limit the accessibility to selected cases (whenever the data obtained in a wakefulness state are insufficient to formulate a therapeutic approach), must be considered.

There are no absolute contraindications for sleep endoscopy except pregnancy, propofol allergy, and a high anesthetic risk (ASA 4).

Conclusions

The presence of morphological alterations reducing the upper airway lumen is one of the main factors responsible for OSAS.

The identification of the obstructive sites and pattern and the appropriate selection of surgical patients and surgical techniques depend on otolaryngologists. Several diagnostic tools are available for these purposes, and the use of these tools and the collected data must be considered based on specific competence.

A thorough diagnostic approach and the collection of as much information as possible about morphological and functional anomalies underlying the obstructive respiratory disorder are key elements to identify the macrocategories of patients and formulate individualized therapeutic approaches.

REFERENCES

Bassetti C, Aldrich MS. Sleep apnea in acute cerebrovascular disease: final report on 128 patients. *Sleep*. 1999;22:217-223.

Berry S, Roblin G, Williams A, Watkins A, Whittet HB. Validity of sleep nasendoscopy in the investigation of sleep related breathing disorders Laryngoscope. *Department of Otorhinolaryngology-Head and Neck Surgery, Singleton Hospital, Swansea, UK*. 2005 Mar;115(3):538-540.

Bonsignore MR, Marrone O, Insalaco G, Bonsignore G. The cardiovascular effects of obstructive sleep apnoeas: analysis of pathogenic mechanisms. *Eur Respir J*. 1994 Apr;7(4):786-805.

Boot H, Poublon RM, Van Wegen R, et al. Uvulopalatopharyngoplasty for the obstructive sleep apnoea syndrome: value of polysomnography, Mueller manoeuvre and cephalometry in predicting surgical outcome. *Clin Otolaryngol Allied Sci*. 1997 Dec;22(6):504-510.

Coccagna G, Capucci A, Bauleo S, Boriani G, Santarelli A. Paroxysmal atrial fibrillation in sleep. *Sleep*. 1997 Jun;20(6):396-398.

Coccagna G, Lugaresi E. Haemodynamics during sleep: old results and new perspectives. *J Sleep Res*. 1995 Jun;4(S1):2-7.

den Herder C, van Tinteren H, de Vries N. Sleep endoscopy versus modified Mallampati score in sleep apnea and snoring. *Laryngoscope*. 2005 Apr;115(4):735-739.

Eckert DJ, Malhotra A. Pathophysiology of adult obstructive sleep apnea. *Proc Am Thorac Soc*. 2008;5:144-153.

Eckert DJ, White DP, Jordan AS, Malhotra A, Wellman A. Defining phenotypic causes of obstructive sleep apnea. Identification of novel therapeutic targets. *Am J Respir Crit Care Med*. 2013 Oct 15;188(8):996-1004.

Fernandez-Julian E, Garcia-Perez MA, Garcia-Callejo J, Ferrer F, Marti F, Marc J. Surgical planning after sleep versus awake techniques in patients with obstructive sleep apnea. *Laryngoscope*. 2014 Aug;124(8):1970-1974.

Friedman M, Ibrahim H, Bass L. Clinical staging for sleep disordered breathing. *Otolaryngol Head Neck Surg*. 2002;127:13-21.

FRIEDMAN M, TANYERI H, LAROSA M, ET AL. Clinical predictors of obstructive sleep apnea. *Laryngoscope*. 1999;109:1901-1907.

FRIEDMAN NR, PRAGER JD, RUIZ AG, KEZIRIAN EJ. A Pediatric grading scale for lingual tonsil hypertrophy. *Otolaryngology Head and Neck Surgery*. 2015 Aug 25;1-4.

HEDNER J, GROTE L. Cardiovascular consequences of obstructive sleep apnoea. In: McNicholas WT. *Respiratory Disorders during sleep*. European Respiratory Monograph, 1998 Dec, Vol. 3, pag. 245.

HESSEL NS, DE VRIES N. Results of uvulopalatopharyngoplasty after diagnostic workup with polysomnography and sleep endoscopy: a report of 136 snoring patients. *Eur Arch Otorhinolaryngol*. 2003 Feb;260(2):91-95. Epub 2002 Sep 4.

HUNG J, WHITFORD EG, PARSONS RW, HILLMAN DR. Association of sleep apnea with myocardial infarction in men. *Lancet*. 1990;336:2611-2264.

KEZIRIAN EJ, HOHENHORST W, DE VRIES N. Drug-induced sleep endoscopy: the VOTE classification. *Eur Arch Otorhinolaryngol*. 2011 May;268:1233-1236.

KILIC K, AKTAN B, SEDAT-SAKAT M, KIZILTUNÇ A, YORUK O. Vascular Endothelial Dysfunction Caused by Oxidative Stress is a Predictor Factor for Complications of Obstructive Sleep Apnea Syndrome. *West Indian Med J*. 2016 Feb 15;DOI:10.7727/wimj.2015.383.

KRIBBS NB, PACK AI, KLINE LR, ET AL. Objective measurement of patterns of nasal CPAP use by patients with obstructive sleep apnea. *Am Rev Respir Dis*. 1993;147:887-895.

KRIEGER J, SFORZA E, APPRIL M, LAMPERT E, WEITZENBLUM E. Pulmonary hyprtension, hypoxemia and hypercapnia in obstructive sleep apnea patients. *Chest*. 199;96:729-737.

LAVIE P, HERER P, PELED R, ET AL. Mortality in sleep apnea patients: a multivariate analysis of risk factors. *Sleep*. 1995;18:149-157.

LIISTRO G, ROMBAUX PH, BELGE C, ET AL. High Mallampati score and nasal obstruction are associated risk factors for obstructive sleep apnoea. *Eur Respir J*. 2003;21:248-252.

LYBERG T, KROGSTAD O, DJUPESLAND G. Cephalometric analysis in patients with obstructive sleep apnoea syndrome. I. Skeletal morphology. *J Laryngol Otol*. 1989 Mar;103(3):287-292.

MALLAMPATI SR, GATT SP, GUGINO LD, ET AL. A clinical sign to predict difficult tracheal intubation: a prospective study. *Can Anaesth Soc J*. 1985;32:429-434.

MARAIS J. The value of sedation nasendoscopy: a comparison between snoring and non-snoring patients. *Clin Otolaryngol Allied Sci*. 1998 Feb;23(1):74-76.

MILLMAN RP, CARLISLE CC, ROSENBERG C, KAHN D, MCRAE R, KRAMER NR. Simple predictors of uvulopalatopharyngoplasty outcome in the treatment of obstructive sleep apnea. *Chest*. 2000 Oct;118(4):1025-1030.

NG AT, DARENDELILER MA, PETOCZ P, CISTULLI PA. Cephalometry and prediction of oral appliance treatment outcome. *Sleep Breath*. 2012;16:47-58.

NG AT, QIAN J, CISTULLI PA. Oropharyngeal collapse predicts treatment response with oral appliance therapy in obstructive sleep apnea. *Sleep*. 2006;29:666-671.

PAOLI JR, LAUWERS F, LACASSAGNE L, TIBERGE M, DODART L, BOUTAULT F. Craniofacial differences according to the body mass index of patients with obstructive sleep apnoea syndrome: cephalometric study in 85 patients. *Br J Oral Maxillofac Surg*. 2001 Feb;39(1):40-45.

PARRA O, ARBOIX A, BECHIC S, ET AL. Time course of sleep-related breathing disorders in first-ever stroke or transient ischemic attack. *Am J Respir Crit Care Med*. 2000;161:375-380.

PARTINEN M, GUILLEMINAULT C, QUERA-SALVA MA, JAMIESON A. Obstructive sleep apnea and cephalometric roentgenograms. The role of anatomic upper airway abnormalities in the definition of abnormal breathing during sleep. *Chest*. 1988 Jun;93(6):1199-1205.

PEPPARD PE, YOUNG T, PALTA M, SKATRUD J. Prospective study of the association between sleep-disorder breathing and hypertension. *N Engl J Med*. 2000;342:1378-1384.

PORTERFIELD JG, PORTERFIELD LM, NESTOR JR. Daily variations in the occurrence of symptomatic supraventricular tachycardia as determined by ambulatory event monitoring. *Am J Cardiol*. 1997;80:889-891.

POWELL NB, GUILLEMINAULT. Obstructive sleep apnea syndrome: a review of 306 consecutively treated surgical patients. *Otolaryngol Head Neck Surg. Riley RW*. 1993 Feb;108(2):117-125.

PRINGLE MB, CROFT CB. A grading system for patients with obstructive sleep apnoea—based on sleep nasendoscopy. *Clin Otolaryngol Allied Sci*. 1993 Dec;18(6):480-484.

RILEY R, GUILLEMINAULT C, HERRAN J, POWELL N. Cephalometric analyses and flow-volume loops in obstructive sleep apnea patients. *Sleep* 1983;6(4):303-311.

SFORZA E, BACON W, WEISS T, THIBAULT A, PETIAU C, KRIEGER J. Upper airway collapsibility and cephalometric variables in patients with obstructive sleep apnea. *Am J Respir Crit Care Med*. 2000 Feb;161(2 Pt 1):347-352.

SHER AE, SCHECHTMAN KB, PICCIRILLO JF. The efficacy of surgical modifications of the upper airway in adults with obstructive sleep apnea syndrome. *Sleep*. 1996 Feb;19(2):156-77. Review.

SHER AE, THORPY MJ, SHPRINTZEN RJ, SPIELMAN AJ, BURACK B, MCGREGOR PA. Predictive value of Müller maneuver in selection of patients for uvulopalatopharyngoplasty. *Laryngoscope*. 1985 Dec;95(12):1483-1487.

SKATVEDT O. Localization of site of obstruction in snorers and patients with obstructive sleep apnea syndrome: a comparison of fiberoptic nasopharyngoscopy and pressure measurements. *Acta Otolaryngol*. 1993 Mar;113(2):206-209.

SORRENTI G, LATINI G, BONETTI M, ET AL. *Caratteristiche cefalometriche ed endoscopiche nei pazienti affetti da roncopatia cronica e sindrome delle apnee ostruttive: valutazione statistica*. 27-30 Settembre 1999. Caserta: IX congresso nazionale A.I.M.S.

Sorrenti G, Piccin O, Latini G, et al. Cephalometric and endoscopic features in snores and patients with obstructive sleep apnea. A multivariate analysis. Surgery for Snoring and Obstructive Sleep Apnea Syndrome. Atti "Roma OSAS 2000", pp. 315-320.

Terris DJ, Hanasono MM, Liu YC. Reliability of the Müller maneuver and its association with sleep-disordered breathing. *Laryngoscope*. 2000 Nov;110(11):1819-1823.

Vicini C, De Vito A, Benazzo M, et al. The nose oropharynx hypopharynx and larynx (NOHL) classification: a new system of diagnostic standardized examination for OSAHS patients. *Eur Arch Otorhinolaryngol*. 2012 Feb;269:1297-1300.

Woodson BT, Conley SF, Dohse A, Feroah TR, Sewall SR, Fujita S. Posterior cephalometric radiographic analysis in obstructive sleep apnea. *Ann Otol Rhinol Laryngol*. 1997 Apr;106(4):310-313.

Woodson TB, Wooten MR. Comparison of upper-airway evaluations during wakefulness and sleep. *Laryngoscope*. 1994;104:821-828.

Zucconi M, Ferini-Strambi L, Palazzi S, Orena C, Zonta S, Smirne S. Habitual snoring with and without obstructive sleep apnoea: the importance of cephalometric variables. *Thorax*. 1992 Mar;47(3):157-156.

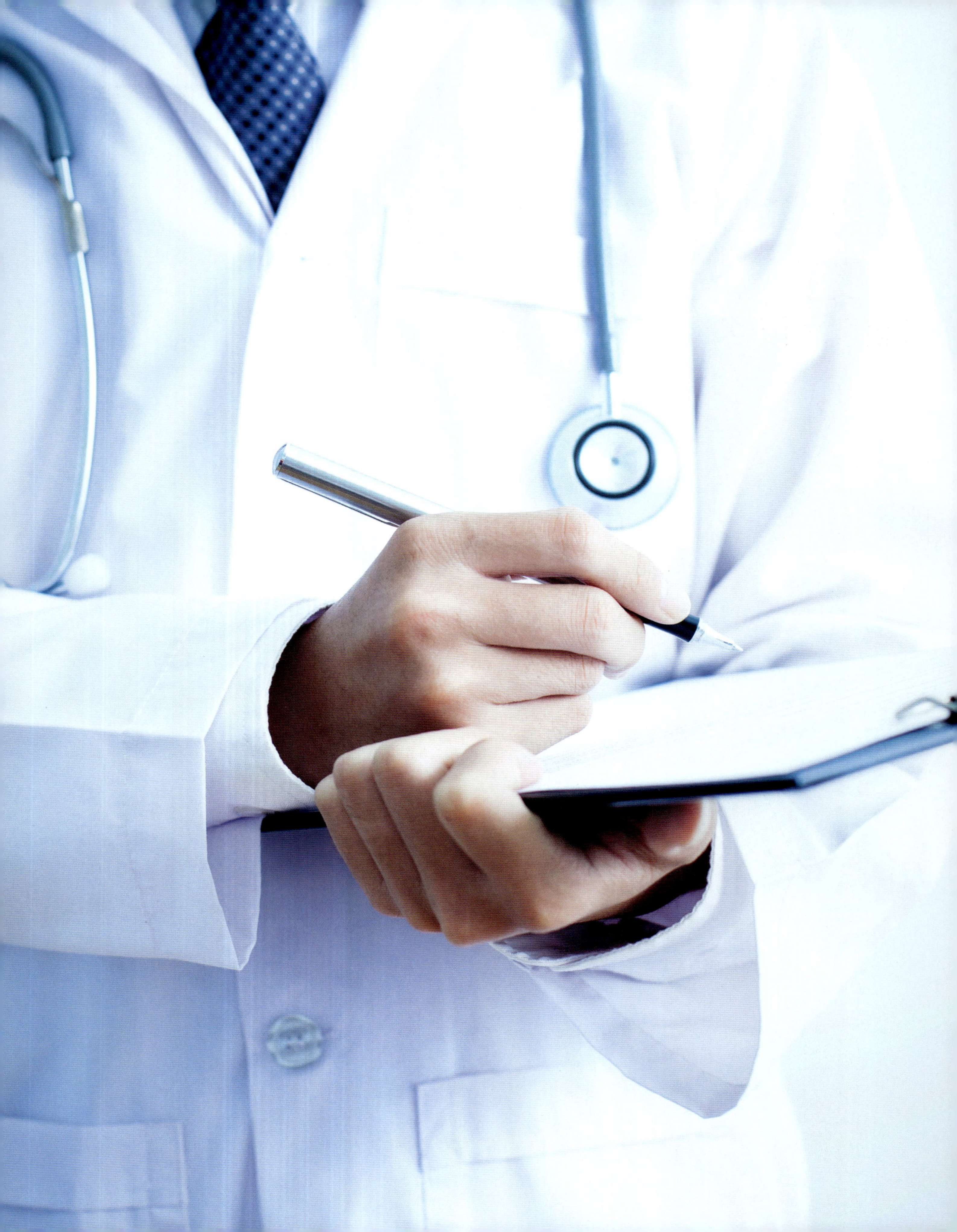

Therapeutic choice

Fabio Cirignotta

Objectives

- Identifying patients who require treatment
- Defining the most adequate therapeutic option
- Understanding the components to evaluate the efficacy of the therapy

Introduction

At the end of the diagnostic procedure (■ 4.1) a series of clinical and instrumental information is available to establish the diagnosis of obstructive sleep apnea syndrome (OSAS). The overall evaluation of this information enables to decide whether to initiate treatment and choose among a range of therapeutic options (■ 4.2).

■ **4.1** Clinical and instrumental information.

Personal data	Age and sex Profession
Anamnesis data	Snoring history Awakening with choking sensation, insomnia Road accidents Ear, nose, and throat (ENT) surgery
Clinical data	Body mass index (BMI), neck circumference, facial morphometry Daytime sleepiness [Epworth sleepiness scale (ESS)] Cognitive disorders ENT and cephalometric evaluation Comorbidities
Polysomnographic data	Sleep structure, arousals Apnea-hypopnea index (AHI) [respiratory disturbance index (RDI) or respiratory event index (REI)]: total and in lateral/supine position Saturometry [oxygen desaturation index (ODI), mean SaO_2 of the minimum values, minimum SaO_2, CT < 90, mean SaO_2] Periodic limb movement during sleep

■ **4.2** Therapeutic options.

Lifestyle changes	Weight loss Positional therapy Oropharyngeal exercise Avoiding alcohol and drugs, which depress the muscular tone and respiratory drive, particularly tranquilizers and hypnotics
Specific therapy	Continuous positive airway pressure (CPAP) [Bilevel, C-Flex, automatic positive airway pressure (APAP)] Endo-oral devices ENT surgery, maxillofacial and bariatric surgery Tracheotomy Oxygen therapy with CPAP

The fundamental **preliminary components** involved in the therapeutic choice decision-making are natural history of OSAS, correct definition of the disease severity, and clarity regarding identifying patients who require treatment, defining the most adequate therapeutic options, and understanding how to evaluate the efficacy of treatment.

Natural history of OSAS

After diagnosing OSAS, we should investigate whether all patients should be treated immediately or if, in at least some patients, spontaneous healing or improvement can be expected.

Few controlled studies have evaluated the natural history of OSAS over time and often reported conflicting results. A study on 32 patients who refused treatment at the time of being diagnosed with OSAS reported no significant changes in polysomnographic parameters in the absence of BMI variations or pulmonary functionality after a follow-up of 5 years (Sforza et al. 1994).

Other studies have suggested a tendency of disease worsening in patients with mild to moderate OSAS aged between 40 and 60 years (Fisher et al. 2002; Berger et al. 2009); however, these findings are not applicable to elderly individuals, in whom OSAS manifests specific characteristics (Launois et al. 2007), or to patients with severe OSAS. BMI appears to be the main risk factor associated with disease worsening in all age groups. In terms of spontaneous healing in the absence of BMI variations, to the best of our knowledge, at present, there is no data in the literature suggesting that untreated OSAS can improve spontaneously.

Severity criteria for OSAS

The severity of clinical cases (which depends on two variables: the presence of daytime sleepiness and polysomnographic data) must be considered in the therapeutic choice decision-making. Mild sleepiness is defined if it occurs only during relaxing situations, moderate if it occurs in situations requiring moderate attention, and severe if it occurs during stimulating situations. According to ESS, excessive sleepiness is defined if the ESS score is >14 (Johns 1991).

For the **polysomnographic component**, AHI (or RDI) has been traditionally used as a polysomnographic parameter: mild OSAS, AHI scores between 5 and 14; moderate OSAS, AHI scores between 15 and 29; and severe OSAS, AHI scores of ≥30. The severity of OSAS corresponds to AHI (or RDI) with the most severe component (Fleetham et al. 2006).

Although codified reference values are lacking, the author believes that severity assessment must consider the overnight oxygen saturation level quantified with the mean SaO_2 of the minimum values, the sleeping time spent with $SaO_2 < 90\%$, and the mean SaO_2. A modest number of apneas may have a different prognostic significance if they are associated with significant desaturation.

Comorbidity is another component that must be considered: few apneas [e.g., in rapid eye movement (REM)-related forms] can represent high-risk factors in patients with concurrent cardiac arrhythmia.

Finally, it is essential to consider the possible positionality, namely, cases wherein the respiratory disorder is present exclusively or predominantly in a supine position, representing 60%–80% of mild/moderate OSAS (Oksenberg and Gadoth 2014); moreover, the severity of clinical cases during each night depends on the sleeping time spent in a supine position. This indicates that it would be more logical to establish a classification system of the severity of OSAS that distinguishes AHI in the supine position from AHI in the lateral position. Meanwhile, it is recommended that this aspect always be considered in the overall evaluation.

Objectives of therapy for OSAS

The **short-term objectives** of therapy for OSAS are *normalizing obstructive respiratory events* [apneas, hypopneas, and, in specific cases, respiratory effort-related arousal (RERA)] and *eliminating symptoms*, particularly sleepiness. **The long-term objectives** are *reducing the use of healthcare structures* and related costs, *improving quality of life, and reducing the comorbidity and mortality* associated with cardiovascular diseases as well as road accidents.

To treat or not to treat

According to a study published in 2001, CPAP therapy does not improve quality of life, objective sleepiness, attention, memory, learning, visual-motor coordination, or arterial pressure in patients with AHI scores of >30 in the absence of subjective daytime sleepiness; therefore, this study concluded that CPAP therapy is not indicated for patients with pathological AHI in the absence of daytime sleepiness (Barbé et al. 2001).

This concept has been resumed by the guidelines of the Scottish Intercollegiate Network (2003). According to these guidelines, OSAS treatment must aim at eliminating the symptoms and not reducing the cardiovascular risks in patients without sleepiness or other symptoms, independent of the number of apneas/hypopneas. However, a more prudent approach has been recommended considering the findings of a series of studies published between 2005 and 2008 (Arzt et al. 2005; Marin et al. 2005; Yaggu et al. 2005; Marshall et al. 2008), which investigated the increased cardiovascular risks and mortality in patients with OSAS, the endothelial damage and proinflammatory activity caused by apneas (Steiner et al. 1985; Ryan et al. 2005), the relationship between OSAS and metabolic syndrome (Bonsignore et al. 2013), the evidence regarding increased risks of road accidents in patients with OSAS (Tregear

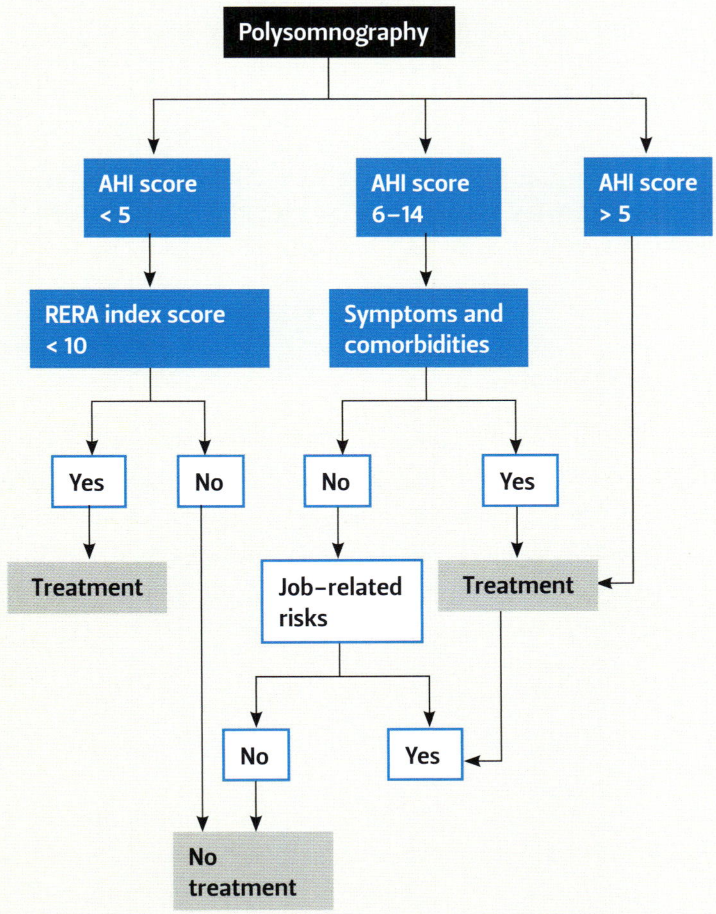

4.1 Therapeutic choice decision-making in patients with OSAS (modified by Kryger and Malhotra

et al. 2009; Tregear et al. 2010), and the difficulties in establishing a subjective definition of the symptoms and the variability in the self-assessment of sleepiness.

The American Academy of Sleep Medicine (AASM) guidelines (Epstein et al. 2009) simply recommend that all patients with a diagnosis of OSAS be treated. Kriger and Malhotra proposed an algorithm suggesting treatment for all patients with AHI scores of >5 (or RERA index scores of >10), those with sleepiness or comorbidity, or those whose jobs are associated with risks of road accidents (commercial vehicle drivers and pilots). Contrary to that recommended by the AASM guidelines, treatment is not expected for a selected group of patients with AHI or RDI scores between 5 and 15 in the absence of daytime sleepiness, comorbidity, and particular risks associated with their jobs (4.1). This setting reflects a revision of the Canadian Thoracic Society guidelines, which state that there is limited evidence on the utility of treatment for OSAS in asymptomatic patients with AHI scores of <15 (Fleetham et al. 2011).

Informing the patient

Whether the decision is to treat or not to treat, it is essential to inform the patient by explaining the results of the analysis, the nature of the disease, the possible risks associated, the advantages of treatment (or no treatment), the probability of success, and the possible inconveniences associated with the therapy. The patients must understand and agree with the therapeutic choice. Patients with excessive daytime sleepiness should be prevented from driving and must be informed about the high risks associated with it.

Therapeutic options

In general, the guidelines agree on the therapeutic strategy with minimal and nonsignificant differences. The data reported below represent a summary of the recommendations provided by the main international guidelines (Fleetham et al. 2006; Epstein et al. 2009; Remmelink and Hoeke 2010; Fleetham et al. 2011; Nigiam et al. 2013; Qaseem et al. 2013), which are based on evidence from randomized and controlled studies; however, there is no evidence from reviews or specific experimental studies.

The strength and significance of the indications are generally moderate or low, and we can distinguish between "change of behavior" and "specific" strategies.

A therapy requiring lifestyle changes can usually be recommended to all patients with OSAS, and a single therapeutic strategy could be sufficient for mild OSAS; however, for moderate and severe OSAS, treatment strategies must always be associated with a specific therapy.

In evidence-based terms, there are no definitive predictive criteria for demonstrating the specific efficacy of different therapeutic options for individual patients (Qaseem et al. 3013). To ensure correct adherence to the treatment, patient characteristics and preferences must be considered.

Therapy adopting lifestyle changes

1. All obese or overweight patients should be advised to lose weight by following a diet under medical supervision. Unfortunately, from a practical viewpoint, the significance of this recommendation is strongly reduced by difficulties in losing weight and maintaining the achieved results.
2. Positional therapy comprises devices that help patients to maintain a lateral position while sleeping (alarms, special pillows, sleeping backpack, tennis balls, etc.). This therapy should be applied only under specific conditions, such as in mild OSAS without comorbidities or when the positional characteristic is clear. This therapy should be associated with other strategies such as weight loss; however, its long-term compliance is limited.

3. Alcoholic drinks and medications (e.g., benzodiazepines), which depress the respiratory drive and increase the arousal threshold, are contraindicated.
4. Oropharyngeal exercise can be performed by playing particular wind instruments (e.g., the didgeridoo). It has been proven to be effective in reducing (but not completely eliminating) overnight apneas/hypopneas. Similar results have been achieved with daytime electric stimulation of the genioglossus muscles. However, data on the efficacy of "pharyngeal training" are not yet sufficient for it to be provided as an evidence-based recommendation.

Specific therapy

1. **CPAP** therapy has provided the best therapeutic results. Except for some limitations, it represents the first therapeutic choice for patients with OSAS. However, patients with OSAS should always be informed about the possible alternatives that can be considered according to the clinical case severity, anatomical factors, and individual preferences. Regarding the variants of CPAP (APAP, C-Flex, Bilevel), there is no evidence that APAP is better than fixed CPAP in terms of outcomes. Thus, APAP is currently being used as a cost-effective and useful titration method. Similarly, there is no sufficient evidence suggesting that solutions, such as Flexible Bilevel or C-Flex CPAP, reduce the pressure at the initiation of expiration as well as improve the comfort and compliance of patients.
2. **Endo-oral mandibular advancement devices** (MAD) are recommended, irrespective of the clinical case severity, in cases wherein patients cannot tolerate CPAP or prefer them. Some guidelines propose MAD as the first therapeutic choice for mild and moderate OSAS (Fleetham et al. 2006). The efficacy of MAD has been demonstrated to be comparable yet slightly inferior to the efficacy of CPAP; therefore, CPAP remains the first therapeutic choice for patients with severe OSAS. In contrast, tongue-retaining devices (TRD) are not recommended for such patients. All the above-mentioned guidelines agree that MAD should be used by specialized dentists who have undergone adequate training in the field of sleep medicine. These endo-oral devices are effective therapeutic options for OSAS, although it is necessary to consider that a significant percentage of patients do not respond or respond only partially to these devices. Long-term efficacy and compliance are based on key points such as clinical and polysomnographic follow-ups to monitor the efficacy of the treatment, the comfort and compliance with the devices, and their side effects. Furthermore, integration of medical competences from physicians and doctors who are experts in sleep medicine must be integrated in managing such patients (Gauthier et al. 2012; Ngiam et al. 2013).
3. **ENT and maxillofacial surgical treatment** (note that the objective of this chapter is not to examine the different methods thoroughly) is not ri-

sk-free, and the current evidence regarding its efficacy (probably because of the high heterogeneity of the interventions) is limited and insufficient to demonstrate clear benefits in the treatment of OSAS. It is the first therapeutic choice only when OSAS is clearly caused by factors that can be surgically corrected (i.e., tonsillar hypertrophy, microgenia). In the majority of cases, this treatment strategy should be considered as a choice to be reserved only for patients in whom CPAP or endo-oral devices cannot be applied, those who refuse this treatment, or those in whom this treatment is not effective, such as young, slim, and asymptomatic patients who refuse chronic treatment with CPAP or MAD because of the associated reduced quality of life. Tracheotomy represents an extreme intervention to be reserved for very severe and life-threatening cases of OSAS, in which other therapeutic methods either cannot be performed or are intolerable.

4. **Bariatric surgery** can be used to achieve weight loss in patients with pathological obesity (BMI > 40 kg/m2) or obesity (BMI > 35 kg/m2) and associated comorbidities when all other attempts of weight loss have failed.

5. The genioglossus is one of the most important dilator muscles of the upper airways. It can be stimulated directly via transcutaneous genioglossal stimulation or indirectly via apnea-triggered **hypoglossal nerve stimulation**. Some studies have reported that this method can improve OSAS, whereas other studies have reported that it is ineffective and presents several side effects. The current evidence in the literature about this method is insufficient for it to be to be recommended.

6. Several **medicaments** have been evaluated for the treatment of apneas (e.g., mirtazapine, paroxetine, protriptyline, pantoprazole, xanthine, steroids, and estrogens). However, studies performed to date have not achieved sufficient evidence to recommend pharmacological treatment, with the exceptions for hypothyroidism and acromegalia when these pathologies are a cause of OSAS.

7. **Nocturnal oxygen therapy** is not recommended as a specific treatment for OSAS because it can prolong apneas and potentially aggravate nocturnal hypercapnia, particularly in patients with pulmonary comorbidities. When necessary, this oxygen therapy can be used in combination with CPAP or other treatments under specific pulmonary control.

Follow-up

Whatever the therapeutic choice is, its efficacy must be documented with a polysomnographic recording and a clinical follow-up within 3 months after initiation of the treatment. Given that patients with OSAS are chronically ill, the importance of follow-ups in the therapeutic management should be highly emphasized. The immediate success of any treatment does not absolutely indicate that its efficacy will be maintained over time; thus, periodic controls (at least once a year) are fundamental.

The components for evaluating the efficacy of the therapy are sleepiness reductions and polysomnographic data. During the follow-up, the adherence to the therapy must always be evaluated; in cases of CPAP, it must be documented with the reports provided by the CPAP machine. In case of poor adherence, it is necessary to talk to the patient to determine the associated reasons. Frequent informative meetings led by experienced paramedical personnel considerably improve the adherence to the therapy. When the therapy is ineffective or intolerable, despite correct management of the follow-up, **another therapeutic modality** must be recommended.

Conclusions

The therapeutic choice decision-making in patients with OSAS is a complex process that:

- Starts from the diagnosis and assessment of the clinical case severity;
- Must consider patient characteristics and preferences;
- Requires discussions with patients and informing them about the different possibilities of therapies that require lifestyle changes or therapies that are specific;
- Requires polysomnographic evidence of the achievements of the objectives;
- Requires clinical follow-ups that are both instrumental and informative;
- Must consider that OSAS is a multidisciplinary disease, and therefore, the expert managing the patient needs to coordinate with other specialists.

Therapy with positive airway pressure (i.e., CPAP) is the first therapeutic choice recommended to all patients, except for patients in whom the apneas are clearly caused by anatomical factors, in which a surgical approach is suggested as the first therapeutic choice. MAD, which are comparable with CPAP, represent the second therapeutic choice recommended to patients with mild and moderate OSAS. ENT and maxillofacial surgery is a therapeutic choice reserved for patients who cannot tolerate CPAP and MAD and for those who do not present with comorbidities that may increase the surgical risk.

Therapy involving lifestyle changes can be recommended to all patients, but it can be considered as the standalone therapeutic choice only for patients with mild OSAS. The recommendations of the current guidelines are based on evidence whose strength and quality are modest overall. However, further studies regarding lifestyle changes and their therapeutic results are required for patients with mild OSAS.

In a recent survey, a sample of stakeholders (patients, physicians, politicians, manufacturers, and providers) were asked about their opinions on the primary needs and components to be investigated in further research on OSAS (Patel et al. 2013), and the following list presents their opinions in order of priority:

- (Cost analysis/efficacy) cost-effective solutions for treating mild and moderate OSAS;
- Components of OSAS specific to women and children;
- Importance of the perioperative screening of OSAS;
- Importance of the diagnosis of OSAS by a specialist/expert in sleep medicine compared with that by a nonspecialist;
- Improvements in the prognostic accuracy of patient outcomes.

REFERENCES

American Academy of Sleep Medicine. *Diagnostic and Coding Manual Westchester*. In: *International Classification of Sleep Disorders*. 3rd ed. (ICSD-3). 2014.

Arzt M, Yount T, Finn L, Skatrud JB, Bradley TD. Association of sleep-disordered breathing and the occurrence of stroke. *Am J Respir Crit Care Med*. 2005;172:1447-1451.

Barbé F (1), Mayoralas LR, Duran J, et al. Treatment with continuous positive airway pressure is not effective in patients with sleep apnea but no daytime sleepiness. a randomized, controlled trial. *Ann Intern Med*. 2001,134(11):1015-1023.

Berger G, Berger R, Oksenberg A. Progression of snoring and obstructive sleep apnoea: the role of increasing weight and time. *Eur Respir J*. 2009;33:338-345.

Bonsignore MR1, Borel AL, Machan E, Grunstein R. Sleep apnoea and metabolic dysfunction. *Eur Respir Rev*. 2013 Sep 1;22(129):353-364.

Epstein LJ, Kristo D, Strollo PJ, et al. Clinical guideline for the evaluation, management and long-term care of obstructive sleep apnea in adults. *J Clin Sleep Med*. 2009;5:263-276.

Fisher D, Pillar G, Malhotra A, et al. Long-term follow-up of untreated patients with sleep apnoea syndrome. *Respir Med*. 2002;96:337-343.

Fleetham J, Ayas N, Bradley D, et al. CTS Sleep Disordered Breathing Committee. Canadian Thoracic Society guidelines: diagnosis and treatment of sleep disordered breathing in adults. *Can Respir J*. 2006;13(7):387-392.

Fleetham J, Ayas N, Bradley D, et al. Canadian Thoracic Society Sleep Disordered Breathing Committee. Canadian Thoracic Society 2011 guideline update: diagnosis and treatment of sleep disordered breathing. *Can Respir J*. 2011 Jan-Feb;18(1):25-47.

Gauthier L, Almeida F, Arcache JP, et al. Position paper by Canadian dental sleep medicine professionals on the role of different health care professionals in managing obstructive sleep apnea and snoring with oral appliances. *Can Respir J*. 2012 Sep-Oct;19(5):307-309.

Johns MW. A new method for measuring daytime sleepiness: the Epworth sleepiness scale. *Sleep*. 1991 Dec;14(6):540-545.

Kryger MH, Malhotra A. *Management of obstructive sleep apnea in adults*. Wolters Kluwer healt. www.uptodate.com.

Launois SH, Pépin JL, Lévy P. Sleep apnea in the elderly: a specific entity? *Sleep Med Rev*. 2007;11:87-97.

Marin JM, Carrizo SJ, Vicente E, Agusti AG. Long-term cardiovascular outcomes in men with obstructive sleep apnoea-hypopnoea with or without treatment with continuous positive airway pressure: An observational study. *Lancet*. 2005;365:1046-1053.

Marshall NS, Wong KKH, Liu PY, Cullen SRJ, Knuiman MW, Grunstein RR. Sleep apnea as an independient risk factor for all-cause mortality, The Busselton Health Study. *Sleep*. 2008;31:1079-1085.

Ngiam J1, Balasubramaniam R, Darendeliler MA, Cheng AT, Waters K, Sullivan CE. Clinical guidelines for oral appliance therapy in the treatment of snoring and obstructive sleep apnoea. *Aust Dent J*. 2013 Dec;58(4):408-419.

Oksenberg A, Gadoth N. Are we missing a simple treatment for most adult sleep apnea patients? The avoidance of the supine sleep position. *J Sleep Res*. 2014 Apr;23(2):204-210.

Patel K, Moorthy D, Chan JA, et al. High priority future research needs for obstructive sleep apnea diagnosis and treatment. *J Clin Sleep Med*. 2013 Apr 15;9(4):395-402.

Qaseem A, Holty J-E C, Owens DK, Dallas P, Starkey M, Shekelle P (for the Clinical Guidelines Committee of the American College of Physicians). Management Management of Obstructive Sleep Apnea in Adults: A Clinical practice Guideline From the American College of Physicians. *Annals of Internal Medicine*. 2013;159:471-483.

Randerath WJ, Verbraecken J, Andreas S, et al. European Respiratory Society task force on non-CPAP therapies in sleep apnoea. Non-CPAP therapies in obstructive sleep apnoea. *Eur Respir J*. 2011 May;37(5):1000-1028.

Remmelink HJ1, Hoeke A. Dutch national guidelines for diagnosis and treatment of obstructive sleep apnea syndrome in adults. *Ned Tijdschr Tandheelkd*. 2010 Apr;117(4):227-231.

Ryan S, Taylor CT, McNicholas WT. Selective activation of inflammatory pathways by intermittent hypoxia in obstructive sleep apnea syndrome. *Circulation.* 2005;112:2660-2667.

Scottish Intercollegiate/British Thoracic Society Guideline. *Management of obstructive sleep apnoea/hypopnoea syndrome in adults. Guideline 73.* 2003. http://www.sign.ac.uk/guidelines/fulltext/73/index.html>

Sforza E, Addati G, Cirignotta F, et al. Natural evolution of sleep apnoea syndrome: a five year longitudinal study. *Eur Respir J.* 1994;7:1765-1770.

Steiner DR, Gonzalez NC, Wood JG. Interaction between reactive oxygen species and nitric oxide in the microvascular response to systemic hypoxia. *J Appl Physiol* (1985). 2002 Oct;93(4):1411-1418.

Tregear S, Reston J, Schoelles K, Phillips B. Continuous positive airway pressure reduces risk of motor vehicle crash among drivers with obstructive sleep apnea: systematic review and meta-analysis. *Sleep.* 2010 Oct;33(10):1373-1380. Review.

Tregear S, Reston J, Schoelles K, Phillips B. Obstructive sleep apnea and risk of motor vehicle crash: systematic review and meta-analysis. *J Clin Sleep Med.* 2009 Dec 15;5(6):573-581. Review.

Yaggi HK, Concato J, Kernan WN, Lichtman JH, Brass LM, Mohsenin V. Obstructive sleep apnea as a risk factor for stroke and death. *N Engl J Med.* 2005;353:2034-2041.

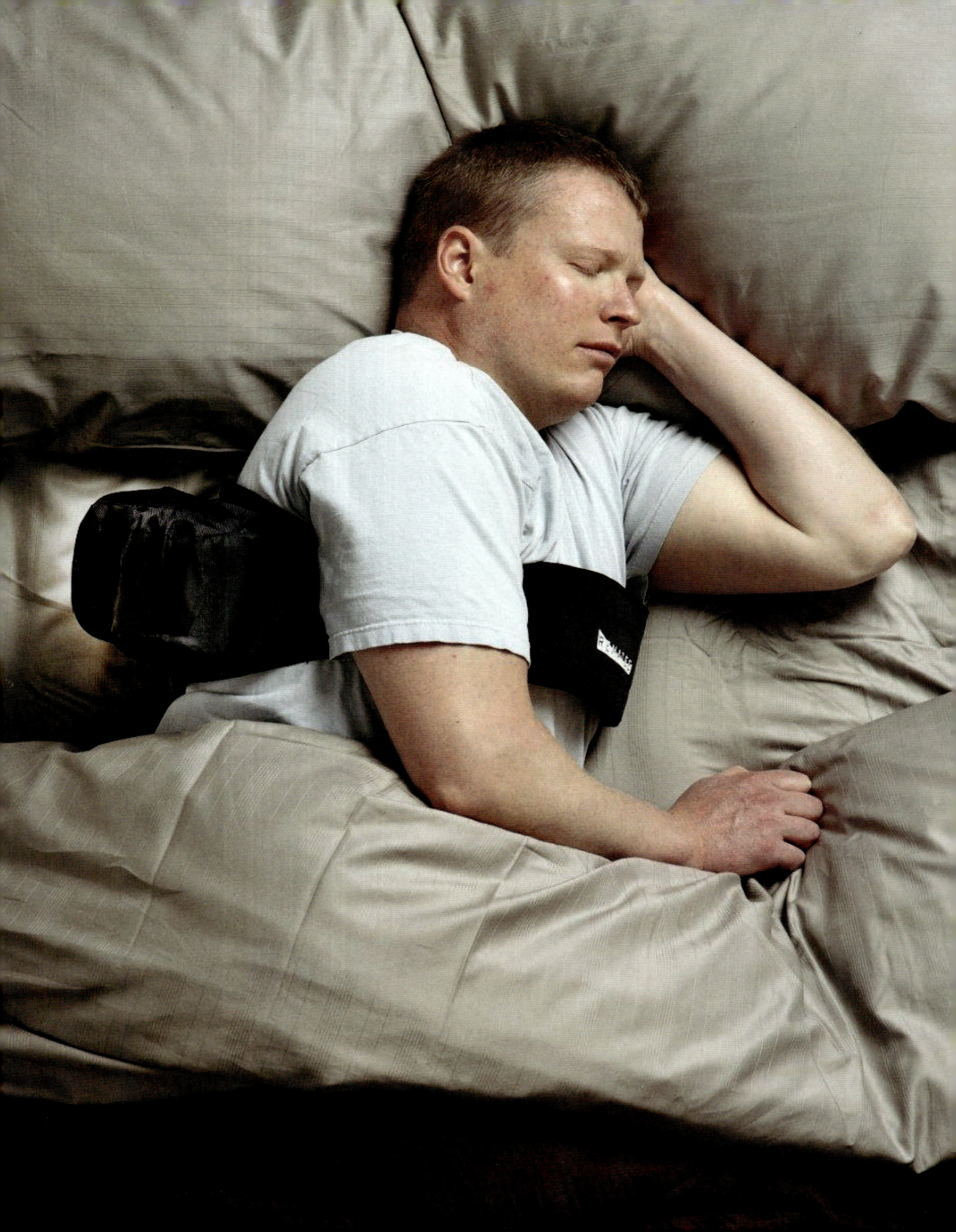

Lifestyle interventions and pharmacological therapy for obstructive sleep apnea syndrome

Susanna Mondini ▪ Simone Baiardi
Luigi Taranto-Montemurro*

* *The author would like to thank Nicole Calianese for her help in redacting the manuscript.*

Objectives

- → Defining the rationale in the most common obstructive sleep apnea syndrome (OSAS)-related lifestyle interventions
- → Illustrating the main lifestyle interventions and their effectiveness
- → Clarifying the state of the art on the possible strategies of a pharmacological approach to obstructive sleep apnea (OSA)

Lifestyle interventions

Some daily habits and behaviors may have an important role in favoring the onset or aggravation of OSAS. The most typical example is represented by changes in body weight: weight gain can turn a primary snorer into a patient with OSAS. In fact, an increase of 32% on the apnea/hypopnea index (AHI) is predictable with a 10% body weight increase and vice versa. The weight loss can significantly reduce AHI and therefore, it is considered to be an effective therapy for some patients with OSAS.

It is thus clear that modifying those behaviors (conditions, life habits, medication, etc.) that have a role in determining OSAS can improve and, in some cases, even solve the sleep-disordered breathing.

Lifestyle interventions means that a set of unspecific, therapeutic approaches (not exclusively typical for OSAS, to distinguish them from specific therapies) intervene to correct or avoid factors favoring the onset or aggravation of OSAS, particularly:

- **positional therapy** to avoid the supine position during sleep;
- **weight loss** and keeping weight under control; and
- **behaviours to be avoided**, such as avoiding assuming substances in the evening that interfere with the function and tonus of the muscles of the upper airways.

Positional therapy

RATIONALE

Sleeping in a supine position is always an unfavorable condition for the patient with OSAS. In fact, this sleeping position is detrimental for the ventilatory capacity and the physiology of the upper airways, especially for the patients with positional OSAS that represent ca. 50%-60% of all patients affected with OSAS and ca. 80% of those patients with a mild-moderate OSAS (Joosten *et al.* 2014).

Positional OSAS is characterized by the number of apneas + hypopneas per hour (AHI) in supine position, which is double compared to the AHI in a nonsupine position. Some authors have proposed to distinguish the patient with positional prevalence (supine AHI ≥ 2 times the nonsupine AHI) from the patient with isolated positional OSAS (supine AHI ≥ 2 times the nonsupine AHI + nonsupine AHI < 5) who presents obstructive apneas/hypopneas only in supine position (Joosten *et al.* 2014).

Compared to patients affected with nonpositional OSAS, the patients with positional OSAS present a less severe sleep-disordered breathing (generally mild or moderate OSAS), and they are slimmer and younger (Joosten *et al.* 2014).

For this group of patients, it is clear that avoiding sleeping in supine position can significantly improve the sleep-disordered breathing.

Hence, the strong rationale is in favor of positional therapy, which should be indicated exactly for that range of patients with a mild or moderate OSAS who find it difficult to accept the continuous positive airway pressure (CPAP) therapy.

For more details about the clinical and polysomnographic characteristics of OSAS, see Chapter 2.

More recently, Frank and his collaborators have proposed a new classification—Amsterdam Positional OSA Classification (APOC)—with the aim to optimize the prescription of the positional therapy. APOC distinguishes the patients with OSAS in three categories:

1. APOC I: the true positional patients with an AHI of 5 in the best sleeping position (nonsupine). They can be treated solely with positional therapy.
1. APOC II: the patients with OSAS severity (established based upon the AHI according to the agreed categories [mild, 5; moderate, > 15 and < 30; and severe, > 30]) in the best sleeping position (nonsupine) compared with the one of the overall respiratory disorder. They can benefit from the positional therapy in association with other therapies.
1. APOC III: the "multifactorial" patients with an overall AHI > 40 and the AHI in the best sleeping position (nonsupine) less than 25% of the overall AHI. Even if these patients do not meet the criteria for the positional OSAS, the severity of OSAS is partially affected by the sleep position. Hence, avoiding sleeping in a supine position (worst sleeping position) can improve the efficacy or acceptability of other treatments (Frank *et al.* 2015).

Furthermore, the application of new criteria recommended by the American Academy of Sleep Medicine (AASM 2012) to identify hypopneas has significantly increased the percentage of subjects with OSAS who can be classified as APOC I and thus, can be cured with the positional therapy, making it look as a more interesting option (Duce *et al.* 2017).

Finally, a new impulse to this kind of therapy and the inherent medical literature has begun with the introduction of a new generation of well-tolerated electronic devices for the positional therapy (positional trainers; see below) that do not disturb the sleep and whose efficacy and use can be documented daily.

TECHNIQUES

Positional therapy includes all those techniques conceived and studied to avoid the supine position during sleep and thus, eliminate the respiratory disorders occurring in such position. The most common techniques are:

- Verbal instructions communicated to the patient (Cartwright 1984; Cartwright *et al.* 1991).
- The tennis ball technique, of tennis balls, which was originally a homemade trick with tennis balls sewn into the backside of pajamas. Now, it has

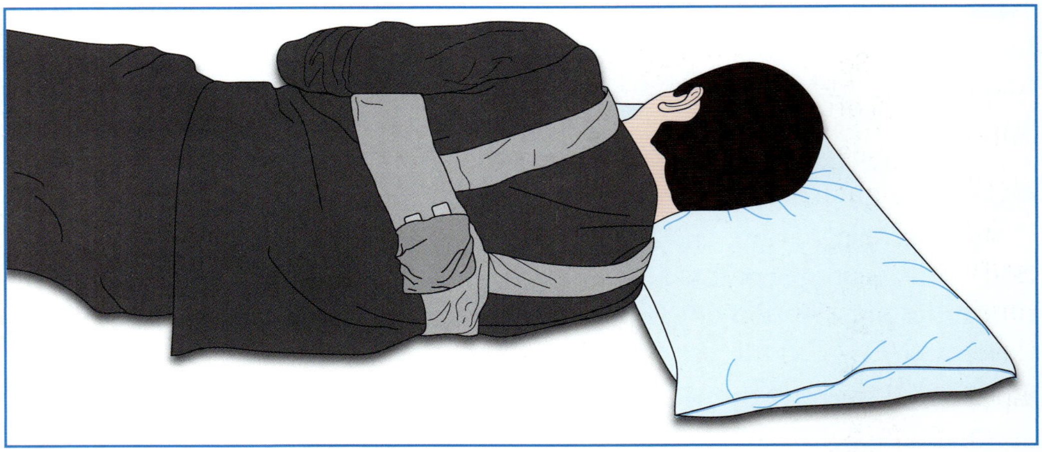

5.1 Positional therapy device using the tennis ball technique. (Modified from Bignold *et al.* 2009)

been replaced by thoracic band with a bulky mass at the back (5.1) (Skinner *et al.* 2008; Bignold *et al.* 2009);

- Specialized pillows that prevent assuming the supine position (Zuberi *et al.* 2004; Loord and Hultcrantz 2007);
- Shirts, vests, or belts with inflatable cushions or a foam block at the back (5.2) (Permut *et al.* 2010);
- Vibrational supine alarm devices strapped to the chest or neck of the patients. These devices start to vibrate when the patient lies in a supine position, causing them to shift the sleeping position (positional trainer; 5.3) (Bignold *et al.* 2011; Van Maanen *et al.* 2013; Levendowski *et al.* 2014).

5.2 Positional therapy device with belt and inflatable airbags.

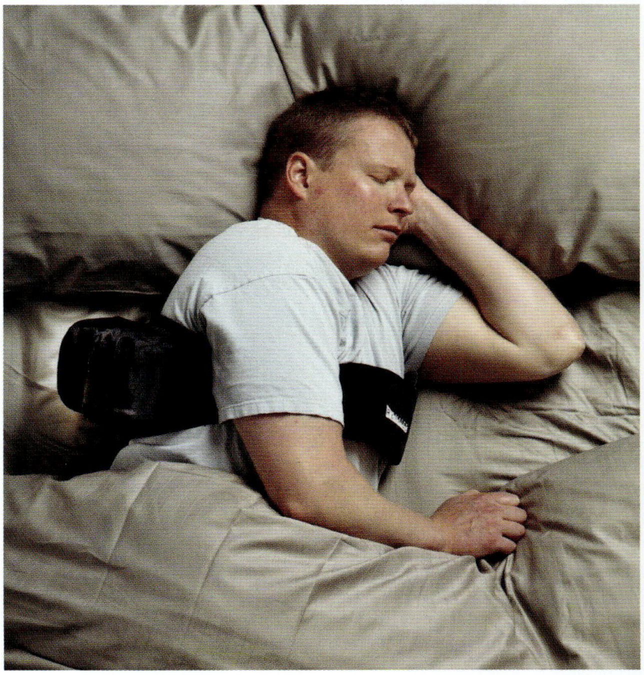

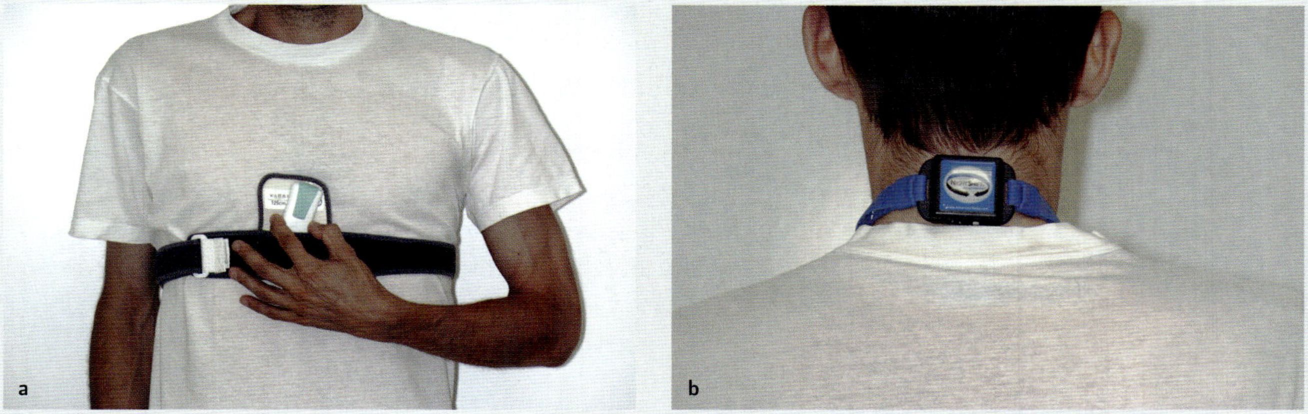

5.3 New generation of position monitoring devices training the patient to avoid supine sleep *(positional trainer)*. These systems have a position sensor that vibrates when the patient sleeps in the supine position. The vibration continues until the patient assumes a nonsupine position. **a**. The position sensor is inside a strap placed around the thorax. **b**. Position sensor is placed around the neck.

The tennis ball technique has been largely used for years because of its simplicity and inexpensiveness. Using the same principle, a series of devices with balls, wedges, and hard foam-rubber or inflatable cylinders have been developed to be worn by the patient and placed at the center of their back, thus making the supine position uncomfortable. The use of these devices every night causes discomfort and, in the long term, the patient markedly reduces their use. To improve comfort and increase the adherence to the treatment, a new set of electronic devices with different characteristics (vibratory alarms placed on the chest or the neck) has been created whose aim is not discouraging the supine position, but training the patient gradually not to sleep in such position. An example of such a device is a vibration alarm that activates each time the patient assumes the supine position; the signal increases in intensity until the patient stays supine and stops when the patient changes the sleeping position. Data about such devices show a more rapid "conditioned" change of position in response to the alarm as the patients gradually reduce the shift to the supine position during sleep. Furthermore, they do not seem to be disturbed by the signal (Bignold *et al.* 2011). To verify the adherence to the treatment, these systems allow recording the hours of use for an extended period of time (≥15 d) and the data concerning the sleeping position, so as to evaluate the progressive learning to avoid the supine position during sleep.

EFFICACY

Although the clinical rationale for the positional therapy is very clear, the studies led on this therapeutic option have scarce evidence due to poor clinical records (mainly case series without control group, cohort studies, and very few randomized and controlled studies); methodology problems (some studies did not control time spent in supine position and AHI per position); and short duration of follow-up.

In spite of being led on a limited number of studies and showing possible bias, the recently published three meta-analyses have clearly shown the efficacy of the positional therapy to reduce the sleeping time in the supine position and the AHI in patients with positional OSAS (Barnes *et al.* 2017; Ravesloot *et al.* 2017; Omobomi and Quan 2018).

All the investigated techniques of positional therapy have proven to be **efficacious** in **reducing the sleeping time in the supine position** n patients with OSAS, this time goes below 15% and with some device it reaches 0% (Permut *et al.* 2010; Ravesloot *et al.* 2013; Joosten *et al.* 2014; Barnes *et al.* 2017; Omobomi and Quan 2018).

The positional therapy is certainly **efficacious in reducing AHI in patients with positional OSAS**, however, the efficacy is **moderate** if AHI decreases to ca. 50%, but the average is 9.59 events/h. It must be highlighted that in some studies, the total AHI for patients having positional therapy falls within the normal limits, perhaps due to a better selection of patients (isolated positional OSAS), which influences the result of the therapy (Permut *et al.* 2010; Randerath *et al.* 2011; Ravesloot *et al.* 2013; Joosten *et al.* 2014; Oksenberg and Gadoth 2014; Barnes *et al.* 2017; Ravesloot *et al.* 2017; Omobomi and Quan 2018).

The new generation of devices with vibrating alarms has proved to be particularly effective according to randomized and controlled studies, which highlighted a considerable reduction in the sleeping time in supine position (only 0%-2%) and a better efficacy on AHI (-11.33 events/h) (Ravesloot *et al.* 2017).

However, the efficacy of positional therapy on the main outcomes of OSAS, especially the daily sleepiness and cardiovascular complications, is not well-defined, even though some data from literature indicate that patients with positional OSAS are less sleepy and hypertensive than those with non-position-dependent OSAS.

Particularly, some studies on small samples seem to show a good efficacy on daytime sleepiness, both subjective (Epworth sleepiness scale [ESS] reduction) and objective (MWT improvement), that overlaps with CPAP. Only one study evaluated the systemic arterial pressure during the 24-h period after one month of positional therapy in patients with OSAS (very limited sample of only 13 patients). They found a reduction in all daytime and nighttime values in both hypertensive and normotensive patients (Berger *et al.* 1997; Jokic *et al.* 1999 Oksenberg *et al.* 2006; Oksenberg and Gadoth 2014).

However, recent meta-analyses that validate the efficacy of the positional therapy have not shown a substantial change in the subjective symptoms and the quality of life in patients treated with positional therapy (evaluated with the ESS and FOSQ specific questionnaires). Also, due to the short-term follow-up, they could not evaluate the metabolic and cardiovascular effects of OSAS in the long term (Barnes *et al.* 2017).

Positive predictive factors for the outcome of the therapy are: young age, respiratory disorder of modest entity, nonsupine AHI < 15, and low body weight.

Only one study compared the tennis ball technique with the use of positional alarms, documenting a greater efficacy of the latter in reducing AHI and oxygen desaturation index (ODI) without detecting differences on daytime sleepiness and the total sleeping time (Eijsvogel *et al.* 2015).

Some studies compared the efficacy of positional therapy with CPAP (the reference therapy for OSAS) showing a greater efficacy of CPAP in reducing AHI and improving SaO_2; whereas, no significant differences were found in the quality of night sleep (arousal index, total sleeping time, and sleep efficiency) (Ha *et al.* 2014; Barnes *et al.* 2017).

Two randomized and controlled trials compared the treatment using positional trainer and endo-oral mandibular advancement device showing the same therapeutic efficacy in terms of AHI reduction and similar adherence to the therapy during a follow-up of 3 and 12 months (Benoist *et al.* 2017; de Ruiter *et al.* 2018).

The positional therapy was also efficacious as a treatment of primary snoring (AHI < 5) determining a significant reduction in the duration and intensity of the noise (evaluated objectively and subjectively). On the contrary, in apneic patients treated with positional therapy, snoring does not improve altogether (some clinical records indicate a worsening of the noise) even if the number of apneas/hypopneas decreases. Therefore, evaluating the efficacy of positional therapy must take into account the clinical evaluation using subjective questionnaires or when the patient's primary complaint is of disturbing the bed partner.

ADHERENCE TO THE TREATMENT

The poor adherence to the treatment seems to be the fundamental problem of the positional therapy. A few follow-up studies after 3 months to 2.5 years show that a very low percentage of patients (between 29% and 38%) continues to use the device to avoid supine position; particularly in a study after 2.5 years, the percentage had decreased to 6% (Bignold *et al.* 2009; Ravesloot *et al.* 2013; Joosten *et al.* 2014; Oksenberg and Gadoth 2014; Omobomi and Quan 2018).

The **reasons for the scarce use** are: physical discomfort caused by the device (indicated as the main cause by many studies) and the forced position; fragmented sleep due to the increase in awakenings; and impossibility to sleep in the favored position. Furthermore, a discreet percentage of patients were reported to have learned to avoid the supine position, but these data have not been proved objectively.

The most recent devices (vibratory alarms) cause fewer disturbances to the patient and have the possibility to objectively monitor the use and sleep position for a longer period. They seem to be associated with a better adherence to the treatment (85% and 97% on follow-up of 3 weeks to 1 months), although the published studies are few and the follow-up period are too short to gain definitive indications (Bignold *et al.* 2011; Van Maanen *et al.* 2013).

INDICATIONS OF THE INTERNATIONAL GUIDELINES

According to the guidelines of AASM (2006) on positional therapy (considered in the field of the Practice Parameters for Medical Therapy of OSAS) such therapy, consisting in an adequate method for the avoidance of supine position during sleep, it is indicated as a second choice or supplementary therapy to another specific therapy of first choice for OSAS in patients with supine AHI higher than the nonsupine AHI (Morgenthaler *et al.* 2006).

The AASM guidelines on the management of patients with OSAS (2009) confirm the measures already stated in the previous guidelines and also specify that it is necessary:

- to document with instrumental methods the effective efficacy of the positional therapy before undertaking it as a primary treatment, taking into consideration that not all patients achieve a normalization of AHI with such therapy;
- to document with instrumental methods the effective efficacy of the positional therapy before undertaking it as a primary treatment, taking into consideration that not all patients achieve a normalization of AHI with such therapy;
- to use a positional device expressly studied to inhibit the supine position (alarm, belt, pajama or tennis ball) and not to provide uniquely verbal instructions on how to make it or how to avoid sleeping in a supine position; and
- to evaluate the answer to the treatment in terms of resolution of symptoms, side effects, and adherence to the therapy, reported subjectively or if possible, monitored objectively (Epstein *et al.* 2009).

The **European Respiratory Society** agrees with the AASM clinical guidelines on the indications to the non-CPAP therapy for OSAS (2011) and specifies that:

- the positional therapy is not recommended for OSAS (when it is generically defined, without specifying the difference between OSAS and positional OSAS), except for patients carefully selected;
- if it is decided to utilize the positional therapy as a primary treatment, it is necessary to document the efficacy with a sleep study; and
- adherence to the treatment in the long run is to be verified with periodical clinical controls (Randerath *et al.* 2011).

The international guidelines about positional therapy as part of clinical practice are all very restrictive as they are affected by the lack of scientific evidences on the efficacy of positional therapy in treating OSAS in terms of primary (significant reduction in AHI) and secondary outcomes (sleepiness, quality of sleep, and cardiovascular complications), as well as adherence to the treatment. Considering the strong rationale of positional therapy, the authors still believe that it is possible to use PT as a primary therapy in clinical practice by always taking into account some of the following fundamental requirements:

- It must be used only for patients with positional OSAS who have been adequately and accurately selected, for example, the patients with isolated positional OSAS who have been identified with an instrumental recording where the position has been adequately monitored also with an appropriate amount of sleeping time spent in different positions.
- It is advisable only in the mild-moderate forms, without comorbidities or significant cardiovascular risk factors and particular occupational risks associated with OSAS.
- The efficacy of the therapy in terms of normalization of AHI on supine and nonsupine positions must be documented with a night sleep recording.
- It is advisable to use the new positional device to monitor both sleep position and use of the device.
- It is necessary to control the patient with periodic follow-up, verifying also the efficacy of the therapy in terms of secondary outcomes (daytime sleepiness, quality of sleep, and evolution or onset of comorbidities) and the adherence to the treatment (this clinical behavior is always indicated in any therapeutic approach to OSAS as this is a chronic pathology).

POSITIONAL THERAPY ASSOCIATED WITH OTHER SPECIFIC THERAPIES

The AASM guidelines agree that positional therapy can be used in association with other specific therapies (CPAP, surgery, or endo-oral devices). In spite of the several data confirming the importance of the positional component in successful or poor outcomes of the specific therapy (fundamental requirement for the supplementary use of PT), specific studies on efficacy of association of PT and specific therapy on the overall result.

Positional therapy and surgery of the upper airways

By analyzing therapeutic good and bad outcomes of the ENT surgery on soft tissues of the upper airways, particularly at the velopharyngeal site, some studies have shown that uvulopalatopharyngoplasty (UPPP) has significantly reduced AHI in lateral position; whereas, AHI in supine position was not significantly modified.

Hence, UPPP may amplify the positional component of OSAS. For such reason, it is indicated that "associating the positional therapy may significantly improve the response to the therapy with UPPP" (Lee *et al.*2011; Ravesloot *et al.* 2013).

Positional therapy and oral devices

There are many evidences showing a higher efficacy of the mandibular advancement device in patients with positional OSAS. However, only one old study evaluated the efficacy of the combined therapy of positional therapy (device + alarm) + oral device (tongue retaining device [TRD]) compared to only positional therapy or device. The study showed a higher efficacy of the combined therapy on the reduction in AHI compared to the two isolated therapies (Cartwright *et al.* 1991). Even if it is encouraging, this information alone is insufficient to assess the efficacy and indications of combined therapy (Ravesloot *et al.*2013).

CONCLUSIONS

As demonstrated by a significant number of recent scientific studies, the interest on positional therapy has gradually increased due to the high prevalence of patients with mainly positional OSAS, the difficulties to adapt to the CPAP therapy for patients with mild-moderate forms of OSAS or without daytime sleepiness, and the clinical guidelines suggesting to choose a tailored therapy that takes into account the requirements of the patient.

Furthermore, the positional therapy has become more standardized and also verifiable; thanks to the availability of new positional devices, which disturb less and are able to provide information about their use.

All the revisions in literature affirm that further studies are necessary, preferably performed with the new positional devices, adequate sample of patients, and a correct method (randomized and controlled trials, and standardized selection of the investigated population) to better clarify the efficacy of the positional therapy and the problems related to the adherence to the treatment (perhaps also due to learning the behaviors to avoid).

It is also necessary to use criteria of classification of positional OSAS that are univocal and agree to correctly identify the patients to be treated.

Only then, it will be possible to define with precision the indications for the application of this therapy for patients with positional OSAS and such treatment may play a role in the tailored therapy for OSAS (Oksenberg and Gadoth 2014).

Weight Loss

RATIONALE

OSAS and obesity are strictly connected pathologies:

- Obesity is the main risk factor for OSAS and 60% of the patients with OSAS are overweight.

- The overweight patients present deposition of adipose tissue both in the muscles and tissues around the upper airways, thus reducing the diameter of the airways and increased collapsibility at the thoracoabdominal level, thus reducing the lung volumes.
- OSAS and obesity are both risk factors for diabetes and cardiovascular pathologies, probably through common inflammatory and endocrine mechanisms (Mehra and Redline 2008; Bonsignore *et al.* 2012).

Epidemiological studies on the overall population have documented that spontaneous changes in the body weight go along with **significant modifications of respiratory events**. For example, a 10% weight gain determines 6 times greater probability to develop OSAS; and with a 10% weight gain, 32% increase in AHI (95% confidence interval [CI], 20%–45%) is predicted; whereas, a 10% weight loss is associated with 26% decrease in AHI (95% CI, 18%–34%) (Peppard *et al.* 2000).

Furthermore, the increase in obesity in the overall population and the consequent increase in OSAS prevalence require not only the specific symptoms of OSAS to be considered as the objective of the treatment, but also obesity, which affects the severity and progression of the disease (Peppard *et al.* 2013).

Hence, weight loss should always be taken into consideration in the therapeutic approach to the patient with OSAS, also remembering its limitations and evaluating the general clinical situation.

OSAS–OBESITY RELATION: FACTORS AFFECTING THE RESULT OF WEIGHT LOSS

By considering weight loss as a therapy for OSAS, it is necessary to keep in mind some fundamental premises of the OSAS–obesity relation that have been highlighted in longitudinal studies on the overall population. These premises that can influence the efficacy of losing weight are:

- Men and women do not respond the same way to weight changes: The correlation between body weight and AHI is linear enough in male individuals; whereas, females tend to develop sleep-disordered breathing only at higher levels of obesity. Furthermore, changes of weight in women (both gain and loss) determine the corresponding modifications in AHI of minor entity compared to men; thus, weight loss is less effective (5.4) (Redline *et al.* 2003; Newman *et al.* 2005).
- The impact of weight in determining OSAS decreases with age and becomes less significant after 60 years (Tishler *et al.* 2003).
- Weight loss contrasts only partially the disease progression in the patients with OSAS: In fact, the improvement in the sleep-disordered breathing (in terms of reduction of events/h) that is obtained with a certain amount of weight loss is minor compared to the worsening of AHI determined by a corresponding weight gain (Peppard *et al.* 2000; Newman *et al.* 2005).

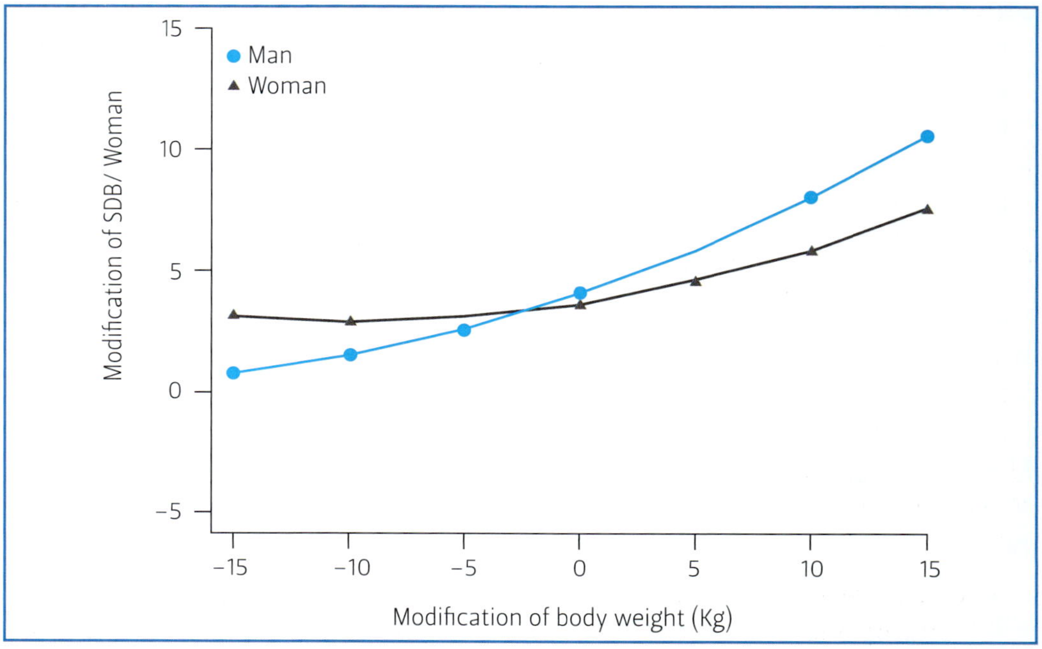

5.4 Modification of the number of respiratory events per hour of sleep (SDB) in relation to the modification of body weight in man and woman (Modified by Newman *et al.* 2005)

- *Obesity and OSAS are correlated bidirectionally by a series of pathophysiological and genetic mechanisms* that reinforce each other reciprocally. Hence, not only obesity favors the respiratory disorder, but also OSAS favors weight gain. This correlation can explain the difficulty in obtaining and maintaining a weight loss when a sleep-disordered breathing persists (5.5) (Brown *et al.* 2011; Tuomilehto *et al.* 2013a).

TECHNIQUES TO OBTAIN WEIGHT LOSS

The methods to obtain weight loss and the criteria to choose among several techniques are the same for both the patients with OSAS and obese patients not affected by OSAS.

The main techniques that have been evaluated in patients with OSAS are:

- *Lifestyle interventions:* These are generally accomplished with techniques to change behavior that include programs for controlling the food intake, hypocaloric diets associated with modifications in eating habits, and programs for regular physical exercise (if necessary, combined together) for patients who are overweight or present a mild-to-moderate obesity (Grade I and II).
- *Bariatric surgery*: It is performed on those patients with moderate obesity (Grade II) and comorbidities (diabetes, hypertension, or cardiopathy) who did not respond to previous lifestyle interventions or in patients with severe obesity (Grade III). We distinguish that:

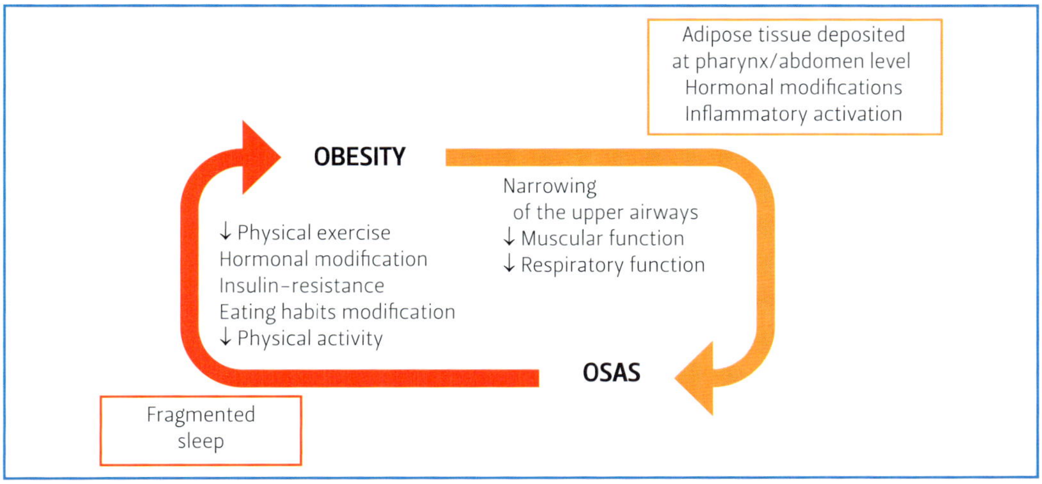

5.5 Mechanisms of bidirectional association between OSAS and obesity (Modified from: Tuomilehto *et al.* 2013a)

- restrictive surgery reduces the gastric volume (gastric bypass, gastric banding, and plastic surgery) by limiting the amount of food the stomach can hold, thus resulting in earlier satiety;
- malabsorptive surgery causes an intestinal malabsorption by reducing the surface of the small intestine (intestinal bypass); and
- mixed surgery procedures combining elements of the previous ones (biliopancreatic diversion).

- *Weight loss achieved with medication.* Few studies have assessed the effects of medication to lose weight in patients with OSAS. Two studies utilized sibutramine, a drug that was withdrawn from the market in Europe due to the adverse cardiovascular effects. One study assessed orlistat, a drug that reduces the absorption of fat and is used for weight maintenance. Due to the scarcity of scientific data at hand, we refer you to the specific literature (Yee *et al.* 2007; Phillips *et al.* 2009; Svendsen and Tonstad 2011).

EFFICACY OF WEIGHT LOSS OBTAINED WITH LIFESTYLE INTERVENTIONS

Weight loss obtained with lifestyle interventions has a minor entity compared to what is achieved with bariatric surgery. Studies have been performed in patients with OSAS and the diabetic patients affected with OSAS (longitudinal studies on diabetes) presenting a sleep-disordered breathing of variable severity, from mild-to-moderate-severe, and with mild-moderate obesity (BMI < 40).

Considering that the association between OSAS and obesity has always been known, weight loss obtained with lifestyle interventions has been one of the first applied therapeutic modalities. Hence, the related literature is abundant, although the main part of the studies has an observational character. It did not imply control groups and led on samples that were selected inadequately; therefore, it has **low levels of scientific evidence**. The most recent studies (randomized and controlled trials) provide conflicting results on its efficacy, and therefore, new randomized and controlled studies are required to be performed by following adequate protocols (Randerath *et al.* 2011; Bakker and Patel 2013).

The revision studies on the related literature show that the entity of weight loss obtained from lifestyle interventions was variable with a mean weight reduction between 3% and 18%, and a reduction of $4{,}7 \pm 2{,}5$ kg/m^2 considering the BMI. A recent meta-analysis (methodologically correct: 21 adequate studies with 893 patients) highlighted a 2.3 kg/m^2 BMI reduction in controlled studies and a 4.9 kg/m^2 reduction in noncontrolled studies. Hence, altogether weight loss obtained with these techniques is modest (5.1) (Randerath *et al.* 2011; Cowan and Livingston 2012; Araghi *et al.* 2013; Tuomilehto *et al.* 2013a).

Weight loss determines a **reduction in AHI/respiratory disturbance index (RDI)**, but the entity varies and the heterogeneity of the samples and studies (some with negative results) do not enable to gather precise information on the degree of efficacy. The revision studies highlight a reduction in AHI/RDI between 3% and 63%, and a mean reduction in AHI of 21 13 events/h (equal to 44%); whereas, the meta-analysis by Araghi and collaborators shows that the reduction in AHI has a modest entity (reduction to 6 events/h in controlled studies and 12 events/h in noncontrolled studies) (see 5.1) (Randerath *et.al* 2011; Cowan and Livingston 2012; Araghi *et al.* 2013; Tuomilehto *et al.* 2013).

The **improvement of nocturnal oxygenation**, is more significant, with a reduction of ODI to 18.9 events/h, most likely justified by the impact of weight loss on nocturnal ventilation (Araghi et al. 2013).

A linear correlation has been demonstrated between the entity of weight loss and the improvement of sleep-disordered breathing, although the studies do not often agree at indicating the exact reduction in AHI with a certain amount of weight loss. Two recent randomized and controlled studies (one on 81 patients with mild OSAS and the other on 264 diabetic patients with moderate OSAS) have both verified an improvement in AHI by 0.4 events/h per each kilogram of weight loss (Randerath *et.al* 2011; Araghi *et al.* 2013; Kuna *et al.* 2013; Tuomilehto *et al.* 2013b).

The meta-analysis by Araghi and collaborators indicates (even without the significant clinical records for the heterogeneity of the studies) that it is necessary to achieve a 10% weight loss from the initial weight to obtain an improvement in OSAS (Araghi *et al.* 2013).

The reduction in AHI with weight loss is greater in patients with a higher basal AHI, for example, with a higher risk of cardiovascular complications; in such a situation, losing weight may have a beneficial effect (Araghi *et al.* 2013).

In literature, the number of patients with OSAS to be considered "cured" with weight loss is variable because the reference parameters are different (a 50% reduction of AHI; AHI <20; AHI <15; AHI <10; AHI ≤ 5). The European

5.1 Studies that evaluated the efficacy of weight loss obtained with lifestyle interventions on OSAS (in terms of AHI/RDI/ODI)

Author	Study design	nr	% Male	GStudy group	Technique of intervention	Follow-up (months)	ΔBMI	ΔAHI	Treated Patients with OSAS
Johansson *et al.*, 2011	Prospective cohort study	63	100	BMI 30–40, AHI ≥15	VLCD and programme of weight maintenance	12	35→31	36→19	10
Nerfeldt *et al.*, 2010	Prospective cohort study	33	73%	BMI ≥30, AHI ≥10 and/or ODI ≥6, OSAS symptoms	LCD and support to lifestyle interventions	24	40→35	43→28	?
Johansson *et al.*, 2009	Randomized and controlled parallel group	63	100	BMI 30–40, AHI ≥15	VLCD	2	34→29 *vs* 35→35	37→12 *vs* 37→35	17 vs 0
Tuomilehto *et al.*, 2009	Randomized and controlled parallel group	72	74	BMI 28–40, AHI 5–15	VCLD, supervision of lifestyle	12	33→? *vs* 31→?	10→6 *vs* 9→10	63% *vs* 35%
Barnes *et al.*, 2009	Cohort study	12	25	BMI >30, AHI 10–50	VLCD and physical activity	12	36→30	25→18	0
Foster *et al.*, 2009	Randomized and controlled parallel group	264	41	BMI ≥25, AHI ≥5, Type 2 diabetes	Intensive intervention on life style (diet/ physical activity)	12	37→? *vs* 37→?	23→18 *vs* 24→28	14 vs 4
Kemppainen *et al.*, 2008	Randomized and controlled parallel group	52	79	BMI 28–40, AHI 5–15	VCLD, supervision of lifestyle	3	33→? *vs* 32→?	11→8 *vs* 9→8	?
Kajaste *et al.*, 2004	Cohort study	31	100	BMI >35, ODI >10	VCLD, CBT for weight loss	24	44→40	51→32 (ODI)	?
Kansanen *et al.*, 1998	Prospective cohort study	15	93	Overweight patients with OSAS	VLCD	3	38→35	31→19 (ODI)	20
Suratt *et al.*, 1992	Cohort study	8	62	Obese patients with OSAS	VLCD	?	54→46	90→62	
Ferland *el al.*, 2009	Non-randomized and parallel group	40	88	BMI ≥30, OSAS	Sibutramine, diet and physical activity vs CPAP	12	37→35 *vs* 36→36	40→37 *vs* 44→4	
Phillips *et al.*, 2009	Cohort study	93	100	BMI 30–38, RDI ≥15	Sibutramine, diet and physical activity	6	34→32	46→30 (RDI)	?
Yee *et al.*, 2007	Cohort study	87	100	BMI 25–35, AHI ≥10	Sibutramine *vs* placebo	1	?	28→27 *vs* 28→28	?

ΔAHI, Apnea/Hypopnea Index (events/hour) before and after the treatment; ΔBMI, Body Mass Index (kg/m²) before and after the treatment; CBT, Cognitive Behavioural Therapy; CPAP, Continuous Positive Airway Pressure; n, number; ODI Oxygen Desaturation Index (events/hour); RDI, Respiratory Disorder Index (events/hour). (V)LCD, (Very) Low Calorie Diet. (Source: Cowan and Livingston 2012).

Respiratory Society reviewed 24 studies and concluded that the treatment results of 39% of the patients were "improved" and 23% were "cured"; whereas, the meta-analysis by Araghi and collaborators highlighted a modest efficacy of weight loss, with only 5 of 21 studies showing a normalization of the nocturnal respiratory situation (considering AHI < 10) in patients with OSAS varying from 17% to 60%.

However, both revisions conclude that the clinical records are overall scant, especially those presenting the more favorable results and also that the scientific evidences are too scarce to draw the exact conclusions on the efficacy of weight loss on OSAS (Randerath *et al.* 2011; Araghi *et al.* 2013).

The effects of losing weight on the main outcomes of OSAS (daytime sleepiness and cardiovascular complications) have been investigated less and the results have been scantily defined, perhaps because obesity and OSAS are independent risk factors both for excessive daytime sleepiness and for cardiocerebrovascular pathologies and this point can be a confusing factor.

The studies evaluating sleepiness with subjective scales (e.g., ESS) have observed significant variations in the scoring. However, these variations have a modest entity (reduction of 1 score on controlled studies and 2.8 scores in noncontrolled ones) and are not clinically important (Araghi et al. 2013).

MAINTENANCE AND EFFICACY OF WEIGHT LOSS OBTAINED WITH LIFESTYLE INTERVENTIONS AT FOLLOW-UP

Maintaining weight loss obtained with lifestyle interventions is always a key problem and requires continual therapeutic counseling intervention for a longer period of time. It has been considered a further limitation for the OSAS patients who obtained weight loss with such techniques as it requires considerable financial and professional efforts against the modest results on the sleep-disordered breathing.

The follow-up studies on weight loss as a therapy for OSAS, with a duration varying from 1 to 4 years, generally included an initial low-calorie diet followed by integrative programs for weight maintenance, change in eating habits, and physical activity combined in various forms. The therapeutic counseling support was always kept with close meetings during the active phase of the treatment, which then reduced to 1.2 meetings per month for the whole duration of the follow-up (Kuna *et al.* 2013; Tuomilehto *et al.* 2013b).

In all the cases, the initial weight loss obtained at the end of an active diet intervention was followed by a partial weight recovery, which corresponded to about 50% of the lost weight in longer follow-up studies (4 years). However, the final weight at the follow-up was still significantly lower compared to the pre-treatment weight (Cowan and Livingstone 2012; Araghi *et al.* 2013; Kuna *et al.* 2013; Tuomilehto *et al.* 2013b).

The AHI reduction obtained with a weight loss persisted in spite of the partial weight recovery as if the weight loss had also favored a redistribution of the adipose tissue at upper airways level with an improvement in the neuromuscular control (5.6) (Kuna *et al.* 2013; Tuomilehto *et al.* 2013a and b).

The efficacy of losing weight on OSAS remains evident at follow-up in terms of reduction of AHI as well as regression or failed progression of the disease. This condition is more obvious in the randomized and controlled studies comparing the patients with OSAS who lost weight and those who did not (5.7) (Cowan and Livingstone 2012; Kuna *et al.* 2013; Tuomilehto *et al.* 2013a and b).

The only follow-up study at 5 years (with very small clinical records of 57 patients) indicates that the disease does not progress in patients with mild

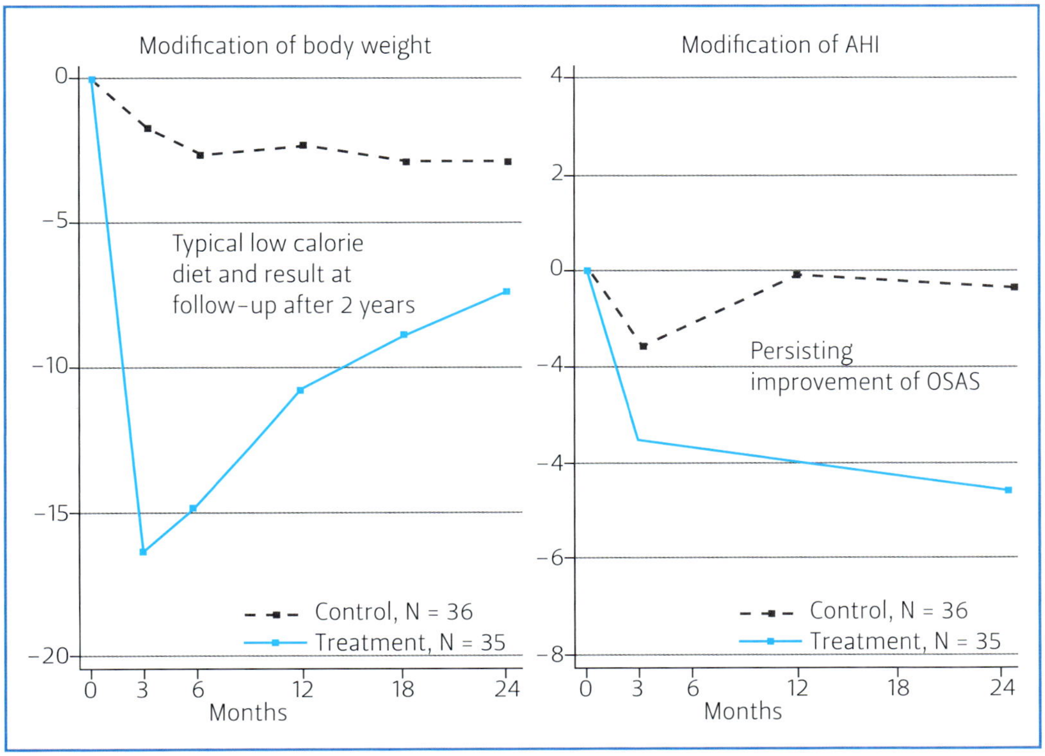

5.6 Maintenance and efficacy of weight loss obtained with behavioural techniques on weight and OSAS. Efficacy a 3, 6, 12 and 24 months of lifestyle interventions with low calories diet on body weight *(left)* and AHI *(right)*. (Modified from: Tuomilehto *et al.* 2013a)

OSAS who maintain a weight loss of ≥ 5% (reduction of AHI after 5 years equals to 3.5 events/h) (Tuomilehto *et al.* 2014).

Although the results of weight loss on OSAS at follow-up are so interesting, we should not forget that they are based on few studies; very few of them are randomized and controlled, and some of them present limited clinical records. Therefore, definitive indications cannot be drawn on the efficacy of weight loss obtained with behavioral techniques on OSAS, as reaffirmed by the international guidelines (see below).

Hence, all the authors, including the more convinced about the importance of weight loss, agree on the necessity of new studies on this field to be developed with the evidence-based criteria of medicine to be able to define the role of weight loss in the therapeutic planning for the patients with OSAS (Araghi et al. 2013; Bakker and Patel 2013; Tuomilehto and Uusitupa 2014).

EFFICACY OF WEIGHT LOSS OBTAINED WITH BARIATRIC SURGERY

Unlike weight loss obtained with lifestyle interventions, the surgical approach to obesity determines important weight loss, especially in the first months, that continues for at least 1-2 years and can be maintained over time with follow-up at 15 years.

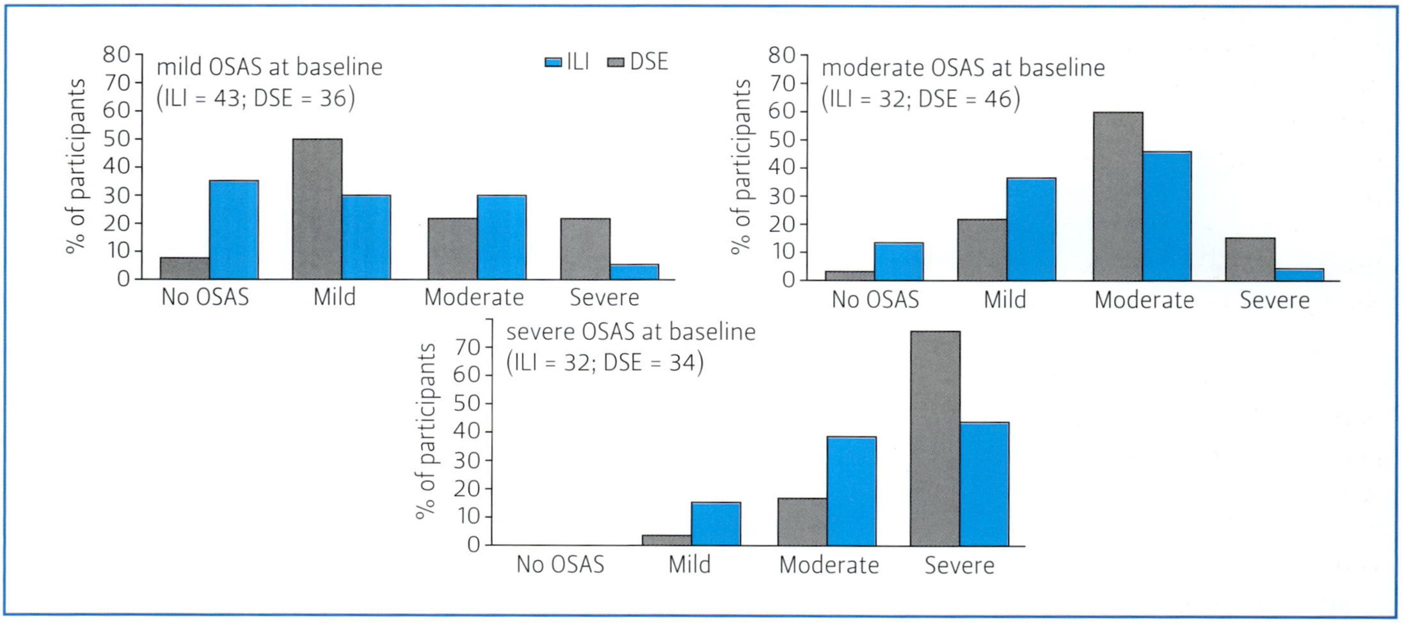

5.7 Modification of the severity of OSAS after weight loss at 4 years follow-up. Comparison with diabetic subjects with OSAS treated with weight loss through behavioural techniques (intensive Lifestyle interventions [ILI], blue bars) and diabetic subject with OSAS treated with educational support (Diabetes Support and Education [DSE], grey bars). The subjects are subdivided in groups according to the severity of OSAS before the treatment: note that 30% of the patients with mild OSAS and circa 10% of those with moderate OSAS result cured (absence of OSAS) with weight loss (ILI) (Modified from: Kuna *et al.* 2013)

Bariatric surgery is effective in reducing metabolic and cardiovascular complications of obesity and decreasing mortality in super-obese patients. However, they are surgical interventions involving risks of peri-and-post operation complications and a mortality rate of 0.3% after 30 d. Both complications and death risk are significantly greater when the patient is affected with OSAS (Sjöström *et al.* 2007; Colquitt *et al.* 2009; Flum *et al.* 2009; Athyros *et al.* 2011).

Among the candidates for bariatric surgery, the prevalence of OSAS is about 70% and ca. 30%–40% of the patients present a severe form of OSAS, although only a small percentage (13%) presents already a diagnosis of OSAS when they register in the list for the surgery.

The failed identification and treatment of OSAS in the pre-operatory phase exposes these patients to higher risks of complications during general anesthesia and the peri-operatory period. It is thus necessary that the candidates for the bariatric surgery undergo an instrumental night recording to evaluate a possible presence of OSAS, which must be treated before the surgery (O'Keeffe and Patterson 2004; Ravesloot *et al.* 2012).

For ethical reasons, there are no randomized and controlled studies on the efficacy of bariatric surgery for OSAS (it is not ethical to randomize who has the clinical indication to undergo surgery); therefore, the data on the efficacy of bariatric surgery on OSAS are based on studies with **low levels of scientific evidence**, retrospective or prospective cohort studies, with scant clinical records, selection bias (for instance, including only symptomatic patients or patients with other respiratory sleep disorders, particularly the obesity hypoventilation syndrome) and bias at post-operatory polysomnographic follow-up. The best results are to be found in retrospective studies, with more selection bias and minor levels of scientific evidence. However, more recent prospective studies present correct criteria for selection and show less evident and more controversial results. For this reason, the international guidelines consider bariatric surgery as a treatment aimed to reduce the risks correlated to obesity rather than a treatment for OSAS in obese patients as it was originally indicated (Morghentaller *et al.* 2006; Greenburg *et al.* 2009).

Bariatric surgery determines a **significant weight loss** with a BMI reduction between 10 and 24.4 kg/m2 in the 24 studies that were reviewed by the European Respiratory Society (mean reduction of 17.9 kg/m2 [95% CI 16.5-19.3]); whereas, the meta-analysis of Greenburg and collaborators (5.2) shows a BMI reduction between 55.3 and 37.7 kg/m^2, independent of the kind of interventions (Greenburg *et al.* 2009; Randerath *et al.* J 2011).

Surgical weight loss involves a **remarkable reduction of AHI** of 44 ± 22 events/h in the revision of Randerath and collaborators, corresponding to a decrease of 77% of the basal AHI, and of 38.2 events/h (95% CI 31.9-44.4) in the meta-analysis from 2009, equal to a decrease of 71% of the basal AHI diminishing from 54.8 to 15.8 events/h (Greenburg *et al.* 2009; Randerath *et al.* 2011).

Some authors have calculated that the reduction of one unit to the BMI (kg/m^2) obtained with surgery determines a reduction of 2.3 respiratory events/h (Romero-Corral *et al.* 2010).

The different techniques of bariatric surgery in terms of efficacy on OSAS have been compared in literature by a recent meta-analysis where the **biliopancreatic diversion** proved to be the most effective procedure to decrease AHI; whereas, the laparoscopic adjustable gastric banding proved to be the least effective, only determining a minor weight loss (Sarkhosh *et al.* 2010).

All studies confirm the impact on OSAS by weight loss achieved with surgical techniques and the substantial reduction of AHI (75% of the treated patients according to a recent revision on the literature of the different surgical techniques). However, it is important to underline that the decrease in the absolute value of AHI does not necessarily mean being "cured" and protected by OSAS' complications (Greenburg *et al.* 2009; Sarkhohsh *et al.* 2013).

Data from the literature on the percentage of obese patients with OSAS treated with bariatric surgery are discordant: a meta-analysis of Buchwald and collaborators from 2004 estimated an 80% of cured patients with OSAS, but the examined studies were flawed with important bias of selection of the patients and methods problems (nonverifiable polysomnography at follow-up) with consequent poor meaning of the obtained data (Buchwald *et al.* 2004).

Greenburg and collaborators' methodologically correct meta-analysis (2009) has instead shown that results of only 25% of the patients with OSAS

5.2 Description of the characteristic of the studies included in the metanalysis of Greenburg *et al.* (2009)

					Pre-surgery			Post-surgery			Differenza			
Author	Year	Nation	Nr.	Type of surgery	BMI	Weight (kg)	AHI	BMI	Weight (kg)	AHI	BMI	Weight (kg)	AHI	Note
Charuzi	1992	Israel	47	Different techniques		139 (24.6)	60.8 (35.5)			8.0 (11.8)			52.8	Retrospective. Follow-up at 1 and 7 years, 92% of the patients with OSAS had a PSG of control. Sample: 7 women and 44 men
Sugerman	1992	USA	40	Different techniques	58 (13.0)	166 (35)	61.1 (39.0)	39.0 (8.0)	110.0 (23.0)	26.0 (26.0)	19	56	38	Retrospective. Unclear inclusion criteria. Potential bias in follow-up: only 34% of the patients with pre-surgery OSAS did a PSG of post-surgery control. Unknown distribution of women/men
Pillar	1994	Israel	14	Different techniques	45 (7.2)	131 (22.5)	40 (28.8)	35.0 (6.0)		24.0 (23.0)	10		16	Retrospective. Unclear inclusion criteria. Sample: 3 women and 11 men
Scheuller	2001	USA	15	Billio-pancreatic diversion or gastroplastic		160 (26.6)	96.9 (44.3)		105.0 (21.2)	11.3 (15.0)		54.6	85.6	Retrospective. Unclear inclusion criteria. No pre-established criteria for control PSG. Wide range at follow-up (1-12 years). Sample: 5 women and 10 men
Guardiano	2003	USA	8	Roux-en-Y	49 (12.0)		55.0 (31.0)	34.0 (12.0)	105 (22.0)	14.0 (17.0)	15		41	Retrospective, modest sample size. Potential bias at follow-up: only 24% of the patients with pre-surgery OSAS did a post-surgery control PSG. Patients that did not adhere to CPAP were excluded. Sample:7 women and 1 man
Rasheid	2003	USA	11	Gastric bypass	62 (3.0)		56.0 (13.0)	40.0 (2.0)		23.0 (7.0)	22		33	Prospective study. Modest Potential bias in the follow-up, only 12% of the patients with OSAS in pre-surgery has done a post-surgery control PSG. Unknown distribution between women/men

Valencia-Flores	2004	Mexico	28	Different techniques	56,7 (2,3)	56,5 (12,3)	51,7 (19,6)	39,2 (1,6)		13,4 (12,8)	17		33	Retrospective. Potential bias at follow-up: only 45% of the patients with OSAS in pre-surgery did a post-surgery control PSG. Sample: 16 women and 13 men. Results expressed only as presence/absence of OSAS
Dixon	2005	Australia	25	Laparoscopic gastric banding	53 (9,5)	154 (35,0)	61,6 (31,9)	37,2 (7,2)	105 (22,0)	13,4 (13,0)	15,5	49	48,2	Prospective. Potential bias at follow-up: only 51% of the patients with OSAS at pre-surgery did a post-surgery control PSG. Sample: 8 women and 17 men
Kalra	2006	USA	17	Gastric bypass	58 (7,2)	163 (30,3)	22,2 (33,6)	43,8 (8,2)		5,6 (11,0)	14,5		16,6	Retrospective. Sample limited to adolescents. Potential bias at follow-up: only 50% of the patients with OSAS at pre-surgery did a post-surgery control PSG. Women/men distribution is not reported
Haines	2007	USA	101	Roux-en-Y	56 (1,0)		51,0 (4,0)	38,0 (1,0)		15,0 (2,0)	18		36	PProspective with clear inclusion criteria. Potential bias at follow-up: only 35% of the patients with OSAS at pre-surgery did a post-surgery control PSG. Women/men distribution is not reported
Fritscher	2007	Brasil	12	Roux-en-Y	55,5 (10,0)	151,9 (22,6)	66 (33,4)	34,1 (8,1)	100,7 (18,9)	23,7 (24,3)	21	50,2	42,3	Prospective with clear inclusion criteria. Only 1 patient did do the PSG at follow-up. Sample: 3 women, 9 men
Lettieri	2008	USA	24	Laparoscopic gastric banding	51 (10,4)	147 (29,0)	47,8 (33,8)	24,5 (18,1)	93,0 (18,5)	24,5 (18,1)	18,9	54	23,3	Prospective with clear inclusion criteria. All the patients surviving the perioperative period did the PSG at follow-up. Sample: 18 women and 6 men

BMI, Body Mass Index; AHI. indice di apnea/ipopnea; PSG, polisonnografia.I valori sono espressi come medie (deviazioni standard).

are cured (AHI < 5) after weight loss obtained with surgery; 44% presents a residual AHI < 10 events/h; and overall 62% of the patients shows a residual OSAS after the surgical weight loss, with a mean AHI > 15 events/h, which involves the risk of cardiometabolic complications and requires an extra treatment (Greenburg *et al.* 2009).

Finally, the revision in the literature from Randerath and collaborators for the European Respiratory Society lead on 24 studies with low levels of evidence (mainly level 4) indicates that the percentage of obese patients with OSAS cured from bariatric surgery was 64% (Randerath *et al.* 2011).

The patients with OSAS results as "cured" are younger and slimmer: a weight <100 kg at follow-up is a predictive factor for AHI < 5; whereas, gender and a pre-treatment AHI do not affect the result (Greenburg *et al.* 2009).

Few studies have evaluated the effect of bariatric surgery on patients with OSAS on different outcomes than AHI; the positive results report thus a scarce scientific evidence but indicate an **improvement on all indexes of nocturnal saturation** (events of desaturation per hour of sleep, sleeping time with SaO_2 < 90%, mean SaO_2, minimum SaO_2), improvement on quality of night sleep and a decrease of **daytime sleepiness** assessed with ESS (Cowan and Livingstone 2012).

Upon these data, it should be highlighted that clinically the patients with OSAS treated with bariatric surgery obtained an adequate weight loss, which is usually associated with an improvement of the subjective symptoms, of quality of sleep, and nocturnal respiratory disorder (in terms of reduction of AHI); in spite of all this, a moderate-mild OSAS often persists and this may require a further treatment (Greenburg *et al.* 2009).

Hence, within a year after obtaining an adequate weight loss with surgery, it is important to plan a polysomnography, a cardiorespiratory monitoring or a polygraphy to verify the entity of the achieved improvement. If the patient was already being treated with CPAP or other devices, it is not advisable to interrupt the treatment before having ascertained the severity of the residual night respiratory disorder.

When it is necessary to maintain the therapy with CPAP, it suffices to the use of minor pressures (in average 4 cm H2O) than to those used before surgery (Greenburg *et al.* 2009; Fleetham *et al.* 2011).

MAINTENANCE OF THE EFFICACY OF BARIATRIC SURGERY AT FOLLOW-UP

Weight loss due to bariatric surgery occurs generally within 12-24 months, then the weight stabilizes until 5-6 years after the treatment, and henceforth, it may remain stable or increase again. Few studies, however, with low scientific evidence and conflicting results have evaluated the efficacy of bariatric surgery on OSAS with follow-up at 5 and 7.5 years, detecting often a worsening of AHI (sometimes consequent to weight recovery and sometimes independent from weight gain) (Cowan *et al.* 2012).

Hence, further prospective studies are necessary with adequate clinical records and without selection bias to obtain sufficient clinical information about the long-term efficacy of this therapeutic modality for patients with OSAS.

INDICATION OF INTERNATIONAL GUIDELINES

The AASM guidelines on weight loss (considered as part of the Practice Parameters for Medical Therapy of OSAS) report that:

- weight loss obtained through a "diet" can significantly improve AHI in obese patients with OSAS (*guideline*);
- weight loss obtained with a diet should always be associated with specific treatments of first choice for OSAS (CPAP, oral device, or oropharyngeal surgery) and cannot be considered as a prominent treatment (*option*); and
- bariatric surgery can be considered as an additional treatment to other first-choice specific therapies for patients with OSAS (*option*) (Morgenthaler *et al.* 2006).

In the indications for the non-CPAP therapy for OSAS, the **European Respiratory Society**, guidelines (2011) specify that:

- weight loss (generically considered, without distinguishing between lifestyle interventions and bariatric surgery) is always recommend for obese or overweight patients to reduce the risks correlated with obesity; and
- weight loss is always considered as an acceptable first-choice therapy for OSAS, considering the scarce scientific evidence and conflicting results reported in literature (Randerath *et al.* 2011).

The **Canadian Thoracic Society** guidelines on diagnosis and therapy for respiratory sleep disorders (*update* 2011) take into consideration only the bariatric surgery (and not weight loss obtained through other methods) among the different modalities of therapy for OSAS. They affirm that:

- bariatric surgery should be considered as part of the therapy for OSAS in obese patients falling in the criteria for obesity surgery (BMI ≥40 or BMI > 35 with comorbidity, or previous failure of dietary therapy) (grade 1 C); and
- a sleep study must also be performed for asymptomatic patients when the maximum weight loss is achieved (usually 1 year after the surgery) to evaluate the severity of the residual OSAS, especially before interrupting the ongoing therapy.

It is also specified that such indications are only based upon studies with low scientific evidence and experts' discussion.

In 2013, the **American College of Physicians** published practice guidelines on the management of adult patients with OSAS where they take into consideration the efficacy of weight loss on OSAS specifying that:

- weight loss should always be encouraged for obese or overweight patients (recommendation 1; *strong recommendation, low-quality evidence*);
- the physician should always encourage weight loss for the obese patient because obesity favors the progression of OSAS and weight loss improves the symptoms of OSAS and determines other beneficial effects (*high-value care*); and
- the therapy, particularly weight loss, must be discussed with the patients according to their clinical characteristics (*clinical considerations*) (Qaseem *et al.* 2013).

CONCLUSIONS

In patients with OSAS, obesity is one of the main factors of disease aggravation or progression. It is also an important metabolic and cardiovascular risk factor increasing the probability of complications of OSAS. For these reasons, all the international guidelines affirm that weight loss should always be associated with the specific therapy for OSAS, not only for the obese patient but also for the overweight patient.

The role of weight loss is to reduce the severity of OSAS, slow down the disease progression, and diminish the risk of complications due to obesity. However, weight loss cannot be viewed as a first-choice treatment for OSAS, considering the conflicting results in literature on its efficacy due to scarce scientific evidence on the topic.

Weight loss obtained with **behavioural techniques** of lifestyle interventions is significant but modest and it presents an efficacy of mild entity on the respiratory sleep disorder that although seems to stay constant over time. For this reason, some authors suggest that it could be considered as a first-choice treatment for obese patients with a mild OSAS, when the disease is still at an initial phase and the body has the capacity to recover by contrasting the progression of the pathological process and disease (Tuomilehto and Uusitupa 2014).

Although to validate this suggestion (ensued from some recent randomized and controlled studies), it is necessary to lead further scientific studies that are correctly planned according to evidence-base medicine.

Weight loss obtained with **bariatric surgery** determines a rather important reduction of body weight and a significant decrease in AHI; yet in a discreet percentage of patients, the respiratory sleep disorder persists even after the surgery, although in a less severe way. This makes necessary maintaining the therapy for OSAS set before pre-surgery. For these reasons, bariatric surgery is recommended only for those obese patients who are eligible for this kind of surgery and with maintenance of the ongoing therapy until verifying the resolution of OSAS with weight loss.

Behaviours to avoid

For patients with snoring or OSAS it should be a good rule to avoid behaviors that can aggravate the sleep-disordered breathing, particularly the assumption of medication or substances (as alcoholic drinks) that can worsen OSAS. Cigarette smoking should also be avoided as it can act as an irritating factor on the upper airways mucosa and favors a condition of inflammation and edema.

Literature studies on behaviors to avoid, also named withdrawal behaviors are very outdated, with small clinical records, scarce levels of evidence, and often conflicting and nonconclusive results.

Nevertheless, the international guidelines on managing patients with OSAS highlight the importance to always educate the patients on behaviors to avoid even if they are already following a specific therapy since an incorrect behavior (such as an excess of alcoholic drinks consumed in the evening at social events or the wrong hypnotic drug to treat insomnia) may significantly aggravate the severity of the respiratory sleep disorder or reduce the efficacy of the ongoing therapy (Epstein *et al.* 2009).

Below, we report summarily the effects of some common-use substances and medication on OSAS in daily life and clinical practice referring partially to more thorough text of sleep medicine. We refer completely to these publications for the description of the less-used drugs, such as opioids, barbiturates, anesthetic, and others (Kryger *et al.* 2011).

MEDICATION AND ALCOHOL

Sedative-hypnotic drugs (benzodiazepines) and alcohol, through a GABAergic inhibitory mechanism, determine:

- a respiratory depression with reduced ventilatory response to hypoxemia (and hypercapnia) acting directly on the respiratory centers;
- a reduction of the muscular tone with consequent hypotonia of the dilator muscles of the upper airways; and
- an increased arousal threshold (Cohn 1983; Vecchio *et al.* 2010).

Hence, through these mechanisms, the severity of OSAS can be influenced by increasing the number and extending the duration of the obstructive respiratory events, with consequent impact on the nocturnal oxygenation and quality of sleep.

Effects of alcohol on patients with OSAS

The studies on the effects of alcohol are all very outdated and with considerable methodologic limits. It is controversial whether alcohol can cause the onset of an obstructive respiratory disorder during sleep in normal nonsnoring patients. It is instead demonstrated that alcohol can determine the onset of pathological numbers of obstructive apneas/hypopneas in snorer patients, aggravate the severity of the disorder in patients with OSAS diagnosis, and increase the duration of the obstructive respiratory events and consequent hypoxemia (Kryger *et al.* 2011).

Furthermore, alcohol worsens the quality of sleep favoring its fragmentation in the second-half of the night. In patients with OSAS, this effect overlaps with the sleep disorder that is secondary to apneas/hypopneas (Kryger *et al.* 2011).

The interaction between the sedative effect of alcohol and daytime sleepiness in patients with OSAS is particularly **dangerous for driving**; in fact, in the patient with OSAS, small amounts of alcohol cause mistakes in simulated driving tests similar to those caused by considerable quantities in healthy patients (Roehrs *et al.* 1994).

In conclusion, the patients with OSAS should always avoid alcohol consumption due to the possible interaction with daytime sleepiness and the consequent increased risk of road accidents (particularly at evening hours) as well as the overall detrimental effect on breathing during sleep and on the quality of sleep.

Effects of the sedative-hypnotic drugs on patients with OSAS

Only some sedative-hypnotic drugs have been investigated in patients with OSAS. However, also in this case, the conducted studies are very outdated; particularly the old generation of long half-life benzodiazepines as flurazepam (hypnotic) and diazepam (sedative) are to be avoided as they worsen OSAS in patients with mild-moderate respiratory disorder (Kryger *et al.* 2011).

On the contrary, hypnotic benzodiazepines with intermediate half-life, such as temazepam and triazolam do not seem to worsen the respiratory sleep disorder in patients with mild OSAS or snoring (Kryger *et al.* 2011).

Particularly, zolpidem, zopiclone, eszopiclone, and short half-life non-benzodiazepine hypnotics (Z-drugs/hypnotics) have a greater selective hypnotic action and minor myorelaxant effects (they act selectively on the α subunit of GABA-A receptor). At the clinical evaluation in patients affected by OSAS and insomnia, they improve the quality of sleep and do not determine significant changes of AHI and nocturnal oxygenation (Zhang *et al.* 2014).

A controlled study has even shown that eszopiclone (not sold in Europe, but very similar to zopiclone, which is available in Europe), a half-life non-benzodiazepine hypnotic, significantly improves AHI in patients with OSAS through an increase in the arousal threshold by interacting with the chemoreceptor in control of breathing and muscle tone of the upper airways (Eckert *et al.* 2011).

The therapy for insomnia associated with mood disorders sometimes uses other drugs with a sedative antidepressant effect. At the clinical evaluation, these drugs proved to be effective in improving AHI through several mechanisms. These drugs are preferable in comparison to benzodiazepines for patients with OSAS and insomnia and/or anxiety (Mason *et al.* 2013, 2015).

In conclusion, the effects of benzodiazepine sedative-hypnotic drugs in patients with OSAS have been evaluated in few studies that are outdated and present with small clinical records and nonconclusive results. However, considering the myorelaxant effect (on respiratory centers and ventilation), it is safer to avoid their use for such patients.

When it is necessary to administer a hypnotic drug to a patient with OSAS, it is recommendable to resort to the non-benzodiazepine Z-drugs/hypnotics, which improve the quality of sleep and do not have adverse effects on OSAS. If these drugs are ineffective, it is advisable to shift to short half-life benzodiazepines or to send the patient to a specialist in Sleep Medicine for the diagnosis and etiological therapy for insomnia associated with OSAS.

When an anxiolytic therapy is indicated, it is recommended to avoid the use of benzodiazepine sedatives; instead, other category of drugs that have been proved as does not worsen OSAS or even produce a certain improvement are preferred (see "Pharmacologic therapy of OSAS").

CIGARETTE SMOKING

Smoking disturbs sleep because of the stimulating effects of nicotine, which causes difficulty in falling asleep, sleep fragmentation, and reduction in deep sleep. Furthermore, cigarette smoking may cause daytime sleepiness as a secondary effect of withdrawal of nicotine stimulation (Phillips and Danner 1995; Jaehne *et al.* 2009).

The effect of smoking on the upper airways determines an increase of the resistance during sleep because of hypotonia and a major collapsibility due to the "rebound effect" of the nightly nicotine withdrawal (nicotine increases the tone of the upper airways), to inflammation and edema of the rhinopharyngeal mucosa with subsequent reduction of the air space.

Smoking is often mentioned among the risk factors of OSAS, but the related studies are few and present discording results. Some studies have observed that the smokers have an increased risk (4–5 times) to develop OSAS compared to nonsmokers as correlated to the entity of cigarette consumption (pack/year [number of cigarettes/day × years of smoking/20]); however, few other studies have not identified a significant correlation between AHI (5) and cigarette smoking by comparing current smokers, ex-smokers, and nonsmokers and also considering pack/year (Wetter *et al.* 1994; Conway *et al.* 2008).

Some studies indicate the presence of a correlation between cigarette smoking and **night hypoxemia** (sleep time with $SaO_2 < 90$ higher than 5%), which was detected on current smokers but not on ex-smokers and the results were significantly correlated to cigarette smoking (>15 pack/year) (Conway *et al.* 2008).

Some studies also investigated the curative effect of nicotine (administered as a gum or transdermal patch) on OSAS, speculating a mechanism of increased upper airway muscle tone; however, the results are contrasting and do not have a clear clinical meaning (Kryger *et al.* 2011).

In conclusion, in spite of the paucity of scientific evidences about the correlation between OSAS and cigarette smoking, the patients with OSAS should always be recommended smoking cessation to avoid the disturbing effects of nicotine on night sleep, the possible increase in daytime sleepiness, and the irritating effects on the rhinopharyngolaryngeal mucosa and especially, to reduce the cardiovascular risk (already high in patients with OSAS).

INDICATIONS OF INTERNATIONAL GUIDELINES

The AASM *clinical guidelines* point out that in addition to instructing the patients with OSAS about the specific therapy, it is essential to always associate a teaching program about the behaviors to be avoided/stopped (alcohol consumption, sedative-hypnotics, and smoking); however, there are no specific protocols or standardized recommendations that the experts can share probably because of the poor and inconsistent indications from scientific literature (Epstein *et al.* 2009).

OSA PHARMACOTHERAPY

OSA is a common and harmful medical condition that remains undertreated due to the poor compliance with the leading therapy, CPAP (Sawyer et al. 2011; Weaver and Grunstein 2008). Currently, there is no approved pharmacotherapy for OSA and the research in this field has been, to date, quite ineffective. Nevertheless, recent developments related to an improved understanding of OSA pathophysiology (Eckert et al. 2013) and the identification of specific pharmacological targets (Horner et al. 2017) has brought new hope to the field for treating this disorder with medications.

Personalized medicine approach

In the last 15 years, researchers have shown that a number of key pathophysiological traits, or endotypes, contribute to the pathogenesis of OSA (Eckert et al. 2013; Younes 2003; Younes 2004; Younes 2008; Wellman et al. 2011; Wellman et al. 2013). These include: 1) an anatomically small, collapsible upper airway; 2) a reduced dilator muscle responsiveness; 3) a reduced arousal threshold; and 4) an oversensitive ventilatory control system (high loop gain). These mechanisms or traits contribute, in different degrees, to the development of the disorder, and while a low muscle compensation may be the main reason for having OSA in one patient, the high loop gain or low arousal threshold may be the cause of the disorder in another patient. CPAP is virtually always efficacious because it can completely abolish the obstructive events by maintaining an open airway regardless of the underlying pathophysiology. To increase the chances of success, a pharmacological approach needs a better understanding of the patient-specific etiology of OSA (📷 5.8).

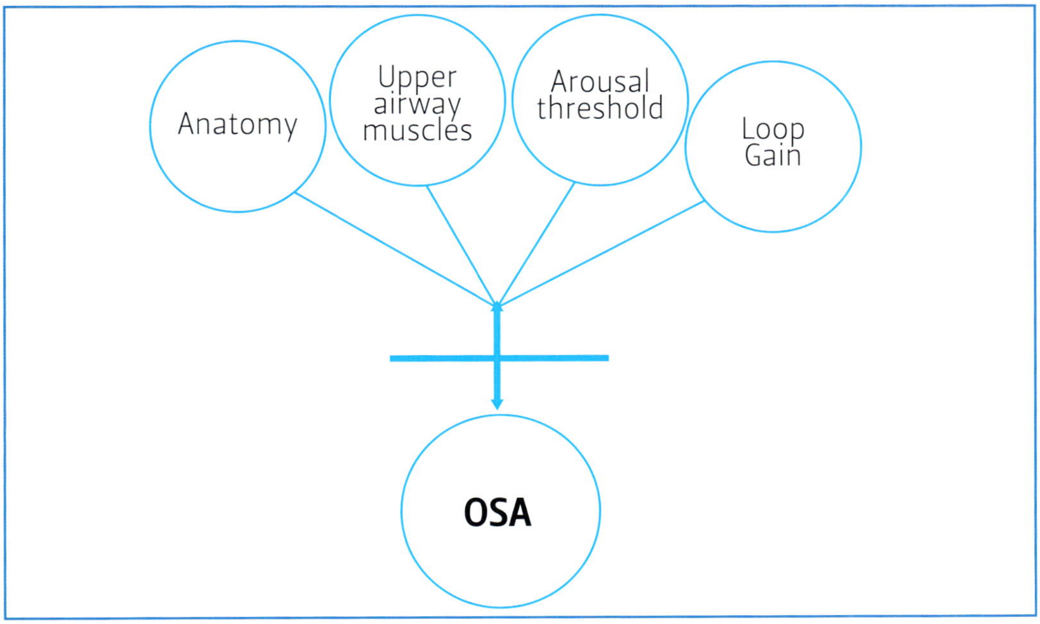

5.8 CPAP is effective regardless of the underlying pathophysiology of OSA because it splints the airway open during sleep and resolve the anatomical predisposition to obstruction.

While this phenotype-based (or endotype-based) approach has so far been limited to the research setting, the recently developed automated analyses allow for the measurement of pathophysiology traits from clinical in-lab polysomnography and will possibly be included in future software packages (Sands et al. 2018a; Sands et al. 2018; Terrill et al. 2015). Measuring the changes in endotypic traits with an intervention will allow researchers to go beyond the usual metric of OSA severity, the AHI, that simply represents the frequency of upper airway obstructive events for every hour of sleep (Rapoport 2018). AHI is currently the main parameter used in research and in clinic to determine OSA severity, and it informs the physician about the necessity of a treatment. However, despite its large use, this metric has several disadvantages: it poorly correlates with subjective patients' symptoms, such as fatigue or sleepiness (Kapur et al. 2005); and it is widely variable from night to night (Bittencourt et al. 2001; White et al. 2015) and for different body positions (Bliwise et al. 1991; Marques et al. 2017; Melania et al. 2016), and poorly predicts health outcomes (Azarbarzin et al. 2019). The efficacy of the medications on OSA severity has been evaluated, to date, using AHI as the main outcome, and less frequently, oxygen desaturation, subjective symptoms, and effects on endotype traits have been used. In the near future, thanks to the developing technologies, we hope that the efficacy of pharmacotherapies and other new treatments will be tested on more articulated metrics, such as the hypoxic burden, arousal intensity, heart rate burden, or the pathophysiologic traits that better characterize the ventilatory burden of sleep apnea (Azarbarzin et al. 2019), its etiology, and its consequences in a patient-specific fashion (Sutherland et al. 2018).

In this chapter, the evidence for the efficacy of medications tested for the treatment of OSA has been analyzed. The medications were divided based on the likely mechanism of action according to the four endotypic traits mentioned previously (i.e., anatomy, upper airway muscle activation, arousal threshold, and loop gain). Most studies mentioned here had enrolled volunteers with OSA regardless of their pathophysiologic traits. Thus, the efficacy of these medications may be higher if administered to the individuals selected according to their endotype.

Upper airway anatomy

All patients with OSA share some anatomic predisposition to upper airway collapse. This condition may be related to an anatomically small or collapsible airway. The possible causes of this anatomic abnormality include fat deposition in the tissues surrounding the airway due to obesity (Isono 2012), a reduced bony skeletal structure (Ito et al. 2016), increased tonsil or adenoid size (Smith et al. 2017), or upper airway edema due to fluid retention (Yadollahi et al. 2014). A chronic nasal congestion (rhinitis) may also increase the likelihood of pharyngeal collapse due to the generation of more negative pressure in the downstream segment of the upper airway (Mahdavinia et al. 2017). Targeting anatomy with medical therapy is challenging, though not impossible. In fact, the reduced size of the upper airway due to a small mandible (micrognatia) or tonsillar hypertrophy possibly needs surgical interventions. On the other end, medical treatments may improve anatomy in select cases, such as weight loss medications associated to a hypocaloric diet may be helpful in the treatment of OSA in obese people; diuretics have been tested for reduction of fluid overload especially in hypertensive patients; and nasal decongestants may be helpful in patients with allergic rhinosinusitis.

WEIGHT LOSS MEDICATIONS

Weight loss has been recently introduced in the guidelines for OSA treatment by the American Thoracic Society as obesity is the most significant risk factor for this disorder (Hudgel et al. 2018). The prevalence of OSA in the obese population is about 50% (Young et al. 2002), and BMI is linearly related with OSA severity. However, a recent meta-analysis about the effects of surgical weight loss on OSA (Wong et al. 2018) showed that there is no relationship between the amount of weight loss and AHI reduction in these patients, likely because other factors are at play in determining AHI even when the anatomical defect has been reduced. In the last 10 years, four weight-loss drugs have been approved by the US Food and Drug Administration, and some of them have already been tested in patients with OSA.

In an uncontrolled cohort study conducted on 87 middle-aged obese patients with OSA, Yee *et al.* (Yee *et al.* 2007) tested the effect of sibutramine, a serotonin and norepinephrine reuptake inhibitor, in combination with a weight loss program on OSA severity. After 6 months, the RDI was reduced by 35% compared to baseline, along with a 10% weight loss and improvement in subjective sleepiness. A subsequent smaller, open-label trial by Ferland *et al.* (Ferland et al. 2009) compared the treatment with sibutramine + weight loss diet to CPAP. Weight loss in sibutramine group was only 5% from baseline and insufficient to cause a significant reduction in AHI.

A hypocaloric diet + liraglutide, a glucagon-like peptide-1 (GLP-1) analog approved for type 2 diabetes and weight loss, was tested by Blackman *et al.* (Blackman *et al.* 2016) in a double-blind trial vs. diet + placebo in a group of 180 vs. 179 moderate-to-severe OSA patients, respectively, for 8 months. The liraglutide group lost 4.2% more weight and had a 12% more reduction in AHI compared to the placebo group.

Finally, in a double-blind, placebo-controlled trial, Winslow *et al.* (Winslow *et al.* 2012) tested the combination of phentermine, a sympathomimetic agent, and topiramate, a GABA-A receptor agonist and inhibitor of carbonic anhydrase, on OSA severity. Fifty-five patients took part in the trial for 28 weeks, 22 in the medication group and 23 in the placebo group. The drug group experienced 5.9% more weight reduction compared to placebo and 36% more reduction in AHI (71% reduction from a baseline of 44.2 events/h, see 5.9).

The other FDA-approved weight-loss drugs that have not been tested for the improvement of OSA severity include orlistat, a lipase inhibitor, and lorcaserin, an appetite suppressant.

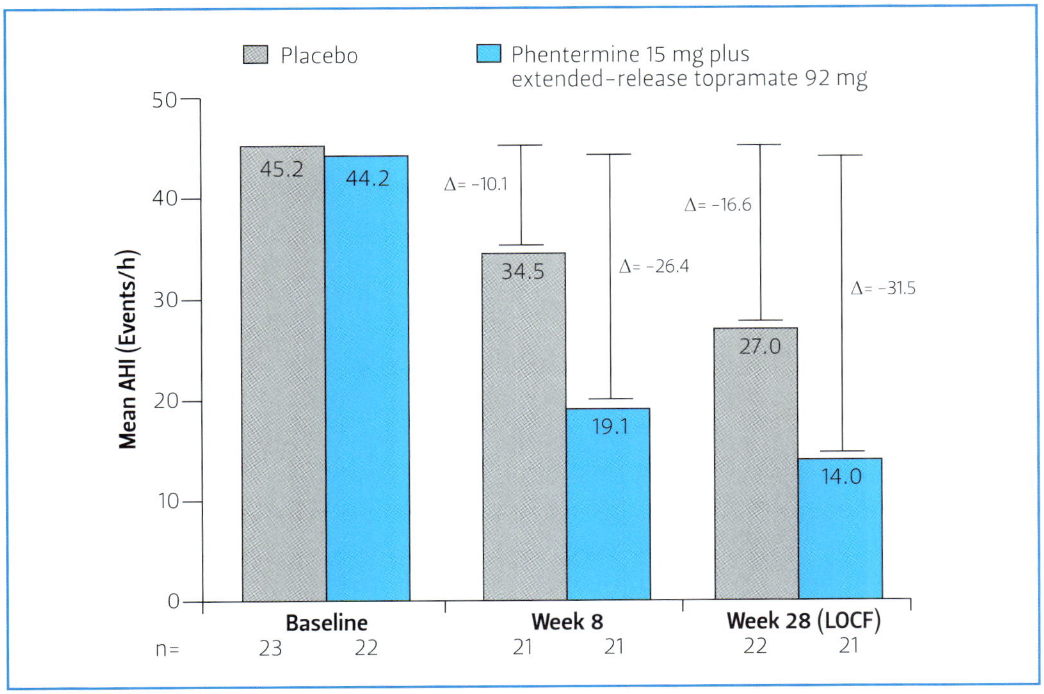

5.9 The combination of Phentermine and Topiramate administered for 28 weeks significantly reduced body weight (not shown) and AHI compared to placebo. Both arms included also a life-style modification counseling. Modified from Winslow *et al.* 2012.

UPPER AIRWAY EDEMA

It has been hypothesized that fluid volume regulation and distribution may be involved in the pathogenesis of OSA (Yadollahi et al. 2014; Redolfi et al. 2015). Several studies have shown a high prevalence of OSA in fluid-retaining states, including hypertension (Pedrosa et al. 2011), heart failure (Yumino et al. 2010), and end-stage renal disease (Lyons et al. 2017). The fluid accumulation in the body may lead to increased parapharyngeal edema and upper airway collapsibility, especially when the patients lay down to sleep and the body fluids redistribute toward the neck from the lower extremities due to gravity (Redolfi et al. 2009).

Medications targeting fluid retention, including diuretics and mineralocorticoid antagonists, have shown potential in reduction of OSA severity at least in certain subgroups of patients. Among the other agents in this group, spironolactone, the inhibitor of mineralocorticoid receptor emerged as a potential agent for OSA treatment when administered alone or in combination with other diuretics. In a group of 12 moderate-to-severe OSA patients with resistant hypertension, Gaddam *et al.* (Gaddam et al. 2010) measured the effect of additional therapy with spironolactone on AHI after 8 weeks of treatment. In this open-label study, there was a reduction in AHI by 45% from baseline, together with improvement in oxygen desaturations and reduced blood pressure. Kasai et al. (Kasai et al. 2014) tested spironolactone in combination with metolazone, a thiazide-like diuretic, during a 2-week, prospective, observational study in a group of 16 patients with resistant hypertension. In this study, the adjunctive treatment caused a 16% reduction in AHI from baseline (57.7–48.5 events/h). In another recent three-arm parallel randomized trial by Fiori *et al.* (Fiori et al. 2018), a combination of furosemide and spironolactone was administered to 18 OSA patients without resistant hypertension and compared to sodium-restricted diet ($n = 18$) or placebo ($n = 18$). Similar to the study of Kasai, in this study, the combination of diuretics caused a 16% reduction in AHI, while the sodium-restricted diet reduced it by 24% compared to placebo.

NASAL DECONGESTANTS

High nasal resistance can contribute to pharyngeal collapse by increasing the negative suction pressure downstream in the velo- and oropharynx. A recent study demonstrated an OSA prevalence as high as 65% in patients with chronic rhinosinusitis (Mahdavinia et al. 2017); therefore, a drug that reduces nasal congestion and pharyngeal edema could potentially improve OSA in some patients. Several nasal decongestants have been trialed for OSA severity. The effect of mometasone alone and in combination with desloratadine, an antihistamine, on AHI was measured in patients with allergic rhinitis by Acar *et al.* (Acar et al. 2013) in a trial including 80 patients. While desloratadine alone or in combination with mometasone did not show significant improvement of OSA severity, mometasone administered alone showed a statistically significant reduction in AHI by 17% compared to placebo.

Another nasal steroid, fluticasone, was tested on 13 patients with rhinitis and OSA for 4 weeks in a randomized, double-blind, placebo-controlled, crossover trial by Kiely *et al.* (Kiely et al. 2004). Patients on fluticasone showed a 21% reduction in AHI compared to placebo. On the contrary, a recent parallel-arm trial performed by Smith *et al.* tested the combination of fluticasone and montelukast in patients with mild OSA but without rhinitis did not find a difference in AHI between the groups, although total sleep time and sleep architecture were improved in the treatment arm (Smith et al. 2019).

A combination of the nasal steroid, dexamethasone, with the decongestant, tramazoline, was tested by Koutsourelakis *et al.* (Koutsourelakis et al. 2013) in a group of 21 OSA patients with normal nasal resistance in a randomized, double-blind, placebo-controlled, crossover trial for 1 week. The treatment reduced AHI by 20% compared to baseline (16% compared to placebo). Similar results were obtained by Clarenbach *et al.* (Clarenbach et al. 2008) with the nasal decongestant, xylometazoline, in 12 patients with chronic nasal congestion. However, AHI was only reduced by 18% in the first part of the polysomnography when the effects of the medication were more pronounced, but not for the rest of the night.

Overall these data show that patients with nasal congestion treated with topical corticosteroid may improve their sleep apnea, especially if they suffer from chronic rhinitis. More studies are needed to confirm these findings, and the studies using more potent anti-inflammatory agents are ongoing (Laidlaw 2018).

Upper airway dilator muscles activation

In humans, there is no fixed bone or cartilage supporting the pharynx. Rather, it is held open by the activation of the surrounding musculature. Relaxation of these muscles during sleep and the lack of sufficient reactivation are the key primary pathophysiological events leading to OSA (Horner et al. 2014). The patients with OSA show higher activation of upper airway muscles during wakefulness compared to healthy controls to maintain their smaller upper airway open while awake. However, at sleep onset, there is a physiological decrease in muscle activation that leads to pharyngeal obstruction (White and Younes 2012). The increase in the epiglottic pressure swings and CO_2 during obstructive events can both reactivate the pharyngeal muscles and eventually restore the upper airway patency during sleep by reflexive recruitment. However, this reflex is widely variable between individuals, with some people showing effective recruitment and the ability to partially reopen the upper airway, and others with only minimal or no upper airway muscle compensation during sleep (Sands et al. 2014; Taranto-Montemurro et al. 2016).

Since the activity of upper airway dilator muscles is regulated by specific neurotransmitters whose concentration varies between wake and sleep, it should be theoretically possible to manipulate the airway muscle tone by identifying the neurotransmitters responsible for muscle activation and administering them during sleep, preventing their withdrawal. In the last decade, many advancements in basic science helped to refine the choice of receptor targets to stimulate the upper airway muscles, and many attempts to translate these findings in the clinical setting are ongoing (Horner et al. 2017).

SEROTONERGIC MECHANISMS

The withdrawal of endogenous serotonin at the hypoglossal nucleus was long thought to be the primary mechanism underlying decreased pharyngeal muscle activity during sleep (Kubin 2016; Veasey 2003). The complexity of the serotonergic system is represented by the presence of seven different receptor families that are distributed in both the peripheral and central nervous systems and can be either excitatory or inhibitory (Veasey 2003).

Serotonin has shown clear *excitatory effects* on respiration when *administered centrally* in mammals. Serotonergic drive is diminished centrally from wakefulness to NREM sleep, and it is minimal during REM sleep, leading to a relative reduction in ventilatory drive. This reduced 5-HT activity may contribute to upper airway collapse in patients with OSA. In contrast, the effects of serotonin *peripherally* are principally *inhibitory*. The key serotonin (5-HT) receptors involved in respiratory control are 5-HT2a/c, 5-HT3, and 5-HT1a (Veasey 2003).

Ondansetron, an antagonist of serotonin receptor 3, reduced the sleep-disordered breathing in the English bulldogs (Veasey et al. 2001) by 54%, but did not have an effect in 10 OSA patients when tested by Stradling et al. in a randomized, controlled, single-night crossover trial at the dose of 16 mg, suggesting that species differences may be at play (Stradling et al. 2003). A pilot trial in five OSA patients using buspirone, a serotonin receptor 1a agonist, was published in the form of a letter by Mendelson et al. (Mendelson et al. 1991), showing an improvement in 4/5 patients' AHI vs. placebo (mean reduction for the whole group was 36%), increased total sleep time, and a tendency for improvement in subjective sleep quality. Besides this small trial, no other data have been published regarding buspirone in the treatment of OSA to our knowledge.

Among the most important serotonergic agents tested in OSA is mirtazapine, a serotonin receptor 3 antagonist, that showed initial positive results on 12 patients (50% reduction of AHI) after 1-week administration (Carley et al. 2007). These results were not confirmed in the two subsequent trials of 2 and 4 weeks on 20 and 26 patients, respectively, in which mirtazapine did not show a significant reduction of OSA severity and was associated to a significant weight increase of 1.4 kg at 4 weeks (Marshall et al. 2008).

Selective serotonin reuptake inhibitors have the potential to reduce OSA severity by increasing the central concentration of serotonin. Paroxetine and fluoxetine were both tested in two small trials. Paroxetine was first evaluated in a double-blind, placebo-controlled, crossover trial by Berry *et al.* (Berry et al. 1999) on eight patients in which the main outcome was the genioglossus activity. Paroxetine significantly increased genioglossus muscle peak activity and muscle responsiveness (by 27%) compared to placebo during the first treatment night; however, AHI remained unchanged. A subsequent study tested the same medication on 17 patients in a similar crossover design showing a significant reduction in AHI by 18% from placebo over a period of 6 weeks.

Specifically, the drug reduced AHI more effectively during NREM sleep (35% reduction), but not during REM sleep, suggesting that two different mechanisms are at play in these sleep states. The most successful results with a serotonergic drug were obtained in two trials testing fluoxetine. One trial by Hanzel *et al.* compared the effects of 4 weeks of fluoxetine vs. 4 weeks of protriptyline in 12 patients in an open-label, randomized crossover trial (Hanzel et al. 1991) (Fig. 3). Both drugs significantly reduced AHI approximately by 40% from baseline, but did not improve oxygen desaturation, with large variability in the response among individuals. Fluoxetine was subsequently tested by Prasad et al. (Prasad et al. 2010) in combination with ondansetron on 10 patients in a parallel group study and again showed a reduction of 40% compared to placebo after 4 weeks of treatment. As ondansetron alone did not have any effect on AHI, and fluoxetine alone showed a similar effect in the trial by Hanzel, we can speculate that most, if not all, of the effects of the combination was due to fluoxetine, although a synergistic effect of the two drugs cannot be excluded.

NORADRENERGIC MECHANISMS

The relatively poor effectiveness showed by serotonergic drugs in OSA required a reinterpretation of the data obtained in the animal model. It was recognized that some of the studies implicating serotonin were conducted in vagotomized animals (a common practice in pharyngeal motor control studies because vagotomy releases the genioglossus from inhibitory vagal afferents). As vagal afferents inhibit serotonin at the hypoglossal nucleus, vagotomy could exaggerate the influence of endogenous serotonin (Kubin 2016).

Subsequent studies showed that the withdrawal of endogenous serotonin has minimal effects on upper airway muscle activation in animals with an intact vagus nerve (Sood et al. 2005; Sood et al. 2006; Fenik et al. 2005). This could explain why serotonergic drugs administered to humans had minimal effects on pharyngeal muscle tone and OSA severity (Berry et al. 1999; Hanzel et al. 1991; Kraiczi et al. 1999). Some evidence has been recently gathered, showing that the loss of noradrenergic activity plays the key role in sleep-related hypotonia of pharyngeal muscles, with serotonergic mechanisms accounting for only about 10% (Fenik et al. 2005). Chan and colleagues (Chan et al. 2006) showed in rats that the noradrenergic antagonist, terazosin, administered at the hypoglossal motor nucleus in the brainstem substantially reduced genioglossus activity during wakefulness and sleep, illustrating the importance of noradrenergic mechanisms. Other studies (Fenik et al. 2005; Lai et al. 2001) also support the notion that progressive withdrawal of noradrenergic tone, from wakefulness to NREM and REM sleep, is the major mechanism causing sleep-related pharyngeal hypotonia.

Translational work performed recently in our laboratory showed that the drugs with noradrenergic stimulant properties, such as desipramine, can increase genioglossus muscle activity (Taranto-Montemurro et al. 2016) and reduce upper airway collapsibility during sleep in humans (Taranto-Montemurro et al. 2016). However, our team and others have also shown that, when taken alone, noradrenergic drugs, such as norepinephrine reuptake inhibitors only mildly reduce overall OSA severity, although interindividual variability was evident in most studies.

The tricyclic antidepressants (TCAs), protriptyline (Brownell et al. 1982; Smith et al. 1983) and desipramine (Taranto-Montemurro et al. 2016), and the selective norepinephrine reuptake inhibitor, atomoxetine (Bart Sangal et al. 2008), have all been tested in patients with OSA with alternate success in reducing the severity of the disorder. Three randomized controlled trials (Hanzel et al. 1991; Brownell et al. 1982; Whyte et al. 1988) and several observational studies (Smith et al. 1983; Conway et al. 1982; Clark et al. 1979) assessed the effects of protriptyline on OSA severity. Brownell and co-workers (Brownell et al. 1982) found no changes in AHI during NREM sleep after 4 weeks of therapy with 20 mg of protriptyline in a group of five obese men with severe OSA, but the patients had improvements in oxygen saturation and referred improved daytime sleepiness.

In another double-blind trial, Whyte and co-workers (Whyte et al. 1988) found that administration of 20 mg of protriptyline for 14 d in 10 moderate-to-severe OSA patients did not change NREM AHI as a group, but generated wide interindividual variability in the response. Only the above mentioned trial by Hanzel *et al.* (Hanzel et al. 1991) showed a statistically significant reduction in AHI by 42% from baseline over 4 weeks of treatment (See 5.10).

Similar to protriptyline, desipramine (another TCA) showed variable results in terms of AHI reduction in a group of 14 patients in which the medication was administered for one night in a placebo-controlled, double-blind, crossover trial performed by our group (Taranto-Montemurro et al. 2016). Although the effect on OSA severity was not significant as a group, patients showed a less collapsible airway on desipramine compared to placebo and a post-hoc analysis identified the subgroup of patients with minimal muscle compensation as the best responders to the treatment. Consistent with these findings, desipramine increased genioglossus activity and reduced upper airway collapsibility in a trial performed in normal patients during sleep (Taranto-Montemurro et al. 2016).

The selective norepinephrine reuptake inhibitor, atomoxetine, was tested by Bart-Sangal *et al.* (Bart Sangal et al. 2008) in a prospective observational study of 15 patients with mild OSA. The drug did not have effects on AHI, but significantly improved daytime sleepiness. A second trial performed in our lab more recently confirmed in nine moderate-to-severe OSA patients that atomoxetine administered alone did not improve OSA severity (Taranto-Montemurro et al. 2019).

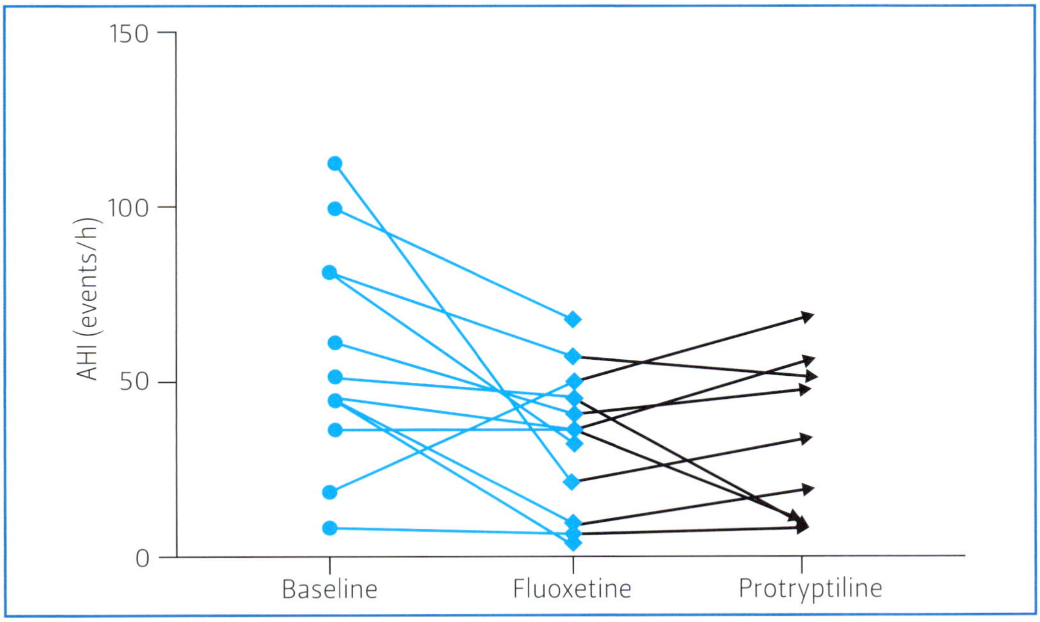

5.10 Fluoxetine 20 mg and protryptiline 10 mg reduced AHI by ~40% from baseline in 12 patients with OSA. Fluoxetine was better tolerated during the 4 weeks of treatment: 3 patients did not complete the protriptyline arm. Graph designed from data by Hanzel et al. Modified from Hanzel *et al.* 1991.

COMBINATION OF NORADRENERGIC AND ANTIMUSCARINIC MEDICATIONS

According to Richard Horner's group, noradrenergic withdrawal is not the only mechanism involved in sleep-related loss of genioglossus activity. For example, noradrenergic stimulation with an alpha-1 adrenergic agonist at the HMN failed to reverse REM sleep-related tongue muscle hypotonia (Chan et al. 2006), indicating that an additional inhibitory mechanism is at work, and this mechanism is likely to be predominantly muscarinic. Grace et al. delivered the muscarinic receptor antagonist, scopolamine, into the HMN in rats and demonstrated that there is progressive muscarinic inhibition of drive to the HMN from wakefulness to NREM and REM sleep (Grace et al. 2013). Muscarinic receptor antagonism had a particularly strong restorative effect on genioglossus activity in REM sleep, but also had important effects on respiratory-related pharyngeal muscle activity in NREM. These findings have been recently applied to humans in a preliminary proof-of-concept study by our laboratory. In 20 OSA patients, the combination of atomoxetine and the antimuscarinic, oxybutynin, was administered before bedtime for one night and results were compared to placebo (Taranto-Montemurro et al. 2019). Atomoxetine-plus-oxybutynin increased by nearly three-fold the genioglossus muscle responsiveness to negative esophageal pressure swings and lowered AHI by 63% (5.11).

The combination reduced the AHI in both REM and NREM sleep and there was an improvement in oxygen saturation parameters as well. The results ob-

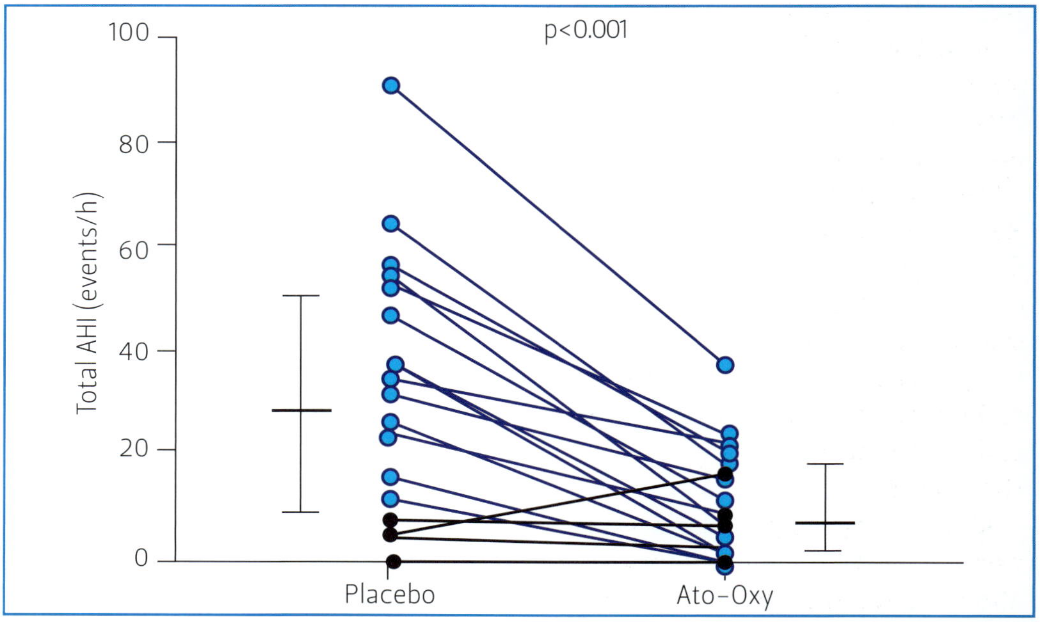

5.11 Ato-oxy reduced the AHI by 63% compared to placebo. Gray lines indicate those patients that had an AHI less than 10 events/h on placebo, despite a previous diagnosis of OSA. All patients improved their AHI except one. Modified from Taranto-Montemurro *et al.* 2019.

tained with this small trial represent one of the most promising steps ahead in the field of OSA pharmacotherapy, although the small sample size and the short duration of the trial limit the generalizability of these findings.

POTASSIUM (K^+) CHANNEL BLOCKERS

The modulation of K^+ channels has been identified as the downstream mechanism through which wake-activating neurotransmitters, such as norepinephrine, serotonin, and acetylcholine modify the motoneuron membrane excitability, both in NREM and REM sleep (Grace et al. 2013). The opening of K+ channels produces a hyperpolarization of neurons due to the increased K+ leak from intracellular space, thereby reducing cell excitability (White and Daigneault 1959).

Studies performed by Grace *et al.* in freely behaving rats have confirmed that blockade of potassium channels with several agents (barium, 4-aminopyridine [4-AP], and tetraethylammonium) constitutes an efficient strategy to increase genioglossus activity and reverse NREM hypotonia and REM atonia during sleep (Grace et al. 2013). Potassium channels are ubiquitous in human cells and the lack of a specific tractable target on the hypoglossal motor nucleus limits the possibility to investigate the effects of this drug class, and thus, the experience in OSA is limited, to date. Suratt et al. (Suratt et al. 1986) tested the effect of one-night intravenous administration of doxapram, a K^+ channel inhibitor used as a respiratory stimulant in a double-blind, placebo-controlled trial on four patients showing the reduction in apnea and hypopnea length and improvement in oxygen desaturation while the patients were on medication. In a pilot study of 10 healthy individuals, our group evaluated the effect on genioglossus muscle activity from 10 mg of extended-release 4-AP administered for a single night before bed (Taranto-Montemurro et al. 2017). Results were inconclusive, despite no improvement in upper airway collapsibility, genioglossus activity was higher during REM sleep on 4-AP compared to placebo. Moreover, 7 out of 10 patients had an improvement in genioglossus responsiveness to negative epiglottic pressure, but the study was likely underpowered to show statistical significance on this outcome. Finally, Bayer Pharmaceuticals is testing a K^+ channel blocker to be administered topically in the upper airway in an ongoing Phase 2 clinical trial in OSA patients (BAY2253651).

Ideally, targeting more specific K^+ receptors that are almost exclusively expressed on cranial motoneurons, such as the recently identified Kir 2.4, would allow a safer and possibly more effective approach for OSA patients (Grace et al. 2014).

CANNABINOIDS

Cannabinoid drugs, which are functionally coupled to K^+ channels (Grace *et al.* 2014; Guo and Ikeda 2004), Cannabinoid receptor (CBR)2 is the third most strongly expressed G protein-coupled receptor at the HMN; it is expressed nearly two-fold more than the adrenergic and muscarinic receptors (Horner *et al.* 2017). Dronabinol is a partial agonist for CBR1 and 2, and it has recently been tested for OSA in a proof-of-concept trial and subsequently, in a Phase 2 clinical trial. In the first trial, 17 patients with moderate-to-severe OSA took increasingly higher doses of dronabinol (from 5 to 10 mg) for 21 d. Data collected on night 21 showed a significant reduction in AHI by 29%.

In the Phase 2, parallel-arm, randomized controlled trial, 73 patients with AHI > 15 events/h received placebo or dronabinol at low or high doses. The interpretation of the results of this trial is problematic because OSA severity in the placebo arm significantly increased by 8 events/h (+35%) compared to baseline, and in the high-dose dronabinol arm, AHI was reduced by 4 events/h from baseline (15%).

So, while the AHI was only reduced by 15% from baseline, it showed a significant improvement by 50% from placebo (📷 5.12).

In a post-hoc analysis adjusted for baseline AHI, age, gender, and race, the authors found that dronabinol at high dose reduced AHI by 8.5 events/h (33%) from baseline. The patients also showed improvement in subjective daytime sleepiness from baseline, but oxygen desaturation was not improved (Carley et al. 2018). Other FDA-approved CBR2 agonists with potential clinical utility are nabilone and cannabidiol.

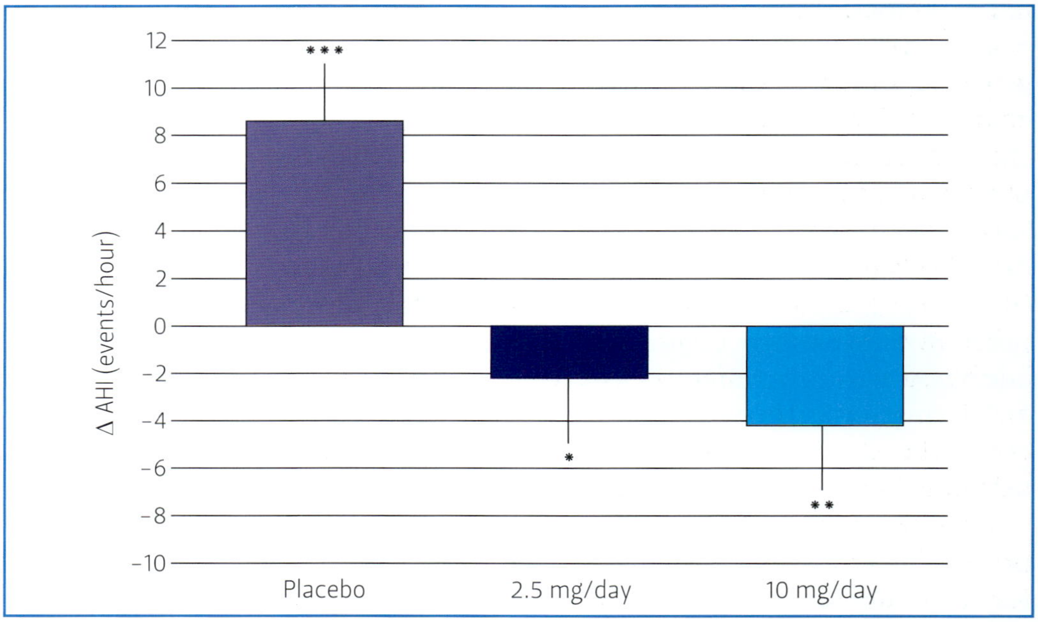

5.12 Dronabinol 2.5 and 10 mg significantly reduced the AHI compared to placebo. Placebo had a significant increase from baseline AHI. See main text for comment. ***p<0.01 vs baseline, *p<0.05 vs placebo, **p=o.03 vs placebo. Modified from Carley *et al.* 2018.

NICOTINE

It is known from animal studies that nicotine has stimulant effects on the genioglossus muscle and ventilatory drive (Haxhiu et al. 1984). Based on these properties, it was hypothesized that nicotine could be useful for OSA treatment; however, the short half-life and small effect size measured in patients did not encourage its clinical investigation, thus far. Nicotine was tested in three small trials. Gothe et al. (Gothe et al. 1985) showed that nicotine administered via chewing gum (14 mg) to eight OSA patients before bedtime reduced the time spent in apnea during the first hour of sleep by 20% and decreased the number of apneas in the first 2 h of sleep after administration. Davila et al. (Davila et al. 1994) subsequently administered a nicotine patch (total dose 11 mg) to 20 patients with OSA in a randomized controlled, crossover trial and found no significant difference in AHI compared to placebo. Finally, Zevin et al. (Zevin et al. 2003) administered 2 and 4 mg of nicotine via a tooth patch over two different nights in a prospective observational study on 10 OSA patients. They found no differences in OSA severity with all of the tested doses.

Arousal threshold

Sedative use in OSA has historically been discouraged because of concerns that delayed arousal would produce further blood gas derangement, and that the drug-driven myorelaxation would worsen obstruction. However, not all studies show worsening of OSA with sedatives (Berry et al. 1995) and some show improvement, even in individuals with moderate OSA (Wang et al. 2011; Höijer et al. 1994). Moreover, recent studies indicate that certain sedatives might improve upper airway dilator muscle recruitment during sleep (Park et al. 2008; Younes et al. 2007; Eikermann et al. 2010).

Therefore, the belief that all sedatives are contraindicated in all patients with OSA is not supported by the literature.

During an obstructive apnea or hypopnea, a reduction in ventilation during sleep leads to a buildup in CO_2, increases the ventilatory drive, and activates the pharyngeal muscles. A low respiratory arousal threshold, however, can preempt this important compensatory mechanism because the patients must be able to stay asleep long enough for these muscles to be recruited, and stable sleep must be present for this to occur (Jordan et al. 2009; Younes et al. 2012). Therefore, while arousal helps protect people from asphyxia, it may be destabilizing for patients with a low arousal threshold because the premature awakening can perpetuate the cycle of repetitive upper airway collapse. Thus, preventing arousals with sedatives in appropriately selected patients with a low arousal threshold could yield more stable breathing and less OSA.

It is still to be determined if the changes in respiratory arousal threshold can modify the severity of sleep-disordered breathing. While the data collected so far do not suggest that raising the arousal threshold can substantially improve OSA severity; only a few trials testing hypnotics on patients with OSA measured the arousal threshold on and off drugs and more data need to be collected on selected patients with low arousal threshold. Moreover, the drugs tested, to date, were unable to increase the arousal threshold by more than 20%–30% (see below for a detailed description). Ideally, a drug that raises the arousal threshold to a point where slow-wave sleep is promoted would also be able to reduce OSA severity, given that this is a protected stage where also patients with severe OSA can spontaneously recover from obstructions by recruiting upper airway muscles (Taranto-Montemurro et al. 2018; Ratnavadivel et al. 2009; Ratnavadivel et al. 2010; Taranto-Montemurro et al. 2017).

BENZODIAZEPINES

Several drugs from benzodiazepine class were tested in OSA patients. Cirignotta *et al.* compared the acute effect of 30 mg of flurazepam vs. placebo in two different placebo-controlled, crossover trials (Cirignotta *et al.* 1988; Cirignotta *et al.* 1992) (including a total of 24 patients) and 0.25 mg of brotizolam vs. placebo (Cirignotta *et al.* 1992) in one trial without showing significant effects on OSA severity for both medications.

Barry et al. (Berry *et al.* 1995), showed that 0.25 mg of triazolam significantly increased the arousal threshold by ~20% in 12 patients with severe OSA during a randomized placebo-controlled trial. The AHI in this group remained unchanged, but the obstructive events were longer and led to lower oxygen saturation. Nitrazepam was tested on 11 patients with mild-to-moderate OSA in the doses of 5 and 10 mg and compared to placebo during one-night treatment in a crossover study by Hoijer et al. (Höijer *et al.* 1994). There was no significant change in AHI or oxygen saturation indices; however, there was high individual variability in the response: three patients had worsening of OSA and six seemed to improve at the highest dose. Phenotypic traits were not measured so it is uncertain if the improvement was in patients with a low arousal threshold. Overall there was a nonstatistical significant reduction in AHI by 33% compared with the placebo group.

Temazepam was tested in two studies. The first one from Camacho *et al.* (Camacho and Morin 1995) included mild OSA patients with insomnia and aged ≥60 years. This trial was placebo-controlled randomized with two parallel groups. The OSA severity on temazepam at the dose of 15 or 30 mg was not significantly different from placebo after 8 weeks of treatment. The second study by Wang et al. (Wang et al. 2011) investigated the one-night effect of 10 mg of temazepam compared to placebo in a crossover trial including 20 patients, mostly with mild-to-moderate OSA. Once again, AHI did not change systematically on the drug, but there was a high interindividual variability in the response. The authors attempted to characterize the patients by the baseline chemosensitivity, but could not find any relationship between the change in AHI and the baseline response to CO_2. Arousal threshold was not determined in this group.

Z-DRUGS

George *et al.* tested zolpidem (10 mg) for a single night in a group of 42 patients with AHI between 10 and 40 events/h in a randomized, crossover trial (George et al. 2010). Compared to placebo, there was no difference in AHI or oxygen saturation. Zolpidem (10 mg) was again recently tested by Carberry et al. (Carberry et al. 2019) in an open-label pilot study, including 12 OSA patients for a single night after a diagnostic polysomnography. There was no systematic effect on the oxygen saturation or on AHI that changed minimally from 29 to 33 events/h, but zolpidem significantly improved sleep efficiency from 77% to 84%. In another recent physiology trial including 21 individuals with and without OSA, the same group showed that not only zolpidem increased the arousal threshold by 25%, but also the genioglossus response to pharyngeal negative pressure increased significantly compared to placebo, suggesting that this medication is not harmful for OSA patients and actually may have beneficial effects on sleep-disordered breathing (Carberry et al. 2017). It is important nonetheless to notice that a previous trial by Cirignotta et al. (Cirignotta et al. 1988) testing the effect of zolpidem at a higher dose of 20 mg in a crossover trial of one night in 12 patients showed a nonsignificant increase in AHI from 17 to 30 events/h ($p = 0.12$), lowered the mean O_2 saturation from 91.7% to 88.6% ($p = 0.02$), and the nadir SaO_2 from 85.2% to 76.8% ($p = 0.02$).

Among other Z-drugs, eszopiclone and zopiclone, were studied in OSA patients to measure their effect on the arousal threshold. Rosenberg *et al.* (Rosenberg et al. 2007) showed that eszopiclone did not change AHI, but improved sleep efficiency and reduced spontaneous arousals compared to placebo in 21 patients enrolled in a double-blind, crossover trial of 2-d treatment. Eckert et al. (Eckert et al. 2011) showed in a one-night crossover trial including 17 OSA patients that eszopiclone increased the arousal threshold by ~30%. Although the group data did not show a significant reduction in AHI, those with a low arousal threshold at baseline (8/17) had their AHI reduced by 43% (5.13). Carter et al. (Carter et al. 2016) showed in a group of 12 OSA patients that zopiclone administered for one night increased the arousal threshold by 20% and did not significantly change the AHI compared to placebo. A subsequent parallel-arm trial from the same group testing zopiclone (14 points) vs. placebo (16 points) showed a nonsignificant reduction in AHI between the two groups after 30 d (Carter et al. 2018).

OTHER HYPNOTICS AND SEDATIVES

Several other sedatives and hypnotics with the potential to increase the arousal threshold were tested in small trials showing minor changes in the arousal threshold or AHI. Tiagabine, a GABA reuptake inhibitor, increased the slow-wave activity (sleep depth), but had no effect on the arousal threshold or AHI (Taranto-Montemurro et al. 2017). Ramelteon, a melatonin receptors agonist, was tested by Kryger et al. (Kryger et al. 2007) in a group of 26 patients with mild-to-moderate OSA for one night in a crossover trial and showed no effect on the AHI or oxygen SaO_2. Melatonin was tested by Deacon et al. (Deacon et al. 2016) in 19 OSA patients over 1 week of treatment and improved sleep consolidation and mean oxygen saturation, but AHI was left unchanged.

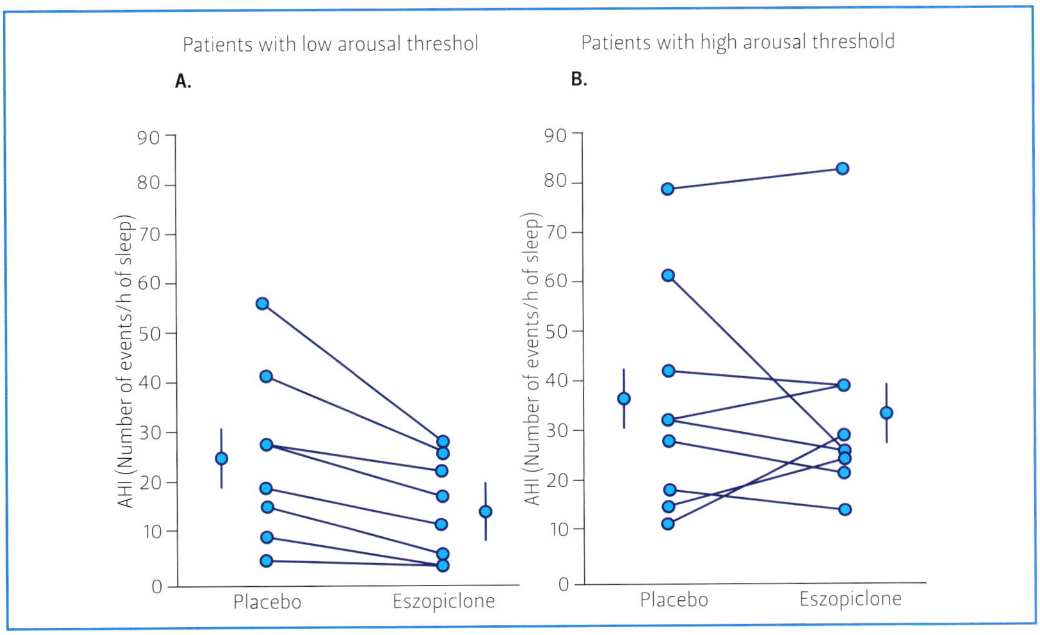

5.13 Patients with low arousal threshold (on the left) showed a 43% reduction in AHI on eszopiclone compared to placebo while patients with high arousal threshold (on the right) did not improve OSA severity. Modified from Eckert *et al.* 2011.

On the other end, gabapentin, an analog of GABA, at a dose of 300 mg was recently tested by Piovezan et al. (Piovezan et al. 2017) in a double-blind, placebo-controlled randomized, crossover trial in eight older (≥60 years) men with no or mild sleep apnea.

The authors found that the medication significantly increased the mean AHI from 12.4 on placebo to 22.2 (84%) during one-night administration, suggesting a potential deleterious effect of this commonly used drug on the population of older OSA patients.

The acute effect of sodium oxybate, a hypnotic prescribed to patients with narcolepsy, was assessed by George *et al.* (George *et al.* 2010) on 42 patients with AHI between 10 and 40 events/h. In this trial, sodium oxybate nonsignificantly reduced AHI by 17% from placebo, although the medication significantly increased the number of central apneas and reduced oxygen saturation parameters in three patients, suggesting different individual responses to the treatment. The same authors subsequently performed a 2-week parallel-arm trial (George *et al.* 2011) testing placebo ($N = 22$) vs. sodium oxybate ($N = 26$). This time there was a significant reduction in AHI by 32% from placebo. Slow-wave sleep was significantly increased by 24%, suggesting that this drug may reduce sleep apnea severity by increasing the time spent in deep sleep and increasing the arousal threshold.

Trazodone is a serotonergic antidepressant with sedative properties and was tested in several trials on OSA patients as a potential non-myorelaxant hypnotic. Heinzer *et al.* (Heinzer *et al.* 2008) showed that the administration of 100 mg of the drug before bedtime to eight OSA patients increased the arousal threshold in response to hypercapnia, allowing tolerance of higher CO2 levels without arousal.

Eckert et al. (Eckert *et al.* 2014) showed in seven OSA patients that trazodone could improve the arousal threshold by 30% in patients with low arousal threshold, but did not affect the AHI compared to placebo. On the contrary, Smales et al. (Smales *et al.* 2015) showed that in 15 patients with AHI ≥ 10 events/h, trazodone (100 mg) reduced AHI by 26% although the arousal threshold was unchanged between nights.

Ventilatory instability (loop gain)

In patients with small and collapsible upper airway, large variations in ventilatory drive in a waxing and waning pattern can increase the propensity for repetitive pharyngeal obstructions when the ventilatory drive is at its nadir. Loop gain is an engineering term that describes the gain of any system controlled by feedback loops. In the case of the respiratory system, the level of CO_2 provides the feedback for the ventilatory drive and regulates its changes. A high respiratory loop gain indicates a control system that disproportionately responds to even small changes in PCO_2. Medical therapies targeting ventilatory instability include carbonic anhydrase inhibitors, such as acetazolamide (Edwards et al. 2012), and oxygen (Wellman et al. 2008).

CARBONIC ANHYDRASE INHIBITORS

It has been shown that acetazolamide influences the changes in PCO_2 for a given change in ventilation (the so-called "plant gain," one of the components of the loop gain) (Edwards et al. 2012), thus lowering the ventilatory instability for a given respiratory disturbance. Acetazolamide at the dose of 250 mg taken four times/d for 2 weeks was tested in a randomized placebo-controlled, crossover trial on 10 moderate-to-severe OSA patients by Whyte et al. (Whyte et al. 1988) Acetazolamide reduced AHI by 52% compared to placebo, but failed to improve the symptoms of sleepiness, morning headache, and sleep disturbance assessed by a visual analog scale. Tojima et al. (Tojima et al. 1988) tested 250 mg/dacetazolamide in nine patients with OSA for 1 week, showing a significant reduction of 28% from baseline and five patients with more severe symptoms of sleep apnea showed improvement. More recently, Edwards *et al.* tested the effect of 500 mg of acetazolamide 2 times/d on phenotypic traits and OSA severity (Edwards et al. 2012). One-week therapy with acetazolamide reduced AHI by 52% compared to baseline in the 12 patients enrolled, and significantly reduced the loop gain by 41%. No other endotypic traits were modified by the treatment. Eskandari et al. (Eskandari et al. 2018) showed that in a group of 13 patients with OSA and hypertension, acetazolamide, in doses ranging from 500 to 750 mg according to patients' tolerance, over a 2-weeks treatment reduced AHI by 40% from baseline. The crossover study also involved a second arm in which acetazolamide was administered with CPAP, and a third arm with CPAP alone. As expected, the arm in which the combination of acetazolamide and CPAP were given had the best improvement in AHI, but only in the two arms including acetazolamide, there was a significant reduction in mean arterial pressure. A summary of the effect of acetazolamide on AHI (📷 5.14) shows a dose-dependent effect size. Given that this medication consistently reduced OSA severity among the studies performed so far, it certainly deserves further evaluation in longer and larger trials as a treatment for OSA.

Zonisamide is another carbonic anhydrase inhibitor that also induces weight loss. It was tested in a parallel-arm trial vs. placebo and CPAP. Although less efficacious than CPAP, zonisamide at the dose of 100 mg 3 times/d ($N = 13$) reduced AHI by ~30% compared to placebo ($N = 15$) during the 4-week treatment period. Zonisamide also caused a small but significant weight reduction compared to CPAP after 24 weeks of treatment.

OXYGEN

It has been shown that oxygen has ventilatory stabilizing properties, mainly related to a reduction in responsiveness of peripheral chemoreceptors (Duffin et al. 2000). The first studies reporting oxygen administration to OSA patients were in the 1980s and results were inconsistent, likely due to the small sample size and differences in patient selection (Mehta et al. 2013). Wellman et al. (Wellman et al. 2008) measured the effect of oxygen on OSA severity in pa-

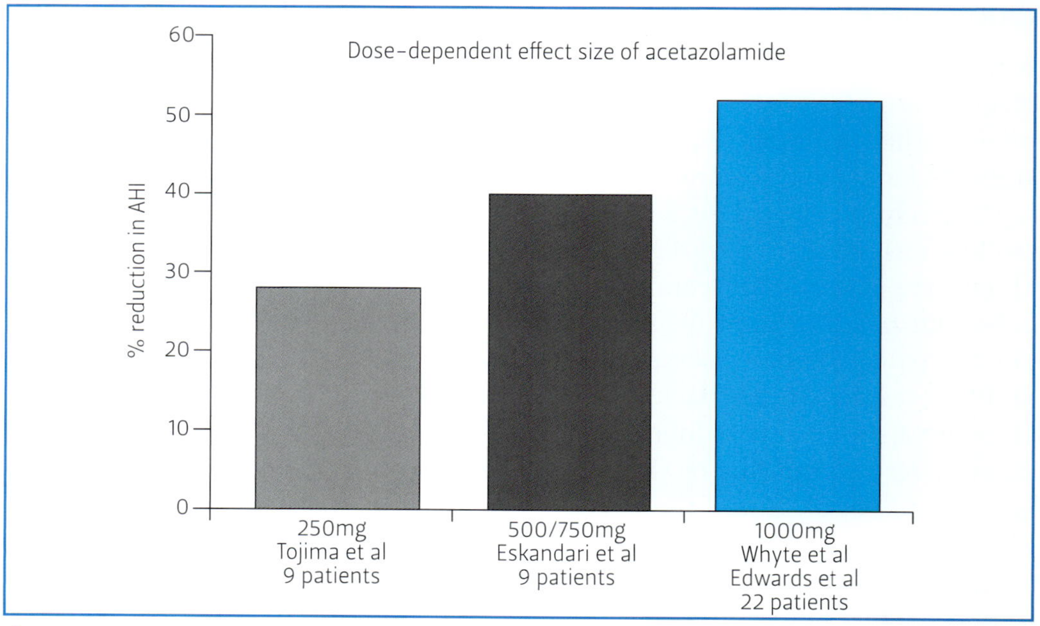

5.14 Acetazolamide consistently caused a significant and dose-dependent reduction in AHI in the studies performed to date in OSA patients.

tients with high (N = 6) and low (N = 6) loop gain showing that in those patients with a high loop gain, administration of oxygen (3–5 L/min) caused a reduction in AHI by 53% compared to room air; whereas, in those with a low loop gain, AHI was only reduced by 8%. Sands et al. (Sands et al. 2018b) showed that loop gain may not be the only predictor of success with oxygen treatment, but other endotypic traits can be important in defining responders to oxygen. In a crossover trial including 36 OSA patients, the presence of higher loop gain, milder collapsibility, and greater upper airway muscle compensation were the best predictors of successful OSA treatment with 40% oxygen. In the group of responders (9/36), AHI dropped by 59% compared to the room air night. Edwards et al. (Edwards et al. 2016) also assessed the effect of the combination of 40% oxygen and eszopiclone (3 mg) vs. room air + placebo in 20 OSA patients to target loop gain and arousal threshold with a combination therapy. The treatment administered for a single night reduced AHI by 43% and responders to therapy were identified among those with low collapsible upper airway, greater upper airway muscle compensation, and less severe OSA (5.15).

Miscellaneous

XANTINES

Xanthines, such as aminophylline, theophylline, or caffeine, increase ventilation by antagonizing adenosine in the central nervous system and improving diaphragm contractility (Lagercrantz et al. 1984). While xanthines have been used effectively to reduce apneas in premature infants (Kassim *et al.* 2009) and seem

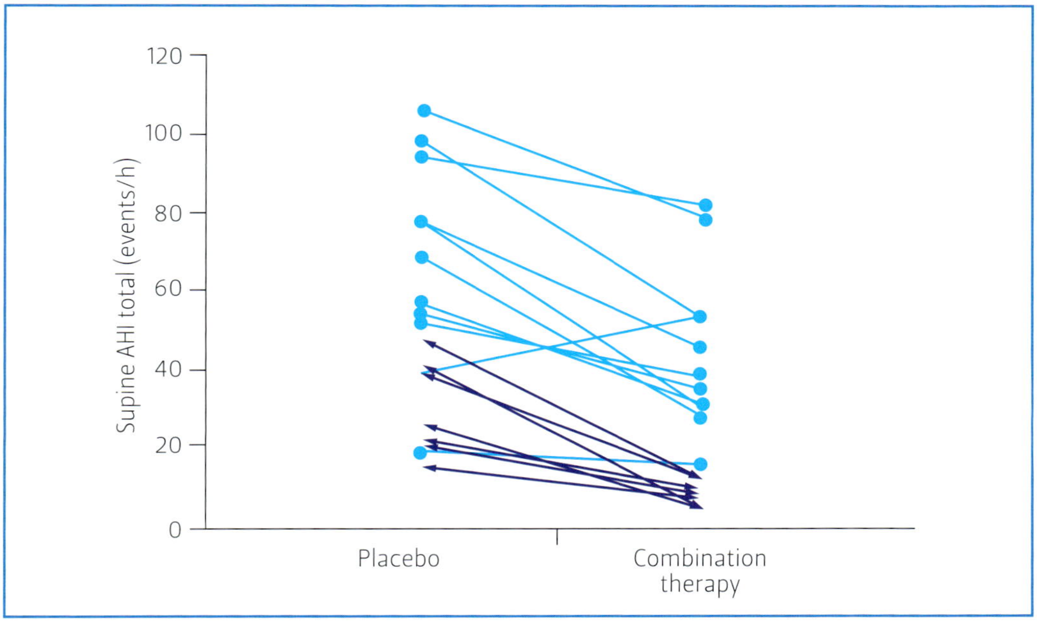

5.15 A combination of oxygen at the concentration of 40% and eszopiclone 3 mg reduced the AHI by 43% in unselected OSA patients. Modified from Edwards *et al.* 2016.

to reduce central apneas in patients with periodic breathing and heart failure (Javaheri et al. 1996), less promising results were obtained in patients with OSA. Mulloy and McNicholas (Mulloy and McNicholas 1992) performed a 1-month crossover trial on 12 patients with moderate-to-severe OSA testing the effect of theophylline (800 mg) vs. placebo. There was a significant but mild reduction in obstructive events (17% from placebo). Hein et al. (Hein et al. 2000) tested theophylline for 1-week treatment in mild sleep apnea patient and showed a reduction by 27% compared to placebo in a group of 14 patients. Espinoza et al. (Espinoza et al. 1987) showed no effect on OSA severity in a group of 10 patients after infusion of aminophylline compared to saline over one-night crossover trial.

OPIOID ANTAGONISTS

Opioid antagonists have been used as ventilatory stimulants for sleep apnea patients. Results were inconsistent among trials. Guilleminault and Hayes (Guilleminault and Hayes 1983) found no effect of naloxone on OSA severity in 28 patients. Atkinson et al. showed improved sleep oxygenation on naloxone when injected intravenously in a group of 10 obese OSA patients. Diamond et al. (Diamond et al. 1982) in a small pilot study of four patients with OSA again found no effect on AHI. Naltrexone (50 mg) administered by mouth was studied in a crossover trial by Ferber et al. (Ferber et al. 1993) on 12 patients with OSA (AHI > 10 events/h). Compared to placebo, the respiratory stimulant significantly reduced AHI by 23% alongside improvements in oxygen indices and an unwanted disruption of sleep architecture, such as increased wakefulness after sleep onset and reduced REM.

ACETYLCHOLINESTERASE INHIBITORS

Donepezil is a reversible inhibitor of the acetylcholinesterase enzyme that enhances cholinergic transmission to both muscarinic and nicotinic receptors. Based on its possible involvement in the ventilatory control during sleep, donepezil was initially tested on OSA severity in a group of 11 patients with Alzheimer disease and compared with placebo (N = 12) in a parallel-arm trial by Moraes et al. (Moraes et al. 2008). Donepezil (10 mg) showed a significant reduction in AHI by ~50% in this population for over 3 months of treatment. A subsequent trial by Sukys-Claudino et al. (Sukys-Claudino et al. 2012) testing the same medication in 11 patients with OSA without Alzheimer for 1 month showed a reduction of 39% compared to placebo. There were also improvements in oxygen saturation and sleepiness, while sleep efficiency was reduced on the medication. In a parallel group trial performed by Hunchaisri et al. (Hunchaisri and Chalermsuwiwattanakan 2016), 21 patients taking donepezil for 2 months were compared to 20 patients taking placebo. There was no significant reduction in AHI on drug and no significant improvement in oxygen saturation or subjective sleepiness. In a single-night, double-blind, crossover trial on 41 sleep apnea patients, Li et al. (Li et al. 2016) tested the effect of donepezil on OSA severity, arousal threshold, and loop gain showing no significant effect on any of these traits as a group. The authors found in a post-hoc analysis that those with a higher loop gain on placebo had a significant reduction of loop gain on donepezil, although this finding may be due to a "regression to the mean" phenomenon. Finally, Hedner et al. (Hedner et al. 2003) tested a continuous infusion of physostigmine, another acetylcholinesterase inhibitor, vs. placebo in a one-night crossover study on 10 patients of OSA and found a 24% reduction in AHI on drug, more prominent during REM and with a trend of improvement of oxygen levels during sleep. In summary these results suggest that donepezil may be selectively helpful in patients with OSA and Alzheimer disease; however, the mechanisms of action on OSA pathophysiology remain uncertain.

SEX HORMONES

Hormonal differences between sexes have been thought to account for the reported increased prevalence of OSA in men compared to women (White and Younes 2012). Supporting this hypothesis is also the fact that postmenopausal women show higher prevalence of sleep apnea compared to premenopausal women. The impact of female sex hormones, that is, estrogen and progesterone, has been investigated in several studies with inconsistent results. Popovic and White reported that the genioglossus muscle activity was positively correlated with progesterone levels and was significantly increased by combined estrogen and progesterone replacement in postmenopausal women (Popovic and White 1998) suggesting a hormonal role in maintaining the upper airway stiffness by dilator muscles recruitment. Other pilot studies investigating the impact of medroxyprogesterone or estrogens alone had alternate results, but generally showed modest or no effects on sleep apnea severity. When both estrogens and progesterone were used, results on OSA severity were more convincing at least in patients with mild OSA (Pickett et al. 1989; Wesström et al. 2005; Keefe et al. 1999) although not all the studies reported significant change in AHI (Cistulli et al. 1994).

SURFACTANT

Following the hypothesis that OSA is partly due to abnormal surface tension forces on the pharyngeal wall, the use of surfactant and topical lubricant was tested to evaluate changes in OSA severity. In particular, Jokic *et al.* (Jokic et al. 1998) topicallyadministered phosphocholinamin twice per night (once every 3.5 h) in the upper airway in 10 males with mild-to-moderate OSA in a randomized, double-blind, placebo-controlled crossover trial. The AHI was reduced by 42% from placebo, suggesting a potential role of this intervention. In another similar trial performed on seven OSA patients, Morrel et al. (Morrell et al. 2002) showed that the administration of surfactant reduced OSA severity by 25% from baseline in the first hour after administration. While these strategies to reduce OSA severity look relatively promising if combined with other treatments, the short half-life of these compounds limit their potential clinical use.

PROTON PUMP INHIBITORS

As for obesity and rhinitis discussed in previous paragraphs, targeting diseases that often are associated with sleep apnea may also reduce OSA severity. Gastroesophageal reflux disease (GERD) and sleep apnea reciprocally affect their pathogenesis. In fact, in OSA patients, the negative intrathoracic pressure generated during an obstructive event can exacerbate GERD by facilitating the displacement of gastric content into the esophagus. In its turn, during episodes of reflux, the upper airway mucosa is exposed repetitively to the acid gastric content that generates inflammation and edema in the pharynx. According to a few small prospective studies, treating GERD may contribute to OSA improvement. Friedman *et al.* (Friedman et al. 2007) found a reduction in AHI after 2–6 months of therapy with esomeprazole in 29 OSA patients in a prospective study and Senior et al. (Senior et al. 2001) found a reduction of 30% after 1-month treatment of GERD with omeprazole. On the contrary, Orr et al. (Orr et al. 2009) found that 8 weeks of treatment of GERD with rabeprazole (20 mg) twice a day reduced pharyngeal edema at the posterior commissure, but did not change AHI, and similar results (i.e., no change in AHI) were found by Steward et al. in a group of 27 mild-to-moderate OSA patients treated with pantoprazole for 3 months (Steward 2004), although a significant improvement in sleepiness and quality of life was reported by the patients. Interestingly, Eryilmaz et al. (Eryılmaz et al. 2012) studied 20 patients with both OSA and GERD and treated half of them with CPAP and half with proton pump inhibitor therapy (lansoprazole [30 mg] twice daily for 3 months). At the end of the treatment period, those who used the CPAP also showed improvements in GERD signs and symptoms, while those treated for GERD did not show improvement in OSA. Thus, there are no conclusive data so far and it is still a matter of debate about the role of GERD in OSA pathogenesis and vice versa.

RESIDUAL SLEEPINESS IN TREATED OSA PATIENTS

Excessive daytime sleepiness is a symptom that worsens the quality of life of several OSA patients. It is estimated that 6%–14% of CPAP-treated patients still experience residual excessive sleepiness even after being treated with CPAP possibly because of irreversible neuronal injury and increased oxidative stress or dopaminergic dysfunctions (Avellar et al. 2016). In selected cases, the prescription of pharmacotherapy is appropriate for patients that experience sleepiness even after being treated for OSA. Modafinil and armodafinil are stimulants that centrally increase the noradrenergic and dopaminergic tone and are approved in the US for residual daytime sleepiness in OSA (Avellar et al. 2016). Solriamfetol is a new medication approved by the Food and Drug Administration with the same indication in 2019. It is a dopamine and norepinephrine reuptake inhibitor that consistently showed a dose-dependent improvement in subjective sleepiness starting from 1 week after the beginning of the treatment (Yang and Gao 2019). Two Phase 3 trials (Schweitzer et al. 2019; Strollo et al. 2019) confirmed its efficacy and safety profile. It is important to note that although this pharmacotherapy is prescribed to OSA patients, it does not treat the underlying disorder but just the symptom of sleepiness and it has to be prescribed to patients compliant with CPAP or other approved treatments.

Conclusion

In the last 40 years, there have been several attempts to find a pharmacotherapy for OSA, with limited success. The research in this field has improved in the last decade, thanks to important discoveries in both the pathophysiology of sleep-disordered breathing and basic science. The recent improvements in technologies and the possibility to apply these discoveries in the clinical setting will allow, in the near future, the possibility to adopt more precise metrics of OSA severity, permitting a better evaluation of the patients and increasing the possibility to find tailored therapies based on more specific pathophysiologic traits, rather than one-size-fits-all treatment, such as CPAP. While we still need agents that can effectively raise the arousal threshold, targeting upper airway muscle activation and loop gain has already given important results and the use of combined therapies targeting more traits at the same time may be a successful strategy. The use of noradrenergic and antimuscarinic drugs combined in a proof-of-concept trial has recently provided new evidence that OSA may be treated with medications at least in a subgroup of patients. While the possibility to translate this therapy in the clinical setting needs to be investigated in a larger trial, new promising tractable targets are already available and await to be tested (Horner et al. 2017).

REFERENCES

Acar M, Cingi C, Sakallioglu O, San T, Fatih Yimenicioglu M, Bal C. The effects of mometasone furoate and desloratadine in obstructive sleep apnea syndrome patients with allergic rhinitis. *Am J Rhinol Allergy*. 2013;27:e113-6.

Araghi MH, Chen YF, Jagielski A, et al. Effectiveness of lifestyle interventions on obstructive sleep apnea (OSA): systematic review and meta-analysis. *Sleep*. 2013;36(10):1553-1562.

Athyros VG, Tziomalos K, Karagiannis A, Mikhailidis P. Cardiovascular benefits of bariatric surgery in morbidly obese patients. *Obes Rev*. 2011;12:515-524.

Avellar AB, Carvalho LB, Prado GF, Prado LB. Pharmacotherapy for residual excessive sleepiness and cognition in CPAP-treated patients with obstructive sleep apnea syndrome: A systematic review and meta-analysis. *Sleep Med Rev*. 2016;30:97-107.

Azarbarzin A, Sands SA, Stone KL, et al. The hypoxic burden of sleep apnoea predicts cardiovascular disease-related mortality: the Osteoporotic Fractures in Men Study and the Sleep Heart Health Study. *Eur Heart J*. 2019;40:1149-57.

Bakker JP, Patel SR. Evaluating behavioral weight loss programs for sleep apnea. *Sleep*. 2013;36(10):1419-1420.

Barnes H, Edwards BA, Joosten SA, Naughton MT, Hamilton GS, Dabscheck E. Positional modification techniques for supine obstructive sleep apnea: A systematic review and meta-analysis. *Sleep Med Rev*. 2017;36:107-115.

Bart Sangal R, Sangal JM, Thorp K. Atomoxetine improves sleepiness and global severity of illness but not the respiratory disturbance index in mild to moderate obstructive sleep apnea with sleepiness. *Sleep Med*. 2008;9:506-10.

BenoistL, de RuiterM, de Lange J, de Vries N. A randomized, controlled trial of positional therapy versus oral appliance therapy for position-dependent sleep apnea. *Sleep Med*. 2017;34:109-117.

BergerM, Oksenberg A, Silverberg DS, Arons E, Radwan H, Iaina A. Avoiding the supine position during sleep lowers 24 h blood pressure in obstructive sleep apnea (OSA) patients. *J Hum Hypertens*. 1997;11(10):657-664.

Berry RB, Kouchi K, Bower J, Prosise G, Light RW. Triazolam in patients with obstructive sleep apnea. *Am j respir crit care med*.1995;151:450-4.

Berry RB, Yamaura EM, Gill K, Reist C. Acute effects of paroxetine on genioglossus activity in obstructive sleep apnea. *Sleep*. 1999;22:1087-92.

Bignold JJ, Deans-Costi G, Goldsworthy MR, et al. Poor long-term patient compliance with the tennis ball technique for treating positional obstructive sleep apnea. *J Clin Sleep Med*. 2009;5(5):428-430.

Bignold JJ, MercerJD, Antic NA, McEvoy RD, Catcheside PG. Accurate position monitoring and improved supine-dependent obstructive sleep apnea with a new position recording and supine avoidance device. *J Clin Sleep Med*. 2011;7(4):376-383.

Bittencourt LR, Suchecki D, Tufik S, et al. The variability of the apnoea-hypopnoea index. *J Sleep Res*. 2001;10:245-51.

Blackman A, Foster GD, Zammit G, et al. Effect of liraglutide 3.0 mg in individuals with obesity and moderate or severe obstructive sleep apnea: the SCALE Sleep Apnea randomized clinical trial. *Int J Obes (Lond)*. 2016;40:1310-9.

Bliwise DL, Benkert RE, Ingham RH. Factors associated with nightly variability in sleep-disordered breathing in the elderly. *Chest*. 1991;100:973-6.

Bonsignore MR, McNicholas WT, Montserrat JM, Eckel J. Adipose tissue in obesity and obstructive sleep apnoea. *Eur Respir J*. 2012;39(3):746-767.

Brown MA, Goodwin JL, Silva GE, et al. The impact of sleep-disordered breathing on body mass index (BMI): the Sleep Heart Health Study (SHHS). *Southwest J Pulm Crit Care*. 2011;3:159-168.

Brownell LG, West P, Sweatman P, Acres JC, Kryger MH. Protriptyline in obstructive sleep apnea: a double-blind trial. *N Engl J Med*. 1982;307:1037-42.

Buchwald H, AvidorY, Braunwald E, et al. Bariatric surgery: a systematic review and meta-analysis. *JAMA*. 2004;292(14):1724-1737.

Camacho ME, Morin CM. The effect of temazepam on respiration in elderly insomniacs with mild sleep apnea. *Sleep*. 1995;18:644-5.

Canova CR, Downs SH, Knoblauch A, Andersson M, Tamm M, Leuppi JD. Increased prevalence of perennial allergic rhinitis in patients with obstructive sleep apnea. *Respiration*. 2004;71(2):138-143.

Carberry JC, Fisher LP, Grunstein RR, et al. Role of common hypnotics on the phenotypic causes of obstructive sleep apnoea: paradoxical effects of zolpidem. *Eur respir j*. 2017;50.

Carberry JC, Grunstein RR, Eckert DJ. The effects of zolpidem in obstructive sleep apnea - an open-label pilot study. *J Sleep Res*. 2019;28:e12853.

Carley DW, Olopade C, Ruigt GS, Radulovacki M. Efficacy of mirtazapine in obstructive sleep apnea syndrome. *Sleep*. 2007;30:35-41.

Carley DW, Prasad B, Reid KJ, et al. Pharmacotherapy of apnea by cannabimimetic enhancement, the pace clinical trial: effects of dronabinol in obstructive sleep apnea. *Sleep*. 2018;41.

Carter SG, Berger MS, Carberry JC, et al. Zopiclone increases the arousal threshold without impairing genioglossus activity in obstructive sleep apnea. *Sleep*. 2016;39:757-66.

Carter SG, Carberry JC, Cho G, et al. Effect of 1 month of zopiclone on obstructive sleep apnoea severity and symptoms: a randomised controlled trial. *Eur respir j*. 2018;52.

Cartwright RD, Diaz F, Lloyd S. The effects of sleep posture and sleep stage on apnea frequency. *Sleep*. 1991;14(4):351-353.

Cartwright RD. Effect of sleep position on sleep apnea severity. *Sleep*. 1984;7(2):110-114.

Chan E, Steenland HW, Liu H, Horner RL. Endogenous excitatory drive modulating respiratory muscle activity across sleep-wake states. *Am j respir crit care med*.2006;174:1264-73.

Cirignotta F, Mondini S, Gerardi R, Zucconi M. Effect of Brotizolam on sleep-disordered breathing in heavy snorers with obstructive apnea. *Curr Ther Res*. 1992;51:360-6.

Cirignotta F, Mondini S, Zucconi M, Gerardi R, Farolfi A, Lugaresi E. Zolpidem-polysomnographic study of the effect of a new hypnotic drug in sleep apnea syndrome. *Pharmacol Biochem Behav*. 1988;29:807-9.

Cistulli PA, Barnes DJ, Grunstein RR, Sullivan CE. Effect of short-term hormone replacement in the treatment of obstructive sleep apnoea in postmenopausal women. *Thorax*. 1994;49:699-702.

Clarenbach CF, Kohler M, Senn O, Thurnheer R, Bloch KE. Does nasal decongestion improve obstructive sleep apnea? *J Sleep Res*. 2008;17:444-9.

Clark RW, Schmidt HS, Schaal SF, Boudoulas H, Schuller DE. Sleep apnea: treatment with protriptyline. *Neurology*. 1979;29:1287-92.

Cohn MA. Hypnotics and the control of breathing: a review. *Br J Clin Pharmacol*. 1983;16(2):245S-250S.

Colquitt JL, Picot J, Loveman E, Clegg AJ. Surgery for obesity. *Cochrane Database Syst Rev*. 2009;(2):CD003641. doi: 10.1002/14651858.

Conway SG, Roizenblatt SS, Palombini L, et al. Effect of smoking habits on sleep. *Braz J Med Biol Res*. 2008;41(8):722-727.

Conway WA, Zorick F, Piccione P, Roth T. Protriptyline in the treatment of sleep apnoea. *Thorax*. 1982;37:49-53.

Cowan DC, Livingston E. Obstructive sleep apnoea syndrome and weight loss: review. *Sleep Disord*. 2012;2012:163296. doi: 10.1155/2012/163296.

Davila DG, Hurt RD, Offord KP, Harris CD, Shepard JW, Jr. Acute effects of transdermal nicotine on sleep architecture, snoring, and sleep-disordered breathing in nonsmokers. *Am j respir crit care med*.1994;150:469-74.

Deacon NL, Smales E, Jen R, Jaiswal S, Malhotra A (2016). Effects of melatonin supplementation in obstructive sleep apnea patients. In: International Conference; 2016; San Francisco. American Thoracic Society.

de Ruiter MHT, Benoist LBL, de Vries N, de Lange J. Durability of treatment effects of the Sleep Position Trainer versus oral appliance therapy in positional OSA: 12-month follow-up of a randomized controlled trial. *Sleep Breath*. 2018;22(2):441-450.

Diamond E, Druz W, D'Sousa V, Sharp JT. Effect of naloxone on obstructive sleep apnoea. *Am Rev Respir Dis*. 1982;125;Suppl 4:235.

Duce B, Kulkas A, Langton C, Töyräs J, Hukins C. Amsterdam positional OSA classification: the AASM 2012 recommended hypopnoea criteria increases the number of positional therapy candidates. *Sleep Breath*. 2017;21(2):411-417.

Duffin J, Mohan RM, Vasiliou P, Stephenson R, Mahamed S. A model of the chemoreflex control of breathing in humans: model parameters measurement. *Respir Physiol*. 2000;120:13-26.

Eckert DJ, Malhotra A, Wellman A, White DP. Trazodone increases the respiratory arousal threshold in patients with obstructive sleep apnea and a low arousal threshold. *Sleep*. 2014;37:811-9.

Eckert DJ, Owens RL, Kehlmann GB, et al. Eszopiclone increases the respiratory arousal threshold and lowers the apnoea/hypopnoea index in obstructive sleep apnoea patients with a low arousal threshold. *Clin Sci (Lond)*. 2011;120:505-14.

Eckert DJ, White DP, Jordan AS, Malhotra A, Wellman A. Defining phenotypic causes of obstructive sleep apnea. Identification of novel therapeutic targets. *Am J Respir Crit Care Med*. 2013;188:996-1004.

Edwards BA, Sands SA, Eckert DJ, et al. Acetazolamide improves loop gain but not the other physiological traits causing obstructive sleep apnoea. *J Physiol*.2012;590:1199-211.

Edwards BA, Sands SA, Owens RL, et al. The combination of supplemental oxygen and a hypnotic markedly improves obstructive sleep apnea in patients with a mild to moderate upper airway collapsibility. *Sleep*. 2016;39:1973-83.

Eijsvogel MM, Ubbink R, Dekker J, et al. Sleep position trainer versus tennis ball technique in positional obstructive sleep apnea syndrome. *J Clin Sleep Med*. 2015;11(2):13 9-147.

Eikermann M, Eckert DJ, Chamberlin NL, et al. Effects of pentobarbital on upper airway patency during sleep. *Eur respir j*. 2010;36:569-76.

Epstein LJ, Kristo D, Strollo PJ Jr, et al. Clinical guideline for the evaluation, management and long-term care of obstructive sleep apnea in adults. *J Clin Sleep Med*. 2009;5(3):263-276.

Eryılmaz A, Erişen L, Demir UL, et al. Management of patients with coexisting obstructive sleep apnea and laryngopharyngeal reflux disease. *Eur Arch Otorhinolaryngol*. 2012;269:2575-80.

Eskandari D, Zou D, Grote L, Hoff E, Hedner J. Acetazolamide reduces blood pressure and sleep-disordered breathing in patients with hypertension and obstructive sleep apnea: a randomized controlled trial. *J Clin Sleep Med*. 2018;14:309-17.

Espinoza H, Antic R, Thornton AT, McEvoy RD. The effects of aminophylline on sleep and sleep-disordered breathing in patients with obstructive sleep apnea syndrome. *Am Rev Respir Dis*. 1987;136:80-4.

Fenik VB, Davies RO, Kubin L. REM sleep-like atonia of hypoglossal (XII) motoneurons is caused by loss of noradrenergic and serotonergic inputs. *Am j respir crit care med*.2005;172:1322-30.

Ferber C, Duclaux R, Mouret J. Naltrexone improves blood gas patterns in obstructive sleep apnoea syndrome through its influence on sleep. *J Sleep Res*. 1993;2:149-55.

Ferland A, Poirier P, Sériès F. Sibutramine versus continuous positive airway pressure in obese obstructive sleep apnoea patients. *Eur respir j*. 2009;34:694-701.

Fiori CZ, Martinez D, Montanari CC, et al. Diuretic or sodium-restricted diet for obstructive sleep apnea-a randomized trial. *Sleep*. 2018;41.

Fleetham J, Ayas N, Bradley D, et al. Canadian thoracic Society Sleep Disordered Breathing Committee. Canadian Thoracic

Society 2011 guideline update: diagnosis and treatment of sleep disordered breathing. *Can Respir J.* 2011;18(1):25-47.

Flum DR, Belle SH, King WC, et al. Longitudinal Assessment of Bariatric Surgery (LABS) Consortium. Perioperative safety in the longitudinal assessment of bariatric surgery. *N Engl J Med.* 2009;361(5):445-454.

Frank MH, RaveslootMJ, van Maanen JP, Verhagen E, de Lange J, de Vries N. Positional OSA part 1: Towards a clinical classification system for position-dependent obstructive sleep apnoea. *Sleep Breath.* 2015;19(2):473-480.

Friedman M, Gurpinar B, Lin HC, Schalch P, Joseph NJ. Impact of treatment of gastroesophageal reflux on obstructive sleep apnea-hypopnea syndrome. *Ann Otol Rhinol Laryngol.* 2007;116:805-11.

Gaddam K, Pimenta E, Thomas SJ, et al. Spironolactone reduces severity of obstructive sleep apnoea in patients with resistant hypertension: a preliminary report. *J Hum Hypertens.* 2010;24:532-7.

George CF, Feldman N, Inhaber N, et al. A safety trial of sodium oxybate in patients with obstructive sleep apnea: acute effects on sleep-disordered breathing. *Sleep Med.* 2010;11:38-42.

George CF, Feldman N, Zheng Y, et al. A 2-week, polysomnographic, safety study of sodium oxybate in obstructive sleep apnea syndrome. *Sleep Breath.* 2011;15:13-20.

Gothe B, Strohl KP, Levin S, Cherniack NS. Nicotine: a different approach to treatment of obstructive sleep apnea. *Chest.* 1985;87:11-7.

Grace KP, Hughes SW, Horner RL. Identification of the mechanism mediating genioglossus muscle suppression in rem sleep. *Am j respir crit care med.*2013;187:311-9.

Grace KP, Hughes SW, Horner RL. Identification of a pharmacological target for genioglossus reactivation throughout sleep. *Sleep.* 2014;37:41-50.

Grace KP, Hughes SW, Shahabi S, Horner RL. K+ Channel modulation causes genioglossus inhibition in rem sleep and is a strategy for reactivation. *Resp Physiol Neurobi.*2013;188:277-88.

Greenburg DL, Lettieri CJ, Eliasson AH. Effects of surgical weight loss on measures of obstructive sleep apnea: a meta-analysis. *Am J Med.* 2009;122(6):535-542.

Guilleminault C, Hayes B. Naloxone, theophylline, bromocriptine, and obstructive sleep apnea. Negative results. *Bull Eur Physiopathol Respir.* 1983;19:632-4.

Guo J, Ikeda SR. Endocannabinoids modulate N-type calcium channels and G-protein-coupled inwardly rectifying potassium channels via CB1 cannabinoid receptors heterologously expressed in mammalian neurons. *Mol Pharmacol.* 2004;65:665-74.

Ha SCL, Hirai HW, Tsoi KF. Comparison of positional therapy versus continuous positive airway pressure in patients with positional obstructive sleep apnea: a meta-analysis of randomized trials. *Sleep Med Rev.* 2014;18(1):19-24.

Hanzel DA, Proia NG, Hudgel DW. Response of obstructive sleep apnea to fluoxetine and protriptyline. *Chest.* 1991;100:416-21.

Haxhiu MA, van Lunteren E, van de Graaff WB, et al. Action of nicotine on the respiratory activity of the diaphragm and genioglossus muscles and the nerves that innervate them. *Respir Physiol.* 1984;57:153-69.

Hedner J, Kraiczi H, Peker Y, Murphy P. Reduction of sleep-disordered breathing after physostigmine. *Am j respir crit care med.*2003;168:1246-51.

Hein H, Behnke G, Jörres RA, Magnussen H. The therapeutic effect of theophylline in mild obstructive sleep Apnea/ Hypopnea syndrome: results of repeated measurements with portable recording devices at home. *Eur J Med Res.* 2000;5:391-9.

Heinzer RC, White DP, Jordan AS, et al. Trazodone increases arousal threshold in obstructive sleep apnoea. *Eur respir j.* 2008;31:1308-12.

Höijer U, Hedner J, Ejnell H, Grunstein R, Odelberg E, Elam M. Nitrazepam in patients with sleep apnoea: a double-blind placebo-controlled study. *Eur respir j.* 1994;7:2011-5.

Horner RL, Grace KP, Wellman A. A resource of potential drug targets and strategic decision-making for obstructive sleep apnoea pharmacotherapy. *Respirology.* 2017;22:861-73.

Horner RL, Hughes SW, Malhotra A. State-dependent and reflex drives to the upper airway: basic physiology with clinical implications. *J Appl Physiol (1985).* 2014;116:325-36.

Hudgel DW, Patel SR, Ahasic AM, et al. The role of weight management in the treatment of adult obstructive sleep apnea. An Official American Thoracic Society Clinical Practice Guideline. *Am J Respir Crit Care Med.* 2018;198:e70-e87.

Hunchaisri N, Chalermsuwiwattanakan W. Efficacy of donepezil in the treatment of obstructive sleep apnea: A placebo-controlled trial. *J Med Assoc Thai.* 2016;99;Suppl 8:S31-5.

Isono S. Obesity and obstructive sleep apnoea: mechanisms for increased collapsibility of the passive pharyngeal airway. *Respirology.* 2012;17:32-42.

Ito E, Tsuiki S, Maeda K, Okajima I, Inoue Y. Oropharyngeal crowding closely relates to aggravation of OSA. *Chest.* 2016;150:346-52.

Jaehne A, Loessi B, Barkai Z, Reiman D, Hornyak M. Effects of nicotine on sleep during consumption, withdrawal and replacement therapy. *Sleep Med Rev.* 2009;13(5):363-377.

Javaheri S, Parker TJ, Wexler L, Liming JD, Lindower P, Roselle GA. Effect of theophylline on sleep-disordered breathing in heart failure. *N Engl J Med.* 1996;335:562-7.

Jokic R, Klimaszewski A, Mink J, Fitzpatrick MF. Surface tension forces in sleep apnea: the role of a soft tissue lubricant: a randomized double-blind, placebo-controlled trial. *Am j respir crit care med.*1998;157:1522-5.

Jokic R, Klimaszewski A, Crossley M, SridharG, Fitzpatrick MF. Positional treatment vs. continuous positive airway pressure in patients with positional obstructive sleep apnea syndrome. *Chest.* 1999;115(3):771-781.

Joosten SA, O'Driscoll DM, Berger PJ, Hamilton GS. Supine position related obstructive sleep apnea in adults: pathogenesis and treatment. *Sleep Medicine Reviews.* 2014;18(1):7-17.

Jordan AS, White DP, Lo YL, et al. Airway dilator muscle activity and lung volume during stable breathing in obstructive sleep apnea. *Sleep*. 2009;32:361-8.

Kapur VK, Baldwin CM, Resnick HE, Gottlieb DJ, Nieto FJ. Sleepiness in patients with moderate to severe sleep-disordered breathing. *Sleep*. 2005;28:472-7.

Kasai T, Bradley TD, Friedman O, Logan AG. Effect of intensified diuretic therapy on overnight rostral fluid shift and obstructive sleep apnoea in patients with uncontrolled hypertension. *J Hypertens*. 2014;32:673-80.

Kassim Z, Greenough A, Rafferty GF. Effect of caffeine on respiratory muscle strength and lung function in prematurely born, ventilated infants. *Eur J Pediatr*. 2009;168:1491-5.

Keefe DL, Watson R, Naftolin F. Hormone replacement therapy may alleviate sleep apnea in menopausal women: a pilot study. *Menopause*. 1999;6:196-200.

Kiely JL, Nolan P, McNicholas WT. Intranasal corticosteroid therapy for obstructive sleep apnoea in patients with co-existing rhinitis. *Thorax*. 2004;59(1):50-55.

Koutsourelakis I, Minaritzoglou A, Zakynthinos G, Vagiakis E, Zakynthinos S. The effect of nasal tramazoline with dexamethasone in obstructive sleep apnoea patients. *Eur respir j*. 2013;42:1055-63.

Kraiczi H, Hedner J, Dahlöf P, Ejnell H, Carlson J. Effect of serotonin uptake inhibition on breathing during sleep and daytime symptoms in obstructive sleep apnea. *Sleep*. 1999;22:61-7.

Kryger M, Wang-Weigand S, Roth T. Safety of ramelteon in individuals with mild to moderate obstructive sleep apnea. *Sleep Breath*. 2007;11:159-64.

Kryger MH, Roth T, Dement WC. *Principle and practice of sleep medicine*, 5th ed., Elsevier, 2011; pp. 1219-1232.

Kubin L. Neural control of the upper airway: respiratory and state-dependent mechanisms. *Compr Physiol*. 2016;6:1801-50.

Kuna ST, Reboussin DM, Borradaile KE, et al. Sleep AHEAD Research Group of the Look AHEAD Research Group. Long-term effect of weight loss on obstructive sleep apnea severity in obese patients with type 2 diabetes. *Sleep*. 2013;36(5):641-649.

Lagercrantz H, Yamamoto Y, Fredholm BB, Prabhakar NR, von Euler C. Adenosine analogues depress ventilation in rabbit neonates. Theophylline stimulation of respiration via adenosine receptors? *Pediatr Res*. 1984;18:387-90.

Lai YY, Kodama T, Siegel JM. Changes in monoamine release in the ventral horn and hypoglossal nucleus linked to pontine inhibition of muscle tone: an in vivo microdialysis study. *J Neurosci*. 2001;21:7384-91.

Laidlaw T. Effect of dupilumab on sleep apnea in patients with rhinosinusitis. In: clinicaltrialsgov: clinicaltrials.gov; 2018:NCT03675022.

Lee CH, Kim SW, Han K, et al. Effect of uvulopalatopharyngoplasty on positional dependency in obstructive sleep apnea. *Arch Otolaryngol Head Neck Surg*. 2011;137(7):675-679.

Levendowski DJ, Seagraves S, Popovic D, Westbrook PR. Assessment of a neck-based treatment and monitoring device for positional obstructive sleep apnea. *J Clin Sleep Med*. 2014;10:863-871.

Li Y, Owens RL, Sands S, et al. The effect of donepezil on arousal threshold and apnea-hypopnea index. A randomized, double-blind, cross-over study. *Ann Am Thorac Soc*. 2016;13:2012-8.

Lyons OD, Inami T, Perger E, Yadollahi A, Chan CT, Bradley TD. The effect of fluid overload on sleep apnoea severity in haemodialysis patients. *Eur respir j*. 2017;49.

Loord H, Hultcrantz E. Positioner-a method for preventing sleep apnea. *Acta Otolaryngol*. 2007;127(8):861-868.

Mahdavinia M, Schleimer RP, Keshavarzian A. Sleep disruption in chronic rhinosinusitis. *Expert Rev Anti Infect Ther*. 2017;15:457-65.

Marques M, Genta PR, Sands SA, et al. Effect of sleeping position on upper airway patency in obstructive sleep apnea is determined by the pharyngeal structure causing collapse. *Sleep*. 2017;40.

Marshall NS, Yee BJ, Desai AV, et al. Two randomized placebo-controlled trials to evaluate the efficacy and tolerability of mirtazapine for the treatment of obstructive sleep apnea. *Sleep*. 2008;31:824-31.

Mehta V, Vasu TS, Phillips B, Chung F. Obstructive sleep apnea and oxygen therapy: a systematic review of the literature and meta-analysis. *J Clin Sleep Med*. 2013;9:271-9.

Melania M, Pedro G, Scott AS, et al. Effect of positional therapy on the pharyngeal structure causing collapse in obstructive sleep apnea patients. In: D57 *Don't* be a do-badder: new interventions for OSA: American Thoracic Society; 2016:A7465-A.

Mendelson WB, Maczaj M, Holt J. Buspirone administration to sleep apnea patients. *J Clin Psychopharmacol*. 1991;11:71-2.

Mehra R, Redline S. Sleep apnea: a proinflammatory disorder that coaggregates with obesity. *J Allergy Clin Immunol*. 2008;121(5):1096-1102.

Moraes W, Poyares D, Sukys-Claudino L, Guilleminault C, Tufik S. Donepezil improves obstructive sleep apnea in Alzheimer disease: a double-blind, placebo-controlled study. *Chest*. 2008;133:677-83.

Morgenthaler TI, Kapen S, Lee-Chiong T, et al. Standards of Practice Committee. Practice parameters for the medical therapy of obstructive sleep apnea. *Sleep*. 2006;29(8):1031-1035.

Morrell MJ, Arabi Y, Zahn BR, Meyer KC, Skatrud JB, Badr MS. Effect of surfactant on pharyngeal mechanics in sleeping humans: implications for sleep apnoea. *Eur respir j*. 2002;20:451-7.

Mulloy E, McNicholas WT. Theophylline in obstructive sleep apnea. A double-blind evaluation. *Chest*. 1992;101:753-7.

Newman AB, Foster G, Givelber R, Nieto FJ, Redline S, Young T. Progression and regression of sleep-disordered breathing with changes in weight: the Sleep Heart Health Study. *Arch Intern Med*. 2005;165(20):2408-2413.

O'Keeffe T, Patterson EJ. Evidence supporting routine polysomnography before bariatric surgery. *Obes Surg.* 2004; 14(1):23-26.

Oksenberg A, Gadoth N. Are we missing a simple treatment for most adult sleep apnea patients? The avoidance of the supine sleep position. *J Sleep Res.* 2014;23(2):204-210.

Oksenberg A, Silverberg D, Offenbach D, Arons E. Positional therapy for obstructive sleep apnea patients: A 6-month follow-up study. *Laryngoscope.* 2006;116(11):1995-2000.

Omobomi O, Quan SF. Positional therapy in the management of positional obstructive sleep apnea-a review of the current literature. *Sleep Breath.* 2018;22(2):297-304.

Orr WC, Robert JJ, Houck JR, Giddens CL, Tawk MM. The effect of acid suppression on upper airway anatomy and obstruction in patients with sleep apnea and gastroesophageal reflux disease. *J Clin Sleep Med.* 2009;5:330-4.

Park E, Younes M, Liu H, Liu X, Horner RL. Systemic vs. central administration of common hypnotics reveals opposing effects on genioglossus muscle activity in rats. *Sleep.* 2008;31:355-65.

Pedrosa RP, Drager LF, Gonzaga CC, et al. Obstructive sleep apnea: the most common secondary cause of hypertension associated with resistant hypertension. *Hypertension.* 2011;58:811-7.

Peppard PE, Young T, BarnetJH, Palta M, Hagen EW, Hla KM. Increased prevalence of sleep-disordered breathing in adults. *Am J Epidemiol.* 2013;177(9):1006-1014.

Peppard PE, Young T, Palta M, Dempsey J, Skatrud J. Longitudinal study of moderate weight change and sleep-disordered breathing. JAMA 2000;284(23):3015-21.

Permut I, Montserrat DA, Wissam C, et al. Comparison of positional therapy to CPAP in patients with positional obstructive sleep apnea. *J Clin Sleep Med.* 2010;6(3):238-243.

Phillips BA, Danner FJ. Cigarette smoking and sleep disturbance. *Arch Intern Med.* 1995;155(7):734-737.

Phillips CL, Yee BJ, Trenell MI, etal. Changes in regional adiposity and cardio-metabolic function following a weight loss program with sibutramine in obese men with obstructive sleep apnea. *J Clin Sleep Med.* 2009;5(5):416-421.

Pickett CK, Regensteiner JG, Woodard WD, Hagerman DD, Weil JV, Moore LG. Progestin and estrogen reduce sleep-disordered breathing in postmenopausal women. *J Appl Physiol (1985).* 1989;66:1656-61.

Piovezan RD, Kase C, Moizinho R, Tufik S, Poyares D. Gabapentin acutely increases the apnea-hypopnea index in older men: data from a randomized, double-blind, placebo-controlled study. *J Sleep Res.* 2017;26:166-70.

Popovic RM, White DP. Upper airway muscle activity in normal women: influence of hormonal status. *J Appl Physiol (1985).* 1998;84:1055-62.

Prasad B, Radulovacki M, Olopade C, Herdegen JJ, Logan T, Carley DW. Prospective trial of efficacy and safety of ondansetron and fluoxetine in patients with obstructive sleep apnea syndrome. *Sleep.* 2010;33:982-9.

Qaseem A, Holty JE, Owens DK, Dallas P, Starkey M, Shekelle P (Clinical Guidelines Committee of the American College of Physicians). Management of obstructive sleep apnea in adults: A clinical practice guideline from the American College of Physicians. *Ann Intern Med.* 2013;159(7):471-483.

Rapoport DM. On beyond zebra (and the apnea-hypopnea index) in obstructive sleep apnea. *Am j respir crit care med.*2018;197:1104-6.

Ratnavadivel R, Chau N, Stadler D, Yeo A, McEvoy RD, Catcheside PG. Marked reduction in obstructive sleep apnea severity in slow wave sleep. *J Clin Sleep Med.* 2009;5:519-24.

Ratnavadivel R, Stadler D, Windler S, et al. Upper airway function and arousability to ventilatory challenge in slow wave versus stage 2 sleep in obstructive sleep apnoea. *Thorax.* 2010;65:107-12.

Ravesloot MJ, van Maanen JP, Hilgevoord AA, van Wagensveld BA, de Vries N. Obstructive sleep apnea is underrecognized and underdiagnosed in patients undergoing bariatric surgery. *Eur Arch Otorhinolaryngol.* 2012;269(7):1865-1871.

Ravesloot MJL, Van Maanen JP, Dun L, de Vries N. The undervalued potential of positional therapy in position-dependent snoring and obstructive sleep apnea-a review of the literature. *Sleep Breath.* 2013;17(1):39-49.

Ravesloot MJL, White D, Heinzer R, Oksenberg A, Pépin JL. Efficacy of the new generation of devices for positional therapy for patients with positional obstructive sleep apnea: a systematic review of the literature and meta-analysis. *J Clin Sleep Med.* 2017;13(6):813-824.

Redline S, Schluchter MD, Larkin EK, Tishler PV. Predictors of Longitudinal change in sleep-disordered breathing in a non clinic population. *Sleep.* 2003;26(6):703-709.

Redolfi S, Bettinzoli M, Venturoli N, et al. Attenuation of obstructive sleep apnea and overnight rostral fluid shift by physical activity. *Am j respir crit care med.* 2015;191:856-8.

Redolfi S, Yumino D, Ruttanaumpawan P, et al. Relationship between overnight rostral fluid shift and Obstructive Sleep Apnea in nonobese men. *Am j respir crit care med.*2009;179:241-6.

Roehrs T, Beare D, Zorick F, et al. Sleepiness and ethanol effects on simulated driving. *Alcohol Clin Exp Res.* 1994;18(1):154-158.

Romero-Corral A, Caples SM, Lopez-Jimenez F, Somers VK. Interactions between obesity and obstructive sleep apnea: implications for treatment. *Chest.* 2010;137(3):711-719.

Rosenberg R, Roach JM, Scharf M, Amato DA. A pilot study evaluating acute use of eszopiclone in patients with mild to moderate obstructive sleep apnea syndrome. *Sleep Med.* 2007;8:464-70.

Sands SA, Eckert DJ, Jordan AS, et al. Enhanced upper-airway muscle responsiveness is a distinct feature of overweight/obese individuals without sleep apnea. *Am j respir crit care med.* 2014;190:930-7.

Sands SA, Edwards BA, Terrill PI, et al. Phenotyping pharyngeal pathophysiology using polysomnography in patients with obstructive sleep apnea. *Am j respir crit care med.* 2018a;197:1187-97.

Sands SA, Edwards BA, Terrill PI, et al. Identifying obstructive sleep apnoea patients responsive to supplemental oxygen therapy. *Eur respir j.* 2018b;52.

Sands SA, Terrill PI, Edwards BA, et al. Quantifying the arousal threshold using polysomnography in obstructive sleep apnea. *Sleep*. 2018;41.

Sarkhosh K, Switzer NJ, El-Hadi M, Birch DW, Shi X, Karmali S. The impact of bariatric surgery on obstructive sleep apnea: a systematic review. *Obes Surg*. 2013;23(3):414-423.

Sawyer AM, Gooneratne NS, Marcus CL, Ofer D, Richards KC, Weaver TE. A systematic review of CPAP adherence across age groups: clinical and empiric insights for developing CPAP adherence interventions. *Sleep Med Rev*. 2011;15:343-56.

Schweitzer PK, Rosenberg R, Zammit GK, et al. Solriamfetol for excessive sleepiness in obstructive sleep apnea (TONES 3). A randomized controlled trial. *Am j respir crit care Med*. 2019;199:1421-31.

Senior BA, Khan M, Schwimmer C, Rosenthal L, Benninger M. Gastroesophageal reflux and obstructive sleep apnea. *Laryngoscope*. 2001;111:2144-6.

Sjöström L, Narbro K, Sjöström CD, et al. Swedish Obese Subjects Study. Effects of bariatric surgery on mortality in Swedish obese subjects. *N Engl J Med*. 2007;357(8):741-752.

Skinner MA, Kingshott RN, Filsell S, Taylor DR. Efficacy of the 'tennis ball technique' versus nCPAP in the management of position-dependent obstructive sleep apnoea syndrome. *Respirology*. 2008;13(5):708-715.

Smales ET, Edwards BA, Deyoung PN, et al. Trazodone Effects on Obstructive Sleep Apnea and Non-REM Arousal Threshold. *Ann Am Thorac Soc*. 2015;12(5):758-764.

Smith DF, Sarber KM, Spiceland CP, Ishman SL, Augelli DM, Romaker AM. Effects of medical therapy on mild obstructive sleep apnea in adult patients. *J Clin Sleep Med*. 2019;15:979-83.

Smith MM, Peterson E, Yaremchuk KL. The role of tonsillectomy in adults with tonsillar hypertrophy and obstructive sleep apnea. *Otolaryngol Head Neck Surg*. 2017;157:331-5.

Smith PL, Haponik EF, Allen RP, Bleecker ER. The effects of protriptyline in sleep-disordered breathing. *Am Rev Respir Dis*. 1983;127:8-13.

Sood S, Morrison JL, Liu H, Horner RL. Role of endogenous serotonin in modulating genioglossus muscle activity in awake and sleeping rats. *Am j respir crit care med*. 2005;172:1338-47.

Sood S, Raddatz E, Liu X, Liu H, Horner RL. Inhibition of serotonergic medullary raphe obscurus neurons suppresses genioglossus and diaphragm activities in anesthetized but not conscious rats. *J Appl Physiol (1985)*. 2006;100:1807-21.

Steward DL. Pantoprazole for sleepiness associated with acid reflux and obstructive sleep disordered breathing. *Laryngoscope*. 2004;114:1525-8.

Stradling J, Smith D, Radulovacki M, Carley D. Effect of ondansetron on moderate obstructive sleep apnoea, a single night, placebo-controlled trial. *J Sleep Res*. 2003;12:169-70.

Strollo PJ, Jr., Hedner J, Collop N, et al. Solriamfetol for the treatment of excessive sleepiness in OSA: A placebo-controlled randomized withdrawal study. *Chest*. 2019;155:364-74.

Sukys-Claudino L, Moraes W, Guilleminault C, Tufik S, Poyares D. Beneficial effect of donepezil on obstructive sleep apnea: a double-blind, placebo-controlled clinical trial. *Sleep Med*. 2012;13:290-6.

Suratt PM, Wilhoit SC, Brown ED, Findley LJ. Effect of doxapram on obstructive sleep apnea. *Bull Eur Physiopathol Respir*. 1986;22:127-31.

Sutherland K, Kairaitis K, Yee BJ, Cistulli PA. From CPAP to tailored therapy for obstructive sleep Apnoea. *Multidiscip Respir Med*. 2018;13:44.

Svendsen M, Tonstad S. Orlistat after initial dietary/behavioural treatment: changes in body weight and dietary maintenance in subjects with sleep related breathing disorders. *Nutr J*. 2011;10:21.

Taranto-Montemurro L, Edwards BA, Sands SA, et al. Desipramine increases genioglossus activity and reduces upper airway collapsibility during non-REM sleep in healthy subjects. *Am j respir crit care med*. 2016;194:878-85.

Taranto-Montemurro L, Messineo L, Sands SA, et al. The combination of atomoxetine and oxybutynin greatly reduces obstructive sleep apnea severity. A randomized, placebo-controlled, double-blind crossover trial. *Am j respir crit care med*.2019;199:1267-76.

Taranto-Montemurro L, Sands SA, Azarbarzin A, et al. Effect of 4-aminopyridine on genioglossus muscle activity during sleep in healthy adults. *Ann Am Thorac Soc*. 2017;14:1177-83.

Taranto-Montemurro L, Sands SA, Edwards BA, et al. Desipramine improves upper airway collapsibility and reduces OSA severity in patients with minimal muscle compensation. *Eur respir j*. 2016;48:1340-50.

Taranto-Montemurro L, Sands SA, Edwards BA, et al. Effects of tiagabine on slow wave sleep and arousal threshold in patients with obstructive sleep apnea. *Sleep*. 2017;40.

Taranto-Montemurro L, Sands SA, Grace KP, et al. Neural memory of the genioglossus muscle during sleep is stage-dependent in healthy subjects and obstructive sleep apnoea patients. *J physiol*. 2018;596:5163-73.

Terrill PI, Edwards BA, Nemati S, et al. Quantifying the ventilatory control contribution to sleep apnoea using polysomnography. *Eur respir j*. 2015;45:408-18.

Tishler PV, Larkin EK, Schluchter MD, Redline S. Incidence of sleep-disordered breathing in an urban adult population: the relative importance of risk factors in the development of sleep-disordered breathing. *JAMA*. 2003;289(17):2230-2237.

Tojima H, Kunitomo F, Kimura H, Tatsumi K, Kuriyama T, Honda Y. Effects of acetazolamide in patients with the sleep apnoea syndrome. *Thorax*. 1988;43:113-9.

Tuomilehto H, Seppä J, Uusitupa M, et al. (Kuopio Sleep Apnea Group). The impact of weight reduction in the prevention of the progression of obstructive sleep apnea: an explanatory analysis of a 5-year observational follow-up trial. *Sleep Med*. 2014;15(3):329-335.

Tuomilehto H, Seppä J, Uusitupa M, Tuomilehto J, Gylling H (Kuopio Sleep Apnea Group). Weight reduction and increased physical activity to prevent the progression of obstructive sleep apnea: A 4-year observational postintervention follow-up of a randomized clinical trial. *JAMA Intern Med.* 2013b;173(10):929-930.

Tuomilehto H, Seppä J, Uusitupa M. Obesity and obstructive sleep apnea--clinical significance of weight loss. *Sleep Med Rev.* 2013a;17(5):321-329.

Tuomilehto H, Uusitupa M. Lifestyle changes aiming at weight loss should always be included in the treatment of obese patients with obstructive sleep apnea. *Sleep.* 2014;37(5):1021.

Van Maanen JP, Meester KA, Dun LN, et al. The sleep position trainer: a new treatment for positional obstructive sleep apnoea. *Sleep Breath.* 2013;17(2):771-779.

Veasey SC. Serotonin agonists and antagonists in obstructive sleep apnea: therapeutic potential. *Am J Respir Med.* 2003;2:21-9.

Veasey SC, Chachkes J, Fenik P, Hendricks JC. The effects of ondansetron on sleep-disordered breathing in the English bulldog. *Sleep.* 2001;24:155-60.

Vecchio LM, Grace KP, Liu H, Harding S, Lê AD, HornerRL. State-dependent vs. central motor effects of ethanol on breathing. *J Appl Physiol.* 2010;108(2):387-400.

Wang D, Marshall NS, Duffin J, et al. Phenotyping inter-individual variability in obstructive sleep apnoea response to temazepam using ventilatory chemoreflexes during wakefulness. *J Sleep Res.* 2011;20:526-32.

Weaver TE, Grunstein RR. Adherence to continuous positive airway pressure therapy: the challenge to effective treatment. *Proc Am Thorac Soc.* 2008;5:173-8.

Wellman A, Eckert DJ, Jordan AS, et al. A method for measuring and modeling the physiological traits causing obstructive sleep apnea. *J Appl Physiol (1985).* 2011;110:1627-37.

Wellman A, Edwards BA, Sands SA, et al. A simplified method for determining phenotypic traits in patients with obstructive sleep apnea. *J Appl Physiol (1985).* 2013; 114:911-22.

Wellman A, Malhotra A, Jordan AS, Stevenson KE, Gautam S, White DP. Effect of oxygen in obstructive sleep apnea: role of loop gain. *Resp Physiol Neurobi.* 2008;162:144-51.

Wesström J, Ulfberg J, Nilsson S. Sleep apnea and hormone replacement therapy: a pilot study and a literature review. *Acta Obstet Gynecol Scand.* 2005;84:54-7.

Wetter DW, Young TB, Bidwell TR, Badr MS, Palta M. Smoking as a risk factor for sleep-disordered breathing. *Arch Intern Med.* 1994;154(19):2219-2224.

White DP, Younes MK. Obstructive sleep apnea. *Compr Physiol.* 2012;2:2541-94.

White LH, Lyons OD, Yadollahi A, Ryan CM, Bradley TD. Night-to-night variability in obstructive sleep apnea severity: relationship to overnight rostral fluid shift. *J Clin Sleep Med.* 2015;11:149-56.

White RP, Daigneault EA. The antagonisms of atropine to the EEG effects of adrenergic drugs. *J Pharmacol Exp Ther.* 1959;125:339-46.

Whyte KF, Gould GA, Airlie MA, Shapiro CM, Douglas NJ. Role of protriptyline and acetazolamide in the sleep apnea/hypopnea syndrome. *Sleep.* 1988;11:463-72.

Winslow DH, Bowden CH, DiDonato KP, McCullough PA. A randomized, double-blind, placebo-controlled study of an oral, extended-release formulation of phentermine/topiramate for the treatment of obstructive sleep apnea in obese adults. *Sleep.* 2012;35:1529-39.

Wong AM, Barnes HN, Joosten SA, et al. The effect of surgical weight loss on obstructive sleep apnoea: A systematic review and meta-analysis. *Sleep Med Rev.* 2018;42:85-99.

Yadollahi A, Gabriel JM, White LH, Taranto Montemurro L, Kasai T, Bradley TD. A randomized, double crossover study to investigate the influence of saline infusion on sleep apnea severity in men. *Sleep.* 2014;37:1699-705.

Yang J, Gao J. Solriamfetol for the treatment of excessive daytime sleepiness associated with narcolepsy. *Expert Rev Clin Pharmacol.* 2019;12:723-8.

Yee BJ, Phillips CL, Banerjee D, Caterson I, HednerJA, Grunstein RR. The effect of sibutramine-assisted weight loss in men with obstructive sleep apnoea. *Int J Obes.* 2007;31(1):161-168.

Yee BJ, Phillips CL, Banerjee D, Caterson I, Hedner JA, Grunstein RR. The effect of sibutramine-assisted weight loss in men with obstructive sleep apnoea. *Int J Obes (Lond).* 2007;31:161-8.

Younes M. Contributions of upper airway mechanics and control mechanisms to severity of obstructive apnea. *Am j respir crit care med.* 2003;168:645-58.

Younes M. Role of arousals in the pathogenesis of obstructive sleep apnea. *Am j respir crit care med.*2004;169:623-33.

Younes M. Role of respiratory control mechanisms in the pathogenesis of obstructive sleep disorders. *J Appl Physiol (1985).* 2008;105:1389-405.

Younes M, Loewen AH, Ostrowski M, Laprairie J, Maturino F, Hanly PJ. Genioglossus activity available via non-arousal mechanisms vs. that required for opening the airway in obstructive apnea patients. *J Appl Physiol (1985).* 2012;112:249-58.

Younes M, Park E, Horner RL. Pentobarbital sedation increases genioglossus respiratory activity in sleeping rats. *Sleep.* 2007;30:478-88.

Young T, Peppard PE, Gottlieb DJ. Epidemiology of obstructive sleep apnea: a population health perspective. *Am j respir crit care med.*2002;165:1217-39.

Yumino D, Redolfi S, Ruttanaumpawan P, et al. Nocturnal rostral fluid shift: a unifying concept for the pathogenesis of obstructive and central sleep apnea in men with heart failure. *Circulation.* 2010;121:1598-605.

Zevin S, Swed E, Cahan C. Clinical effects of locally delivered nicotine in obstructive sleep apnea syndrome. *Am J Ther.* 2003;10:170-5.

Zhang XJ, Li QY, Wang Y, Xu HJ, Lin YN. The effect of non-benzodiazepine hypnotics on sleep quality and severity in patients with OSA: a meta-analysis. *Sleep Breath.* 2014;18(4):781-789.

Zuberi NA, Rekab K, Nguyen HV. Sleep apnea avoidance pillow effects on obstructive sleep apnea syndrome and snoring. *Sleep Breath.* 2004;8(4):201-207.

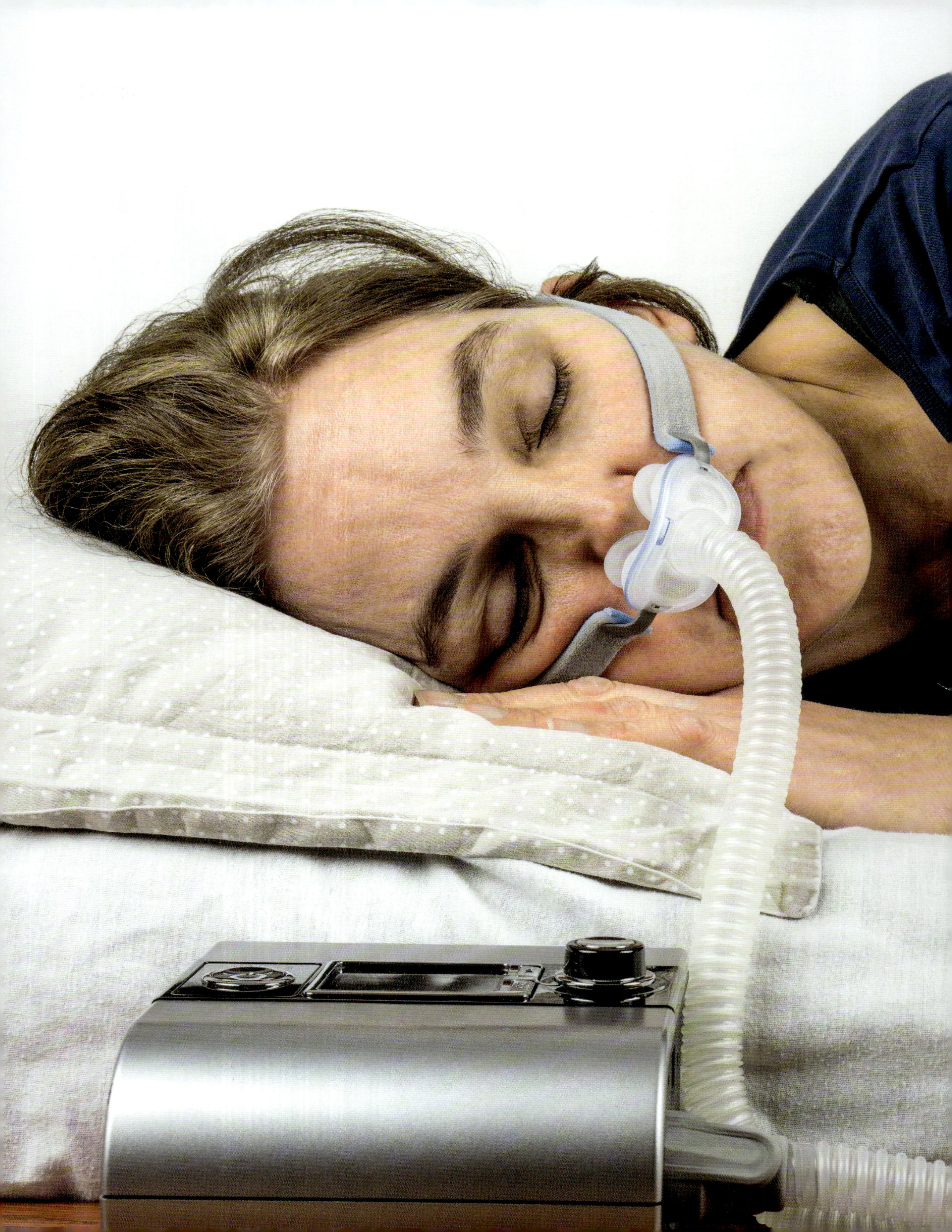

Continuous positive airways pressure therapy and other positive pressure devices

Antonio Sanna

Objectives

- Understanding the therapeutic mechanisms of continuous positive airways pressure (CPAP)
- Evaluating the efficacy of CPAP therapy and its possible side effects
- Describing the methods for CPAP titration
- Learning follow-up management principles for patients treated with CPAP

Introduction

The objectives of all obstructive sleep apnea syndrome (OSAS) treatment strategies are as follows:

- to maintain complete patency of the pharynx during sleep
- to achieve resolution of symptoms
- to mitigate and/or improve comorbidities
- to improve occupational performance
- to reduce the risks of road and occupational accidents

CPAP therapy is the treatment of choice for upper airway obstruction because it can maintain complete patency of the pharynx during sleep, prevent onset of apnea and hypopnea, facilitate resolution of nocturnal and diurnal symptoms, and improve quality of life and life expectancy (Sullivan *et al.* 1981; Jordan *et al.* 2014).

Mechanism of action

CPAP is generated by a medical compressor and is usually applied to the upper airways via a nasal mask (Sullivan *et al.* 1981); therefore, it is considered as pneumatic support (Schwab *et al.* 1996) that prevents pharyngeal narrowing due to turbulent airflow, which subsequently results in snoring as well as collapse of the pharyngeal walls with consequent apnea/hypopnea (Pasterkamp *et al.* 1996; Strohl and Redline 1996). Furthermore, CPAP acts by restoring the normal morphological and functional characteristics of the genioglossus muscles (Carrera *et al.* 1999), indicating that CPAP not only acts as pneumatic support but also has curative effects on the soft tissues of the upper airways, wherein patients with OSAS present with altered muscle fiber and sensorial nerve structures as well as inflammation (Fribert *et al.* 1997; Friberg *et al.* 1998; Boyd *et al.* 2004). This remodeling contributes to the recovery of adequate neurofunctional control of the upper airways muscle.

Effects of CPAP on OSAS symptoms

Habitual (every night) and persistent (lasting at least 6 months) snoring, apnea/hypopnea, and excessive daytime sleepiness (EDS) are the primary symptoms of OSAS (Durán *et al.* 2001). The resolution of snoring, apnea, and hypopnea normalizes respiratory activity during sleep and restores correct sleep posture (Sullivan *et al.* 1981) by eliminating or improving nocturnal symptoms such as awakenings with a choking sensation and nocturia (Cruz *et al.* 2012). Furthermore, it has been demonstrated that the resolution of snoring and apnea/hypopnea improves quality of life as well as sleep in both patients with OSAS and their bed partners (Beninati *et al.* 1999). Randomized controlled studies have demonstrated that CPAP improves EDS as assessed both objectively and subjectively (Giles *et al.* 2006). Such improvements have also been observed in patients with EDS and mild OSAS (Weaver *et al.* 2012). The effects of CPAP on OSAS-associated depression are still controversial (Giles *et al.* 2006), and these effects on cognitive functions have not yet been clearly demonstrated to date (Kushida *et al.* 2012), although CPAP is known to improve cognitive functions in patients with Alzheimer's disease (Ancoli-Israel *et al.* 2008; Cooke *et al.* 2009). Nevertheless, CPAP clearly improves quality of life, particularly in the domains of physical activity, general health, and vitality.

Long-term effects of using CPAP

OSAS is considered an independent risk factor for systemic arterial hypertension (Peppard *et al.* 2000; Marin *et al.* 2012; Parati *et al.* 2013; MacEvoy 2014) and is associated with cardiovascular diseases (Moe *et al.* 1996a; Moe *et al.* 1996b; Peker *et al.* 1999; Kiely and McNicholas 2000; Sanner *et al.* 2001; Javahari 2006; Pratt-Ubunama *et al.* 2007; Yumino *et al.* 2009; Hedner *et al.* 2011) and cerebrovascular diseases (Parra *et al.* 2000; Bassetti *et al.* 2006). Among the available therapeutic options, CPAP has the strongest experimental support for positive effects on cardiocerebrovascular morbidity (Gottlieb *et al.* 2010; Barbé *et al.* 2012) and mortality (Punjabi *et al.* 2009). The reduction in systemic arterial pressure is greater when CPAP is applied for more than 4 hours/night (Barbé *et al.* 2012; Bratton *et al.* 2014), indicating that therapeutic success for hypertension in terms of systemic arterial pressure is dependent on adherence to the therapy.

Long-term observational studies on patients with symptomatic OSAS have indicated that CPAP decreases the incidence of fatal and nonfatal coronary events, although this association has not been observed in patients with asymptomatic OSAS (Barbé *et al.* 2012). Several large-scale studies on patients with OSAS are currently underway to clarify the effects of CPAP therapy on the risk of cardiovascular events (Peker *et al.* 2009; Esquinas *et al.* 2013). It has been demonstrated that CPAP therapy improves the left ventricular ejection fraction and diastolic function in patients with OSAS with cardiac failure (Arias *et al.* 2005; Ryan *et al.* 2010). Observational studies conducted on the same patient population have reported that CPAP reduces the risks of mortality and hospitalization (Kasai *et al.* 2008; Damy *et al.* 2012). Other observational studies have suggested the efficacy of CPAP therapy in preventing the recurrence of atrial fibrillation (Kanagala *et al.* 2003; Fein *et al.* 2013; Naruse *et al.* 2013). Although the relationship between CPAP therapy and stroke is still unclear,

CPAP improves neurological function and motor recovery and prevents or delays the onset of new cardiovascular events in patients with OSAS following stroke (Parra *et al.* 2011; Ryan *et al.* 2011).

OSAS is significantly associated with metabolism-related disorders such as metabolic syndrome, diabetes mellitus, and dyslipidemia (Hedner *et al.* 2011; Kent *et al.* 2014; Nadeem *et al.* 2014). However, recent studies have demonstrated that CPAP therapy does not appear to substantially improve glucose metabolism (Dorkova *et al.* 2008; Surendra *et al.* 2011; Hoyos *et al.* 2012; Myhill *et al.* 2012; Weinstock *et al.* 2012; Chirinos *et al.* 2014) or lipid metabolism (Kohler *et al.* 2011; Phillips *et al.* 2011; Keenan *et al.* 2014).

It is globally well documented that CPAP therapy for OSAS reduces the risks of road and occupational accidents (Garbarino *et al.* 2015; Garbarino *et al.* 2016). Indeed, the risk of road accidents can be reduced by CPAP therapy to the level observed in individuals who have not developed OSAS (George 2001; Strohl *et al.* 2013). Similarly, CPAP therapy appears to reduce occupational accidents that are not associated with motor vehicle operation (Sanna 2013).

Contraindications and adverse effects of CPAP

CPAP therapy is safe and efficacious, and its contraindications and adverse effects are summarized in Table 6.1. While there are no absolute contraindications, relative contraindications include the presence of bubbles in the lungs and the infective pathology of the upper airways and the ear (American Thoracic Society 1994). The most common adverse effects of CPAP therapy are rhinitis symptoms, dryness of nasal and oropharyngeal mucosae, conjunctivitis, wounds and ulcers on the bridge of the nose, choking sensations, and claustrophobia (Kushida *et al.* 2012).

Adherence

Improvements in daytime sleepiness, quality of life, and systemic arterial pressure control increase with CPAP use (Donovan *et al.* 2015). Depending on the criteria used to define it, long-term adherence to this therapy varies from

6.1 Contraindications and adverse effects of CPAP.

Contraindications	Presence of bubbles in the lungs Infective pathologies of the upper airways and the ear
Adverse effects	Rhinitis symptoms Dryness of nasal and oropharyngeal mucosae Conjunctivitis Wounds and ulcers on the bridge of the nose Choking sensation and claustrophobia

46% to 85% (Wozniak *et al.* 2014). It is currently accepted that adherence is good if the therapy is applied for more than 4 hours/night and more than 70% of the night (Schwab *et al.* 2013).

Given this relationship between therapy adherence and efficacy, it is critical to investigate the possible causes of noncompliance. There are two major forms of noncompliance:

1. patients want to follow the therapy but cannot do so because of inadequate or ill-fitted masks, poor humidification of the airways, malfunctioning of the device, or pathologies related to the nose;
2. patients do not want to follow the therapy. In such cases, it is reasonable to propose alternative therapies because adherence is crucial for complete treatment efficacy. Educational interventions, particularly those aimed at improving and maintaining compliance for long term, may also be effective (Donovan *et al.*2015).

Other positive pressure devices

Similar to CPAP devices, automatic positive airway pressure (APAP) devices (or autoCPAP devices) deliver positive pressure to the airways. However, unlike CPAP devices, the pressure delivered by APAP devices is increased or decreased by a specific algorithm according to the severity of pharyngeal obstruction (Teschler *et al.* 1996). This enables the application of the minimal efficacious positive pressure to prevent pharyngeal obstruction, which varies substantially according to body position and sleep phase. Using APAP, it is possible to reduce the therapeutic mean pressure value for the entire night (Kakkar and Berry 2007).

Metaanalyses have concluded that APAP is marginally but significantly superior to CPAP in terms of adherence to the therapy and improvement in daytime sleepiness (Ayas *et al.* 2004; Ip *et al.* 2012). Conversely, CPAP appears to be superior to APAP in terms of reducing cardiovascular risk factors such as hypertension and insulin resistance (Patruno *et al.* 2007; Karasuli *et al.* 2010; Ip *et al.* 2012).

In addition to being an alternative to CPAP, APAP is a valuable tool for defining the optimal therapeutic pressure for CPAP. Based on defined protocols, it is possible to titrate CPAP settings at the patient's home rather than at a sleep laboratory (Planès *et al.* 2003; Morgenthaler *et al.* 2008).

In cases where CPAP does not resolve the instrumental and clinical conditions of OSAS and/or when apnea/hypopnea is associated with another predominant sleep-disordered breathing (e.g., hypoventilation, periodic breathing such as Cheney-Stokes respiration), the first-line treatment includes positive pressure devices other than CPAP such as bilevel positive airway pressure therapy.

In addition to oral devices, the abovementioned devices (Ramar *et al.* 2015) are indicated for patients with OSAS who are intolerant to CPAP (Teschler *et al.* 2001; Kushida *et al.* 2006).

Titration

Prescription of CPAP therapy depends on the results of the titration procedure comprising the identification of the minimal therapeutic pressure value for long-term out-patient CPAP. Titration can be conducted according to different operative standards, but the objective is always to correct pathological respiratory events associated with sleep (apnea, hypopnea, flow limitation, and related indices of saturation) with normalization of polygraphic indices or at least achieve the maximum possible improvement in these events. Manual titration of the CPAP device can be conducted at a sleep laboratory, which is considered the reference method and requires a polysomnographic study (Kushida *et al.* 2008). Here the goal is to normalize arousals associated with respiratory efforts (RERAs) and flow limitation (FL-arousals) or at least achieve the maximum possible improvement. However, APAP devices are often preferred for titration (Morgenthaler *et al.* 2008).
Several additional factors should be considered for CPAP titration and subsequent clinical recommendation:

- CPAP is exclusively indicated for patients presenting with sleep-related respiratory obstructive events alone or predominantly with obstructive events compared with other sleep-related respiratory events such as hypoventilation or periodic breathing (e.g., Cheyne-Stokes respiration)
- patients must adapt to the device for an adequate duration of time under cardiorespiratory monitoring with CPAP to demonstrate normalization of apnea/hypopnea index (AHI) as well as flow limitation and saturation indices or to achieve the maximum possible improvement
- memory card records of the device must be critically analyzed to determine the therapeutic value of CPAP
- the recording night with CPAP must present a satisfying quality of sleep as evaluated using patients' sleep diaries or interviews.

The prescription of a bilevel positive airway pressure device requires different titration strategies, including manual setting at a sleep laboratory by attending personnel (Berry *et al.* 2010). However, similar to CPAP titration, bilevel positive airway pressure titration aims to identify the optimal therapeutic pressure values for long-term home treatment. Similar to the available therapies for OSAS, the objective of these devices is to reduce AHI to <5 with concordant resolution of OSAS symptoms or at least to reduce AHI to <15, which is not possible always. However, even in cases of clear improvement, patients with AHI of >15 still have a considerable risk of metabolic, neurofunctional, and cardiocerebrovascular complications.

Follow-up

The objectives of follow-up are as follows:

- to control disease symptoms, particularly EDS
- to promote correct and consistent use of the prescribed positive pressure device
- to identify possible causes of poor adherence
- to evaluate the necessity for a new titration of the device

The first follow-up must be performed within 3 months from the initiation of treatment at home, whereas subsequent follow-ups can be annually scheduled except when significant changes occur, such as weight gain or loss, surgery of the upper airways, and other clinical events that can modify the clinical situation of OSAS (such as comorbidities of a new diagnosis or aggravation of preexisting conditions and new pharmacologic therapies). The follow-up must comprise interviews with the patients preferably with their bed partners to verify treatment adherence and subjective symptom control. Because of regulatory requirements of the medical fitness of patients with OSAS (such as the European Union Directive on driver licensing in obstructive sleep apnea), objective evaluation of treatment compliance is recommended. This is possible only by analyzing the memory card records of the device, thus enabling to verify the efficacy of the device in real settings.

Conclusions

While CPAP was developed more than 35 years ago, it is still the only treatment with proven therapeutic efficacy independent of OSAS severity. It is also the therapy with the strongest evidentiary support for long-term benefits on quality of life and life expectancy.

REFERENCES

American Thoracic Society. Official statement adopted March 1944. Indications and standards for use of nasal continuous positive airway pressure (CPAP) in sleep apnea syndromes. *Am J Respir Crit Care Med.* 1994;150:1738-45.

Ancoli-Israel S, Palmer BW, Cooke JR, et al. Cognitive effects of treating obstructive sleep apnea in Alzheimer's disease: a randomized controlled study. *J Am Geriatr Soc.* 2008;56:2076-2081.

Arias MA, García-Río F, Alonso-Fernández A, Mediano O, Martínez I, Villamor J. Obstructive sleep apnea syndrome affects left ventricular diastolic function: effects of nasal continuous positive airway pressure in men. *Circulation.* 2005;112:375-383.

Ayas NT, Patel SR, Malhotra A, et al. Auto-titrating versus standard continuous positive airway pressure for the treatment of obstructive sleep apnea: results of a meta-analysis. *Sleep.* 2004;27:249-253.

Barbé F, Durán-Cantolla J, Sánchez-de-la-Torre M, et al.; Spanish Sleep And Breathing Network. Effect of continuous positive airway pressure on the incidence of hypertension and cardiovascular events in nonsleepy patients with obstructive sleep apnea: a randomized controlled trial. *JAMA.* 2012;307:2161-2168.

Bassetti CL, Milanova M, Gugger M. Sleep-disordered breathing and acute ischemic stroke: diagnosis, risk factors, treatment, evolution, and long-term clinical outcome. *Stroke.* 2006;37:967-972.

Beninati W, Harris CD, Herold DL, Shepard JW Jr. The effect of snoring and obstructive sleep apnea on the sleep quality of bed partners. *Mayo Clin Proc.* 1999;74:955-958.

Berry RB, Block AJ. Positive nasal airway pressure eliminates snoring as well as obstructive sleep apnea. *Chest.* 1984;85:15-20.

Berry RB, Chediak A, Brown LK, et al. Best Clinical Practices for the Sleep Center Adjustment of Noninvasive Positive Pressure Ventilation (NPPV) in Stable Chronic Alveolar Hypoventilation Syndromes. NPPV Titration Task Force of the American Academy of Sleep Medicine. *J Clin Sleep Med.* 2010 Oct 15;6(5):491-509.

Boyd JH, Petrof BJ, Hamid Q, Fraser R, Kimoff RJ. Upper airway muscle inflammation and denervation changes in obstructive sleep apnea. *Am J Respir Crit Care Med.* 2004;170:541-546.

Bratton DJ, Stradling JR, Barbé F, Kohler M. Effect of CPAP on blood pressure in patients with minimally symptomatic obstructive sleep apnoea: a meta-analysis using individual patient data from four randomized controlled trials. *Thorax.* 2014;69:1128-1135.

Carrera M, Barbe F, Sauleda J, Tomas M, Gomez C, Augusti AG. Patients with obstructive sleep apnea exhibit genioglossus dysfunction that is normalized after treatment with continuous positive airway pressure. *Am J Respir Crit Care Med.* 1999;159:1960-1966.

Chirinos JA, Gurubhagavatula I, Teff K, et al. CPAP, weight loss, or both for obstructive sleep apnea. *N Engl J Med.* 2014;370:2265-2275.

Cooke JR, Ayalon L, Palmer BW, et al. Sustained use of CPAP slows deterioration of cognition, sleep, and mood in patients with Alzheimer's disease and obstructive sleep apnea: a preliminary study. *J Clin Sleep Med.* 2009;5:305-309.

Cruz IA, Drummond M, Winck JC. Obstructive sleep apnea symptoms beyond sleepiness and snoring: effects of nasal APAP therapy. *Sleep Breath.* 2012;16:361-366.

Damy T, Margarit L, Noroc A, et al. Prognostic impact of sleep-disordered breathing and its treatment with nocturnal ventilation for chronic heart failure. *Eur J Heart Fail.* 2012;14:1009-1019.

Decreto legge – Recepimento della direttiva della Commissione 2014/85/UE recante modifica della direttiva 2006/126/CE del Parlamento europeo e del Consiglio concernente la patente di guida – del 22 dicembre 2015. GU n. 9 del 13 gennaio 2016. www.gazzettaufficiale.it/eli/id/2016/01/13/16A00299.

Decreto ministeriale – Indirizzi medico-legali da osservare per l'accertamento dell'idoneità alla guida dei soggetti affetti da disturbi del sonno da apnee ostruttive notturne, o sospettati di essere affetti da tale malattia – del 3 febbraio 2016. GU n. 41 del 19 febbraio 2016. www.gazzettaufficiale.it/eli/id/2016/02/19/16A01326.

Donovan LM, Boeder S, Malhotra A, Patel SR. New developments in the use of positive airway pressure for obstructive sleep apnea. *J Thorac Dis.* 2015;7(8):1323-1342.

Dorkova Z, Petrasova D, Molcanyiova A, Popovnakova M, Tkacova R. Effects of continuous positive airway pressure on cardiovascular risk profile in patients with severe obstructive sleep apnea and metabolic syndrome. *Chest.* 2008;134:686-692.

Durán J, Esnaola S, Rubio R, Iztueta A. Obstructive sleep apnea-hypopnea and related clinical features in a population-based sample of subjects aged 30 to 70 yr. *Am J Respir Crit Care Med.* 2001;163(3 Pt 1):685-689.

Esquinas C, Sánchez-de-la Torre M, Aldomá A, et al. Spanish Sleep Network. Rationale and methodology of the impact of continuous positive airway pressure on patients with ACS and nonsleepy OSA: the ISAACC Trial. *Clin Cardiol.* 2013 Sep;36(9):495-501.

Fein AS, Shvilkin A, Shah D, et al. Treatment of obstructive sleep apnea reduces the risk of atrial fibrillation recurrence after catheter ablation. *J Am Coll Cardiol.* 2013;62:300-305.

Friberg D, Ansved T, Borg K, Carlsson-Nordlander B, Larsson H, Svanborg E. Histological indications of a progressive snorers disease in an upper airway muscle. *Am J Respir Crit Care Med.* 1998;157:586-593.

Friberg D, Gazelius B, Hokfelt T, Nordlander B. Abnormal afferent nerve endings in the soft palatal mucosa of sleep apneoics and habitual snorers. *Regul Pept.* 1997;71:29-36.

Garbarino S, Guglielmi O, Sanna A, Mancardi GL, Magnavita N. Risk of occupational accidents in workers with obstructive sleep apnea: systematic review and meta-analysis. *Sleep.* 2016 Feb 29. pii: sp-00566-15. Epub ahead of print.

Garbarino S, Pitidis A, Giustini M, Taggi F, Sanna A. Motor vehicle accidents and obstructive sleep apnea syndrome: A methodology to calculate the related burden of injuries. *Chronic Respiratory Disease.* 2015 Nov;12(4):320-328.

George CFP. Motor vehicle collisions are reduced when sleep apnoea is treated with nasal CPAP. *Thorax.* 2001;56:508-512.

Giles TL, Lasserson TJ, Smith BJ, White J, Wright J, Cates CJ. Continuous positive airways pressure for obstructive sleep apnoea in adults. *Cochrane Database Syst Rev.* 2006;(1):CD001106.

Goncalves MA, Paiva T, Ramos E, Guilleminault C. Obstructive sleep apnea syndrome, sleepiness, and quality of life. *Chest.* 2004;125:2091-2096.

Gottlieb DJ, Yenokyan G, Newman AB, et al. Prospective study of obstructive sleep apnea and incident coronary heart disease and heart failure: the sleep heart health study. *Circulation.* 2010;122:352-360.

Hedner J, Grote L, Bonsignore M, et al. The European Sleep Apnoea Database (ESADA): report from 22 European sleep laboratories. *Eur Respir J.* 2011 Sep;38(3):635-642.

Hoyos CM, Killick R, Yee BJ, Phillips CL, Grunstein RR, Liu PY. Cardiometabolic changes after continuous positive airway pressure for obstructive sleep apnoea: a randomised sham-controlled study. *Thorax.* 2012;67:1081-1089.

Ip S, D'Ambrosio C, Patel K, et al. Auto-titrating versus fixed continuous positive airway pressure for the treatment of obstructive sleep apnea: a systematic review with meta-analyses. *Syst Rev.* 2012;1:20.

Javaheri S. Sleep disorders in systolic heart failure: a prospective study of 100 male patients. The final report. *Int J Cardiol.* 2006; 106, 21-28.

Jordan AS, McSharry DG, Malhotra A. Adult obstructive sleep apnoea. *Lancet.* 2014 Feb 22;383(9918):736-747

Kakkar RK, Berry RB. Positive airway pressure treatment for obstructive sleep apnea. *Chest.* 2007;132:1057-1072.

Kanagala R, Murali NS, Friedman PA, et al. Obstructive sleep apnea and the recurrence of atrial fibrillation. *Circulation.* 2003;107:2589-2594.

Karasulu L, Epöztürk PO, Sökücü SN, Dalar L, Altin S. Improving heart rate variability in sleep apnea patients: differences in treatment with auto-titrating positive airway pressure (APAP) versus conventional CPAP. *Lung.* 2010;188:315-320.

Kasai T, Narui K, Dohi T, et al. Prognosis of patients with heart failure and obstructive sleep apnea treated with continuous positive airway pressure. *Chest.* 2008;133:690-696.

Keenan BT, Maislin G, Sunwoo BY, et al. Obstructive sleep apnoea treatment and fasting lipids: a comparative effectiveness study. *Eur Respir J.* 2014;44:405-414.

Kent BD, Grote L, Ryan S, et al. ESADA collaborators. Diabetes mellitus prevalence and control in sleep-disordered breathing: the European Sleep Apnea Cohort (ESADA) study. *Chest.* 2014 Oct;146(4):982-990.

Kiely JL, McNicholas WT. Cardiovascular risk factors in patients with obstructive sleep apnoea syndrome. *Eur Respir J.* 2000;16:128-133.

Kohler M, Stoewhas AC, Ayers L, et al. Effects of continuous positive airway pressure therapy withdrawal in patients with obstructive sleep apnea: a randomized controlled trial. *Am J Respir Crit Care Med.* 2011;184:1192-1199.

Kushida CA, Chediak A, Berry RB, et al. Clinical Guidelines for the Manual Titration of Positive Airway Pressure in Patients with Obstructive Sleep Apnea. *J Clin Sleep Med.* 2008;4(2):157-171.

Kushida CA, Littner MR, Hirshkowitz M, et al. (American Academy of Sleep Medicine). Practice Parameters for the Use of Continuous and Bilevel Positive Airway Pressure Devices to Treat Adult Patients With Sleep-Related Breathing Disorders. *Sleep.* 2006 Mar 1;29(3):375-380.

Kushida CA, Nichols DA, Holmes TH, et al. Effects of continuous positive airway pressure on neurocognitive function in obstructive sleep apnea patients: The Apnea Positive Pressure Long-term Efficacy Study (APPLES). *Sleep.* 2012;35:1593-1602.

Marcus CL, Brooks LJ, Draper KA, et al. (American Academy of Pediatrics). Diagnosis and management of childhood obstructive sleep apnea syndrome. *Pediatrics.* 2012;130(3):576-584.

Marin JM, Agusti A, Villar I, et al. Association between treated and untreated obstructive sleep apnea and risk of hypertension. JAMA. 2012;307:2169-2176.

McEvoy RD. Obstructive sleep apnoea and hypertension: the ESADA study. *Eur Respir J.* 2014 Oct;44(4):835-838.

Mooe T, Rabben T, Wiklund U, Franklin KA, Eriksson P. Sleep-disordered breathing in men with coronary artery disease. *Chest.* 1996a;109:659-663.

Mooe T, Rabben T, Wiklund U, Franklin KA, Eriksson P. Sleep-disordered breathing in women: occurrence and association with coronary artery disease. *Am J Med.* 1996b;101:251-256.

Morgenthaler TI, Aurora RN, Brown T, et al. Standards of Practice Committee of the AASM; American Academy of Sleep Medicine. Practice Parameters for the Use of Autotitrating Continuous Positive Airway Pressure Devices for Titrating Pressures and Treating Adult Patients with Obstructive Sleep Apnea Syndrome: An Update for 2007. *Sleep.* 2008 Jan 1;31(1):141-147.

Myhill PC, Davis WA, Peters KE, Chubb SAP, Hillman D, Davis TME. Effect of continuous positive airway pressure therapy on cardiovascular risk factors in patients with type 2 diabetes and obstructive sleep apnea. *J Clin Endocrinol Metab.* 2012;97:4212-4218.

Nadeem R, Singh M, Nida M, et al. Effect of obstructive sleep apnea hypopnea syndrome on lipid profile: a metaregression analysis. *J Clin Sleep Med.* 2014;10:475-489.

Naruse Y, Tada H, Satoh M, et al. Concomitant obstructive sleep apnea increases the recurrence of atrial fibrillation following radiofrequency catheter ablation of atrial fibrillation: clinical impact of continuous positive airway pressure therapy. *Heart Rhythm.* 2013;10:331-337.

Parati G, Lombardi C, Hedner J, et al. (EU COST Action B26 members). Recommendations for the management of patients with obstructive sleep apnoea and hypertension. *Eur Respir J.* 2013 Mar;41(3):523-538.

Parra O, Arboix A, Bechich S, et al. Time course of sleep-related breathing disorders in first-ever stroke or transient ischemic attack . *Am J Respir Crit Care Med.* 2000;161:375-380.

Parra O, Sánchez-Armengol A, Bonnin M, et al. Early treatment of obstructive apnoea and stroke outcome: a randomised controlled trial. *Eur Respir J.* 2011;37:1128-1136.

Pasterkamp H, Schäfer J, Wodicka GR. Posture dependent change of tracheal sounds at standardized flows in patients with obstructive sleep apnea. *Chest.* 1996;110:1493-1498.

Patruno V, Aiolfi S, Costantino G, et al. Fixed and autoadjusting continuous positive airway pressure treatment are non similar in reducing cardiovascular risk factors in patient with obstructive sleep apnea. *Chest.* 2007;131:1393-1399.

Peker Y, Glantz H, Thunström E, Kallryd A, Herlitz J, Ejdebäck J. Rationale and design of the Randomized Intervention with CPAP in Coronary Artery Disease and Sleep Apnoea—RICCADSA trial. *Scand Cardiovasc J.* 2009;43:24-31.

Peker Y, Kraiczi H, Hedner J, Loth S, Johansson A, Bende M. An independent association between obstructive sleep apnoea and coronary artery disease. *Eur Respir J.* 1999;14:179-184.

Peppard PE, Young T, Palta M, Dempsey J, Skatrud J. Prospective study of the association between sleep-disordered breathing and hypertension. *N Engl J Med.* 2000;342:1378-1384.

Phillips CL, Yee BJ, Marshall NS, Liu PY, Sullivan DR, Grunstein RR. Continuous positive airway pressure reduces postprandial lipidemia in obstructive sleep apnea: a randomized, placebo controlled crossover trial. *Am J Respir Crit Care Med.* 2011;184:355-361.

Planès C, D'Ortho MP, Foucher A, et al. Efficacy and cost of home-initiated auto-nCPAP versus conventional nCPAP. *Sleep.* 2003;26:156-160.

Pratt-Ubunama MN, Nishizaka MK, Boedefeld RL, Cofield SS, Harding SM, Calhoun DA. Plasma aldosterone is related to severity of obstructive sleep apnea in subjects with resistant hypertension. *Chest.* 2007;131:453-459.

Punjabi NM, Caffo1 BS, Goodwin JL, et al. *Sleep-Disordered Breathing and Mortality: A Prospective Cohort Study PLos Med.* August 18, 2009. http://dx.doi.org/10.1371/journal.pmed.1000132.

Ramar K, Dort LC, Katz SG, et al. Clinical Practice Guideline for the Treatment of Obstructive Sleep Apnea and Snoring with Oral Appliance Therapy: An Update for 2015. *J Clin Sleep Med.* 2015 Jul 15;11(7):773-827.

Redline S, Yenokyan G, Gottlieb DJ, Shahar E, O'Connor GT. Obstructive sleep apnea-hypopnea and incident stroke: the sleep heart health study. *Am J Respir Crit Care Med.* 2010;182:269-277.

Ryan CM, Bayley M, Green R, Murray BJ, Bradley TD. Influence of continuous positive airway pressure on outcomes of rehabilitation in stroke patients with obstructive sleep apnea. *Stroke.* 2011;42:1062-1067.

Ryan CM, Floras JS, Logan AG, et al. CANPAP Investigators. Shift in sleep apnoea type in heart failure patients in the CANPAP trial. *Eur Respir J.* 2010 Mar;35(3):592-597.

Sanna A, Bellofiore S, Di Michele L, Marino L, Toraldo D. *Indicazioni per la diagnosi e cura della sindrome delle apnee ostruttive del sonno nell'adulto.* Documento dell'Associazione Scientifica Interdisciplinare per lo studio delle Malattie Respiratorie (AIMAR). www.aimarnet.it. 2014.

Sanna A. Obstructive sleep apnoea, motor vehicle accidents, and work performance. *Chronic Respiratory Disease.* 2013;10:29-33.

Sanner BM, Konermann M, Doberauer C, Weiss T, Zidek W. Sleep disordered breathing in patients referred for angina evaluation-association with left ventricular dysfunction. *Clin Cardiol.* 2001;24:146-150.

Schwab RJ, Badr SM, Epstein LJ, et al. On behalf of the ATS Subcommittee on CPAP Adherence Tracking Systems. An Official American Thoracic Society Statement: Continuous Positive Airway Pressure Adherence Tracking Systems. The Optimal Monitoring Strategies and Outcome Measures in Adults. *Am J Respir Crit Care Med.* 2013;188(5):613-620.

Schwab RJ, Pack AI, Gupta KB, et al. Upper airway and soft tissue structural changes induced by CPAP in normal subjects. *Am J Respir Crit Care Med.* 1996;154:1106-1116.

Seneviratne U, Puvanendran K. Excessive daytime sleepiness in obstructive sleep apnea: prevalence, severity, and predictors. *Sleep Med.* 2004;5:339-343.

Strohl KP, Brown DB, Collop N, et al. ATS Ad Hoc Committee on Sleep Apnea, Sleepiness, and Driving Risk in Noncommercial Drivers. An official American Thoracic Society Clinical Practice Guideline: sleep apnea, sleepiness, and driving risk in noncommercial drivers. An update of a 1994 Statement. *Am J Respir Crit Care Med.* 2013 Jun 1;187(11):1259-1266.

Strohl KP, Redline S. Recognition of obstructive sleep apnea. *Am J Respir Crit Care Med.* 1996;154:279-289.

Sullivan CE, Issa FG, Berthon-Jones M, Eves L. Reversal of obstructive sleep apnoea by continuous positive airway pressure applied through the nares. *Lancet.* 1981 Apr 18;1(8225):862-865.

Surendra KS, Agrawal A, Damodaran D, et al. CPAP for the Metabolic Syndrome in Patients with Obstructive Sleep Apnea. *N Engl J Med.* 2011;365:2277-2286.

Teschler H, Berthon-Jones M, Thompson AB, Henkel A, Henry J, Konietzko N. Automated continuous positive airway pressure titration for obstructive sleep apnea syndrome. *Am J Respir Crit Care Med.* 1996;154:734-740.

Teschler H, Dohring J, Wang Y, Berthon-Jones M. Adaptive Pressure Support Servo-Ventilation. *Am J Respir Crit Care Med.* 2001;164(4):614-619.

WEAVER TE, MANCINI C, MAISLIN G, ET AL. Continuous positive airway pressure treatment of sleepy patients with milder obstructive sleep apnea: results of the CPAP Apnea Trial North American Program (CATNAP) randomized clinical trial. *Am J Respir Crit Care Med.* 2012;186:677–683.

WEINSTOCK TG, WANG X, RUESCHMAN M, ET AL. A controlled trial of CPAP therapy on metabolic control in individuals with impaired glucose tolerance and sleep apnea. *Sleep.* 2012;35:617–625.

WOZNIAK DR, LASSERSON TJ, SMITH I. Educational, supportive and behavioural interventions to improve usage of continuous positive airway pressure machines in adults with obstructive sleep apnoea. *Cochrane Database Syst Rev.* 2014;1:CD007736.

YUMINO D, WANG H, FLORAS JS, ET AL. Prevalence and physiological predictors of sleep apnea in patients with heart failure and systolic dysfunction. *J Card Fail.* 2009;15:279–285.

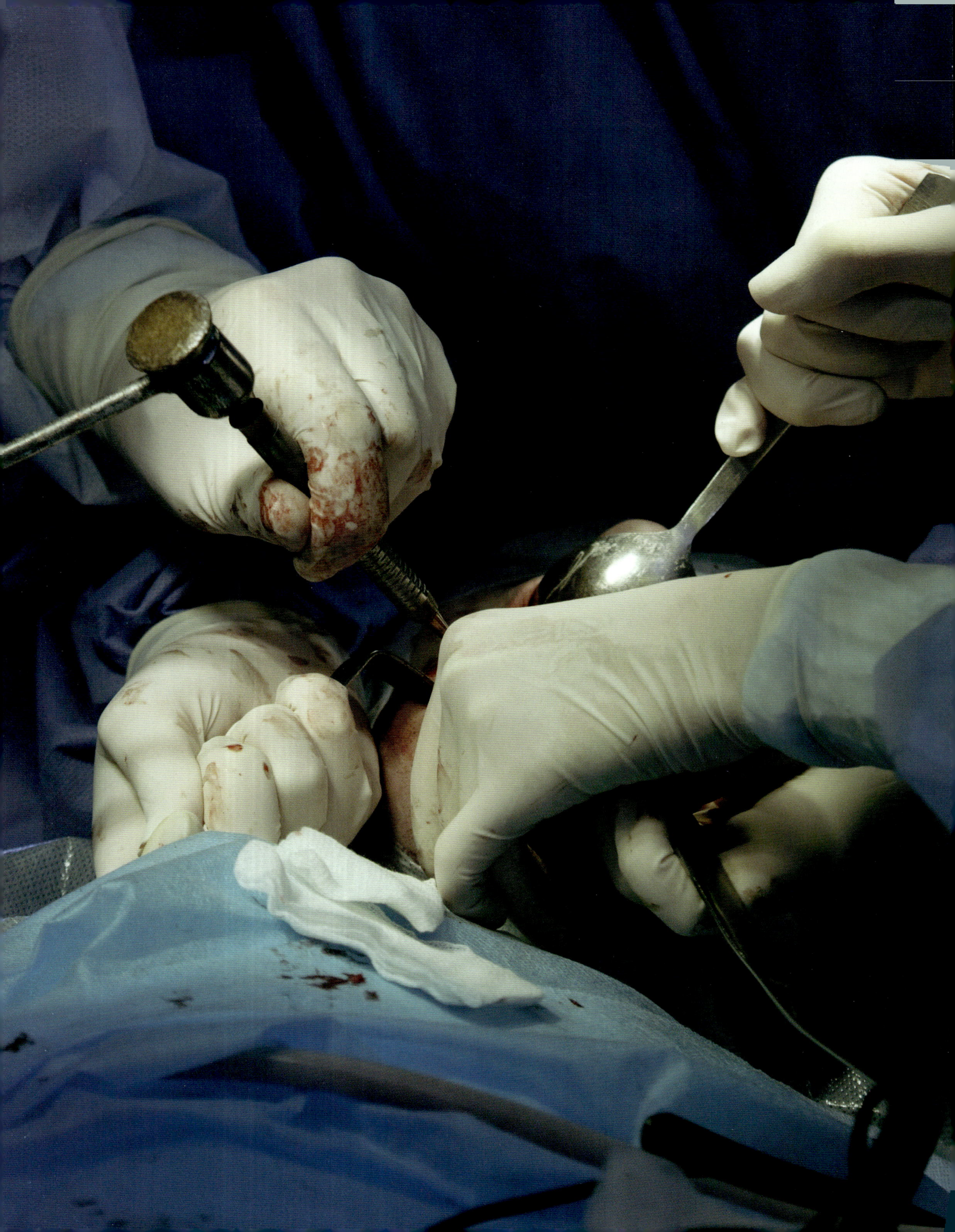

Maxillofacial surgical therapy

Bruno Carlo Brevi · Chiara Copelli · Alberto Di Blasio · Chiara Di Blasio · Francesco Giovacchini

Objectives

- To explain the indications for the use of this method in OSAS management
- To define the physiomechanic basis of the mechanism of surgery
- To explain how to proceed with surgery planning by identifying the most adequate diagnostic tools to be used
- To describe differences between maxillary deformity surgery and maxillomandibular advancement in terms of planning and accomplishing
- To describe the principles of osteodistraction and its role in accomplishing maxillary advancement

Brief history

Surgical therapies for OSAS originated before CPAP, which dates back to 1981, when Sullivan and collaborators tested it for the first time. Tracheostomy had already been employed since 1969. In 1979, Kuo and collaborators described the outcomes of mandibular advancement for the treatment of OSAS through the evaluation of polysomnographic parameters and subjective sleepiness in three patients with OSAS associated with retrognathia who were subjected to this intervention. In the 1980s, isolated mandibular advancement was replaced by combined superior maxilla repositioning and mandibular advancement such that normal maxillomandibular relations and, consequently, dental occlusion could be maintained. Furthermore, this combination amplified functional respiratory outcomes by displacing forward the soft palate and increasing the naso-oropharyngeal volume. Over time, this technique was applied and described by several authors as showing particularly positive functional outcomes (Waite *et al.* 1989; Riley *et al.* 1993; Hochban *et al.* 1997; Prinsell *et al.* 1999). For analyses of results, one of the most complete studies on recommendations for non-CPAP therapies was published by a task force designated for this project by the European Respiratory Society (ERS) (Randerath *et al.* 2011).

Review of reports available in the literature reinstated the efficacy of maxillomandibular advancement (MMA) comparable to that of CPAP in young subjects without particularly excesses of BMI or lung comorbidities.

Indications

Literature reports several indications for the surgical treatment of OSAS (Riley *et al.* 1993; Prinsell 2002; Costello and Posnick 2003). At the beginning, MMA was reserved for patients affected by dysmorphism; however, over time, the indication has been extended to morphic patients as well. This type of facial conformation complicates the planning as it is based on a subtle balance between the necessity of advancing "as much as possible" and maintaining valid aesthetics. According to majority of the authors, this surgical modality is indicated for patients with moderate-to-severe OSAS who cannot adapt to and/or tolerate treatment with CPAP. Particular attention should be paid when dealing with obese patients. In fact, without significant weight loss, the advancement is aggravated by a high risk of partially positive outcomes (7.1).

Mechanism of action

The surgical procedure is aimed at eliminating obstructive apneas is MMA (7.1). The resolution of the obstructive events is linked primarily to the man-

7.1 Maxillomandibular advancement (MMA).

Description	Surgically superior repositioning of the maxilla combined with mandibular advancement
Indications	Patients with moderate-to-severe OSAS who cannot adapt well to and/or tolerate CPAP treatment
BMI	Particular attention should be paid when dealing with obese patients. Without significant weight loss, the advancement is aggravated by a high risk of partially positive outcomes
Advantages	One-time therapy, not affected by patient's compliance Positive modification of the facial aesthetics in retrognathic and biretruded patients
Disadvantages	A potentially unfavorable modification of the facial aesthetic may limit its indication
Technique of execution	Bilateral mandibular sagittal osteotomy Maxillary osteotomy Le Fort I

dible's forward displacement and, hence, to the insertion of different muscles, including the anterior belly of the digastric muscle, mylohyoid muscle, genioglossus, and geniohyoid muscles. All these muscles help bring the tongue forward to increase the retrolingual air space.
In addition to the mandible, the superior maxilla is advanced, with consequent advancement of the insertion line/origin of the soft palate to achieve a similar effect to that obtained with lateral pharyngoplasty (Pang).
On the contrary to ENT surgical methods that correct the structures of the oropharyngeal cavity (tongue, soft palate, tonsils, and uvula, among others), MMA modifies of the oropharyngeal cavity through the expansion of bone structures that constitute the facial skeleton.

In the first case, if the result is strongly influenced by the healing and scarring processes of the affected soft tissues, then in the second case, the stability

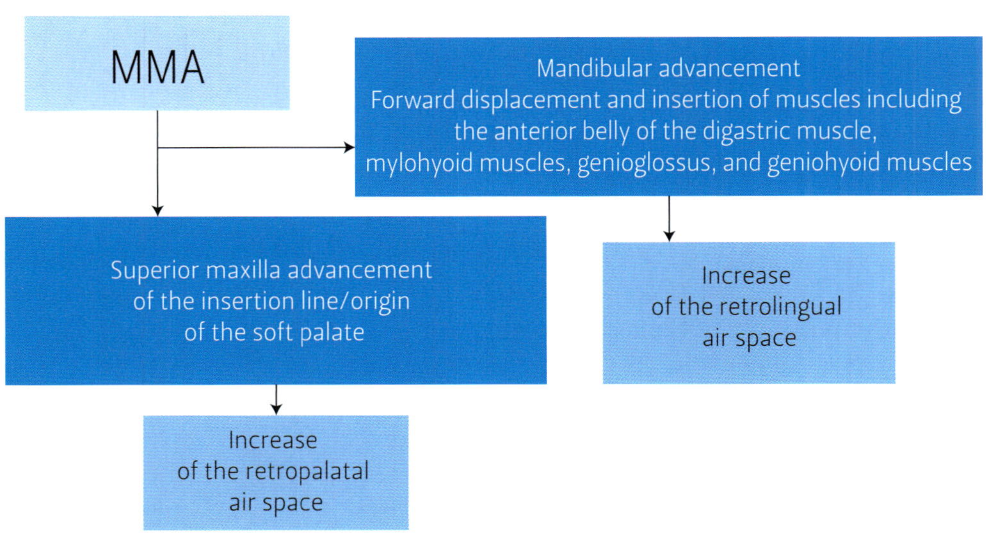

7.1 Bimaxillary advancement: mechanism of action.

and fixation of the involved areas allow for achieving objectives pre-set during planning and better predicting results in the long term. In addition to purely volumetric increases, great functional results are achieved via contracting the aponeurotic muscle structures (and, consequently, the lining mucosa), which constitute the lateral pharyngeal wall. This explains why obstructions due to the fall of the base of the tongue as well as those due to the collapse of the lateral pharyngeal walls are managed with MMA.

Planning

Role of aesthetics in the treatment of OSAS

The aim of MMA in the treatment of OSAS is not to correct facial dysmorphism but to counteract the potentially mortal consequences of night apneas.

Although MMA has been proven to increase the superior air space, the mathematical correlation between the achieved bimaxillary advancement and increase in the dimensions of the upper airways has not yet been identified. Additionally, identifying a threshold value for the airways dimension with corresponding resolution of the clinical situation remains impossible. Furthermore, possible measurements can become even less predictable due to tensioning of the pharyngeal soft tissues, which significantly contributes to preventing nocturnal obstructions.

For this reason, it is normally recommended to advance the mandible as much as possible while maintaining the occlusion and acceptable aesthetics. In addition, a minimal mandibular advancement of at least 10 mm is commonly accepted.

Therefore, we can affirm that the primary limit of this solution is represented by aesthetics. If (and this happens in majority of the cases) a patient exhibits a mandibular retrusion (or, even better, a maxillomandibular biretrusion), this is not a problem as the advancement is both a functional solution (correcting apneas) and an aesthetic improvement associated with a rejuvenating effect (similar to a facelift) due to the disappearance of wrinkles and double chin linked to the contracting of facial soft tissues.

The opposite situation occurs when a patient exhibits normal occlusion or prognathism. In such a case, it is more difficult, if not impossible, to execute MMA while maintaining valid aesthetics.

Role of cephalometric in the treatment of OSAS

The shape of the craniofacial structure can be considered merely a predisposing factor to OSAS. Thus, cephalometry is not indicated to confirm a diagnostic suspicion. Rather, it plays a more important role in

- **providing indications for MMA.** Cephalometry is one of the analyses that can determine indications for MMA when associated with a complete diagnostic framework.
- **planning the intervention.** Planning of MMA in a patient affected by OSAS is not aimed at improving the facial aesthetics but at preventing it from worsening. In the surgical planning phase, it is useful to confirm with the clinician that the project of modification will not go beyond the limits of the structural norm. However, how the structural norm is then translated into a fairly valid facial aesthetic is left to the clinical sense of the surgeon.

Briefly, cephalometry is considered useful in the treatment of patients with OSAS; however, it is recommended to use it rationally and correctly without expecting it to answer what it cannot.

Furthermore, it should be considered that cephalometry

- is a bidimensional evaluation and does not define the transversal width of the airways
- is executed in an awake state, namely at a time when the disorder does not appear

Role of three-dimensional imaging in diagnostics

Through three-dimensional visualization of CT images, it is possible to accurately analyze the air space and determine its volume, with specific measurements feasible in all directions of the space, to understand its development and possible anomalies. This type of imaging allows for a more immediate and direct visualization of the air space than does bidimensional type and can be a vital aid for surgeons, even though it is still an image statically depicting a situation occurring in a wake state without providing any information on the state of tension of the pharyngeal structures or their degree of collapsibility.

CTs are generally executed on the facial and neck skeletons without any contrast medium. The patients are subjected to examination in the supine position with their head in a natural position. Since the volume of the pharyngeal airways changes during breathing, through certain modern radiographic techniques, it is possible to execute dynamic scanning of the same anatomical segment. The images of the transverse section of the airway area at the oropharyngeal and hypopharyngeal sites are obtained in any phase of normal breathing, at the end of a forced inspiration or forced expiration.

The most frequently considered parameters include:

- the transverse section of the retrolingual space, which can be measured by selecting an axial image at the level of the cervicomandibular ring, immediately above the tip of the epiglottis and below the tip of the uvula

- the minimal retropalatal surface, which can be measured in the same way at the level of the axial image of the soft palate
- the height of the respiratory passages
- the maximum anteroposterior diameter
- the maximum lateral diameter between the base of the epiglottis and the soft palate, as measured in the section
- the distance between the posterior nasal spine and the base of the epiglottis
- the length of the neck and laryngeal space, which can be measured using a combination of axial and lateral images of the space included between the foramen magnum, the superior limit of the neck, and the superior limit of the thorax, as identified by the superior pulmonary apex

Visualization of the airways is more direct and easily measurable through three-dimensional reconstruction of CT images of the hard and soft tissues. In recent times, much progress has been made in terms of image-based surgical planning software, which represents a valid tool for surgeons for diagnosis, treatment planning, and possible evaluation of the final results.

This software allows for determining the planned skeletal movements by simulating of the movements of the upper soft tissues and, consequently, the resulting aesthetic effect. The simulation of the change of soft tissues results is more precise but, unfortunately, not yet completely reliable.

Surgical therapy

MMA is executed with a maxillary section reproducing the fracture lines known as "Le Fort I" (7.2), a sagittal mandibular section of the rami (7.3), and repositioning all forward. At the end of this procedure, the displacement of the bone segments is stabilized with screws or plates. Intervention with

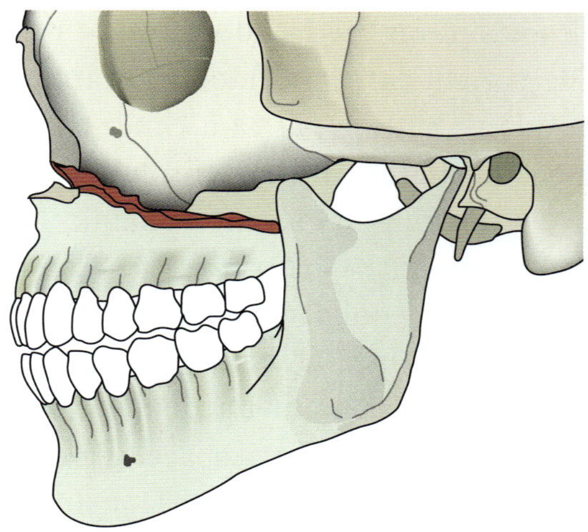

7.2 Le Fort I osteotomy (Modified from Brusati and Sesenna, 1988).

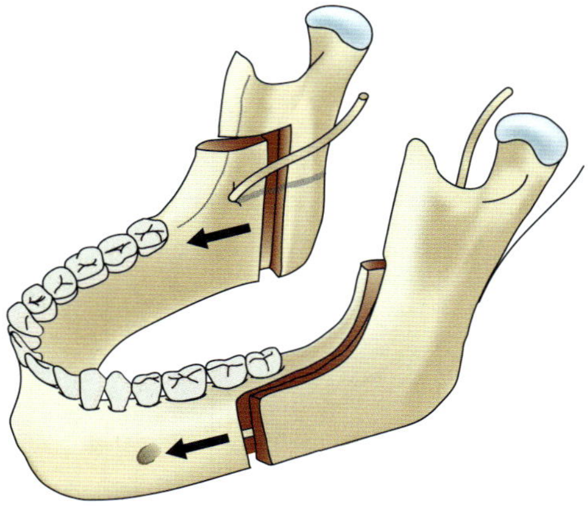

7.3 Mandibular sagittal osteotomy (Modified from Brusati and Sesenna, 1988).

MMA is frequently associated with advancement genioplasty (7.4) aimed at increasing the tension of the genioglossus muscle.
Such procedures were initially devised and expanded to correct maxillomandibular discrepancies with a fundamentally occlusal and aesthetic effect. Only later were they adapted for the management of apneic patients.

Tables 7.2 and 7.3 thoroughly describe the surgical techniques, which do not differ much from the overall standardized technique applied for facial dysmorphic features. Later, we will analyze some technical planning particularities that, according to the authors, may simplify the application of the technique to apneic subjects for the operators.

Bilateral sagittal mandibular osteotomy is described in Tabella 7.2, whereas the technical phases of the maxilla Le Fort 1 osteotomy, which was executed for the first time by Wassmund in 1927 and better defined by Obwegeser in 1969, are illustrated in Tabella 7.3.

In addition to the so-defined classic osteotomy procedure, the authors have adopted certain planning and feasible adjustments to obtain extreme bimaxillary advancement without jeopardizing the aesthetic result.

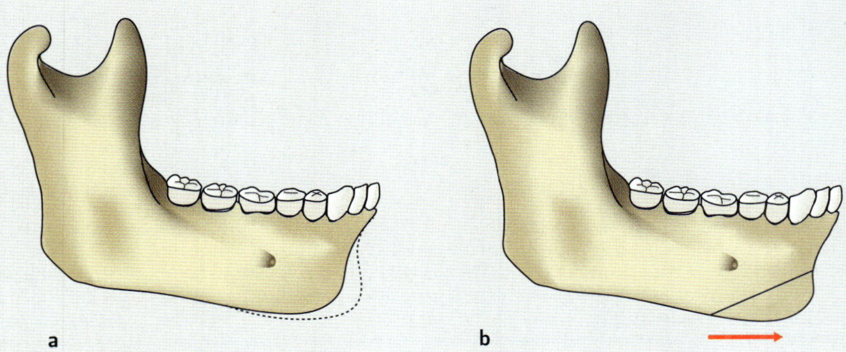

7.4 Advancement genioplasty (Modified from Brusati and Sesenna, 1988).

7.2 Bilateral sagittal mandibular osteotomy: Surgical technique.

1. Infiltration with vasoconstrictor
2. Incision on the anterior surface of the mandibular ramus, starting from the corner and extending downward in the proximity of the second premolar tooth
3. Lateral and medial subperiostal dissection (leaving the masseter muscle inserted)
4. Section of the mandibular cortical bone, starting on the medial side above the mandibular foramen, proceeding downward on the anterior portion of the ramus until reaching the superior part of the mandibular body, and then turning between 6° and 7° on the lateral cortex until reaching the interior edge
5. Splitting the bone stumps
6. Research and visualization of the inferior alveolar nerve block
7. The same procedure must be executed counter laterally
8. Positioning and fixation of the bone segments through two titanium miniplates and monocortical screws. Alternatively, the stabilization can be performed with bicortical transfixed screws (without the miniplate aid); however, considering the entity of advancement, the authors prefer to use two plates per side

The currently employed adjustments include:

- exploitation of the counter-clockwise rotation of the occlusal plan
- use of an inverted planning scheme and a feasible sequence of osteotomies
- mandibular fixation with a double miniplate for each side
- development of management strategies for the original occlusion of the patient
- modification of genioplasty (AIMO type) described by Prinsell

7.3 Maxilla Le Fort I osteotomy: Surgical technique.

1. Infiltration with vasoconstrictor
2. Incision on the vestibule above the mucogingival junction. This incision is made from the first molar on one side to the counter lateral one
3. Subperiosteal dissection of the maxillary anterior and lateral surfaces
4. Exposition of the piriform aperture and subperiosteal separation of the floor of the nose
5. Osteotomy (pterygomaxillary junction, base of zygomatic process of maxilla, lateral maxillary wall, canine fossa, and anterior nasal aperture): during this phase, particular care must be taken in order to not damage the apices of teeth
6. Section of the foot of nasal septum
7. Positioning metallic thread through the nasal spine to allow the following maxillary traction
8. Completing osteotomy by disconnecting the maxilla from the pterygoid processes through a curved osteotome
9. Maxilla downfracturing with digital pressure
10. After the maxilla has been mobilized, it is repositioned and fixed with four titanium plates. In case of important advancement, the bone gap is filled with bone inserts. Sometimes, to optimize the occlusal relation, segmental osteotomy dividing the maxilla into two or more fragments must be performed. Such subdivision generally requires an anterior fragment including canines and incisors and two posterior fragments including premolars and molars

Role of the counter-clockwise rotation of the occlusal plane

Patients affected with OSAS do not always present with facial dysmorphism involving both maxillae. Mandibular underdevelopment often corresponds with a normally developed maxilla. Maxillary advancement is performed to restore the occlusion (modified by mandibular osteotomy), and this may involve an anti-aesthetic result. In the case of a clear Class II malocclusion, it is generally preferable to correct it to a Class I so that it is possible to further advance the mandible compared with the maxilla and, thus, optimize both the mandibular advancement and aesthetic results.

In a case wherein it is required to obtain mandibular advancement without any defect of the maxillary position in the sagittal plane, it is possible to increase the posterior height and/or diminish the anterior height of the superior maxilla, determining a counter-clockwise rotation of the occlusal plane and, thus, achieving mandibular advancement. All this occurs with minimal or no maxillary sagittal displacements. In these cases, the need to resolve the apneic situation in the presence of malocclusion would involve mandibular advancement with maxillary protrusion, which is not considered aesthetically flattering.

By exploiting the counter-clockwise rotation of the occlusal plane, it is possible to limit and, in some cases, to avoid the negative impacts on the aesthetics and occlusion of the maxillary advancement without reducing the efficacy of MMA in terms of increased dimensions of the upper airways.

Inverted planning

In case of bimaxillary osteotomy, surgery for facial dysmorphism has been traditionally preferred by first proceeding with the osteotomy and repositioning of the superior maxillary, followed by those of the mandible.

Inverted planning involves mainly an inversion of this order; hence, the procedure is mandible repositioning (with fixation) followed by maxillary repositioning.

Such modification restores the central role of the mandible on the aesthetic evaluation of complex and extreme movements that must be executed to correct OSAS. The essential leading precept in selecting the method of mandibular advancement is simply "the maximum that can be achieved compatibly with a valid aesthetic."

This procedure allows for the visualization of the aesthetic result before sectioning/dissecting of the maxilla. By itself, this is not a negligible element at all, considering the mean entity of the executed advancement.

Maxillary advancement is simulated by placing a resin prop below the superior lip, which reproduces the desired advancement and is manufactured in the preoperative phase. In case of pre-operation doubts regarding the possible aesthetic result, two or three alternative advancements are planned with their related splints to be tested during the intervention. Once the preferred aesthetic result is obtained, it is possible to proceed with maxillary osteotomic intervention.

Furthermore, mandibular advancement as the first phase simplifies the achievement of a reliable (stable at awakening) intra-operatory occlusion. The tensioning of muscle-tendon structures causes important repositioning of the condyles in the fossae, and the original fixation of the mandible enables its repositioning in three-dimension. The maxilla is then adapted to this position.

Monocortical rigid fixation with double plate

Initially, one of the main problems related to mandibular advancement surgery was the high percentage of relapse, and great instability during the operation and the period following the removal of the intra-maxillary block was one of the main causes.

Therefore, rigid fixation (RF) now plays a fundamental role in guaranteeing an adequate result in both the short and long term. If executed in a particularly stable way, it allows for the removal of the rigid intermaxillary block (RIB) before awakening the patient and, most of the time, even for the avoidance of the use of guiding elastics in the post-operatory phase, with consequent improvements of the mandibular-motor recovery, comfort, nutrition, speech, hygiene, and safety.

Mandibular double plate is the method of fixation that guarantees the most stability in important advancements, as it occurs in the management of OSAS. To position the inferior plate, an angular screwdriver is particularly helpful.

Modified genioplasty

The logical basis of applying genioplasty in the treatment of OSAS stems from the fact that the genioglossus and geniohyoid muscles insert in the mental spine or on its doubling/splitting apophysis geni, which are located on the internal side of the mandibular symphysis. The advancement of this bone segment determines the extent of stretching of the muscles that are inserted on it, resulting in forward movement of the hyoid bone and the base of the tongue. This determines the increase in the anteroposterior dimension of the upper airways. This effect promotes the effect of mandibular advancement; therefore, vertical advancement genioplasty (including the mental spine) is considered an integral part of MMA in OSAS today.

Even in patients whose chin is normally shaped, it is possible to execute advancement genioplasty without causing aesthetic deformities as long as the osteotomy is preceded by the removal of the chin's outer cortex and medulla. The residual internal cortex is dissected, advanced, and fixed to the outer cortex of the symphyseal segment holding the teeth.

Removal of the outer cortex (and a variable portion of the medulla) allows for limiting/eliminating the advancement of the mental soft tissue, whereas advancement of the internal cortex allows for the stretching of the genioglossus and geniohyoid muscles to maintain its efficacy.

Complications

The complications of maxillomandibular surgery overlap those of orthognathic surgery. Abnormal fractures hemorrhage, and infections may complicate the intervention or occur in the immediate postoperative phase; however, they are very rare.

On the contrary, anomalies affecting the temporomandibular joints and inferior alveolar nerve are more frequent. Moderate entity pain and clicks affecting the TM joint are almost always present, although they are generally temporary. They occur due to the tensioning of the over-hyoid muscle-tendon structures with consequent increase of the joint load.

Additionally, the alveolar nerve is subjected to tension because of mandibular elongation with consequent anesthesia of the chin region. Generally, total recovery (or subtotal [paresthesia]) of its function is observed as long as certain limits are not exceeded (12–13-mm elongation).

Osteodistraction and OSAS

The problem of MMA with OSAS lies in the difficulty to execute important advancements. Sometimes, it may be necessary to perform mandibular advancement until 20 mm or even longer. Using the method described above, the achievement of advancement of such an entity may involve some problems including:

- technical execution difficult to implement
- not always predictable occlusion stability during the post-operatory period
- strong stretching of the inferior alveolar nerve (and correlated ischemia), with consequent negative influence on functional recovery. It has, in fact, been reported that mandibular advancements over 12–13-mm difficulty allow for the complete recovery of the inferior lip sensitivity.

Such problems can be overcome by adopting distraction osteogenesis. Patients with severe hypoplasia of the mandibular ramus and body require advancements over 13-14mm; in this case, it is possible to proceed with a mandibular elongation until 35–40 mm while preserving the function of the alveolar nerve by slowly and gradually elongation.

Distraction osteogenesis is a surgical technique using the capability of the bone to regenerate between bone surfaces separated by a gradual elongation.

Planning and surgical technique

To study the mandibular shape (especially the height of the ramus) and estimate the posterior facial height, one must always take into account the clinical aspects (aesthetic and occlusal), radiographic (OPT and teleradiography) evaluation, and models based on the articulator.

This study aims to determine the position of the osteotomy line and, thus, of the distraction device and to establish the necessary inclination to determine the vector of distraction corresponding to the planned advancement. The use of bidirectional distraction appliances permits small degrees of error. In fact, the direction of the vector can be slightly modified during the procedure of distraction.

Compared with the standard osteodistraction techniques, which require a full osteotomy of the mandibular ramus, the authors prefer to execute sagittal osteotomy of the rami. This differs from the classic osteotomy used in dysmorphism osteotomy (Obwegeser Dal Pont), since the outer cortex is implying the angle of the mandible to obtain both sagittal and vertical increases. The vectors of action of the two distraction devices must be parallel to each other as well as to the median line passing through the chin on the transversal plane, representing the vector of distraction.

The distraction devices are activated intra-operationally until an elongation of 8–10 mm is obtained. This has the double objective of immediately increasing the retrolingual airspace (though only partially) and reducing the time of postoperative distraction. The immediate elongation is allowed by the fact that via executing a sagittal section of the ramus, no void space is created during the distraction, so there are two gliding bone surfaces.

Later, during the postoperative course, another elongation of 1 mm a day is performed. Such a procedure is pursued at the patient's home until the maximum possible advancement is reached (dictated by aesthetic and/or mechanical limits) and evaluated with periodical controls. Superior maxillary advancement should correspond with mandibular elongation.

Traditionally, the distraction was always followed by a 2-month consolidation phase to allow for the ossification of the bone callus. In patients with OSAS, it is preferable to eliminate this waiting time for two main reasons:

1. Marked mandibular protrusion with the corresponding occlusal discrepancy performed for the distraction generates significant aesthetic and functional problems (difficult or impossible chewing).
2. Immediate removal of the distraction devices allows one to take advantage of the elasticity of the newly formed bone callus to optimize the mandibular position. In this way, it is then possible to correct possible imperfections concerning the mandibular angles, the chin median, or the occlusal plane line.

For these reasons, the distraction devices are immediately removed at the end of the distraction period, and the mandible is fixed with two plates per side.

Contextually, after the mandibular stabilization, the maxillary advancement osteotomy is then executed according to the Le Fort 1 definition. Due to the nature of the advancement, it is often necessary to insert bone grafts in the obtained gap.

The planning of the second surgical phase consists of using models that are re-applied on the articulator at the end of the distraction. The maxillary will result from its starting point, whereas the mandibular position will be determined through a new wax bite. The position of the maxillary is studied to simulate the necessary movement required to obtain the desired occlusion.

Two factors must always be considered while planning the extension of the maxillary movement:

- mechanical limitation (about 13 mm) due to the palatine arteries;
- the possibility of an unsatisfactory aesthetic result due to excessive advancement.

Therefore, once the necessary entity of the maxillary advancement to the occlusal restoration has been established, this is compared with the aesthetic analysis of the patient.

In cases wherein the optimal occlusion requires an excessive maxillary advancement, it is possible to execute a dentoalveolar retraction osteotomy on the lower incisor level. Such a procedure aims to reduce the maxillary advancement, which is necessary for the occlusal restoration. However, if the limit is due to the traction of the palatine arteries, the problem is solved with some technical devices enabling binding without running the risk of necrosis of the maxillary itself.

The technical particularities described above allow to deal with problems correlated with the use of the classical osteodistraction method.

For instance, the execution of a sagittal osteotomy (rather than the classic full section of the two cortexes) of the rami from the Spix spine to the mandibular angle bisector results in two surfaces of contact between the bone stumps, thus enabling the intra-operative start of the distraction without creating a void. This shortens the time of distraction and, in particular, immediately increases the posterior airspace, benefiting the patient and preventing respiratory problems in the postoperative period. The dissection of the outer cortex is performed much later, and it also allows for increases of the posterior facial height to be obtained.

The immediate removal of distraction devices at the end of the distraction can shorten the total time of the procedure (duration of the classic procedure is about 80 days, while duration of the procedure with the modified technique is about 20 days) and take advantage of the "floating bone" phenomenon to both optimize the mandibular positioning and correct possible anomalies due to imperfect positioning of the distraction devices.

7.4 Osteodistraction versus mandibular sagittal osteotomy.

	Advantages
Osteodistraction	Minor injury affecting the alveolar nerve Major entity of obtainable advancement A more stable result on the treatment of OSAS Adjustable aesthetic result Possibility of planning two separated surgical times Possible reduction of the risk of condylar resorption
Classic technique:	Only one surgical time It does not require the compliance of the patience in managing distraction device

The advantages of osteodistraction and the classic technique are listed in Tabella 7.4.

Occlusion

It may seem that the authors consider the role of occlusion in patients with OSAS as a minor collateral problem. The reason for this likely relies on the fact that the objective of maxillary surgery in OSAS is not to correct dento-skeletal malformations but to eliminate apneas and avoid their complications. In lifesaving surgery, certain not-insignificant problems become less important.

Typically, the aim is to keep the original individual occlusion, except when it affects the final result in a particularly negative way.

Role of orthodontics in pre-surgery

In orthognathic surgery and surgery for patients with OSAS, pre-surgical orthodontic preparation plays an important role in the optimization of the dental arches, often allowing for a major mandibular advancement (Riley *et al.* 1987; Riley *et al.* 1993, Timer, 1996). The orthodontic preparation may enable the planning of a more efficacious intervention, but it significantly delays the surgical time, involving a considerable biological cost to the patients if they are left without adequate therapy for OSAS. It is possible to plan an orthodontic treatment before surgery only for patients who are willing to start or continue treatment with CPAP while waiting for the surgery.

Otherwise, it is preferable not to proceed with pre-surgical orthodontics and not to correct the Class I occlusions and all malocclusions that do not interfere with the mandibular advancement, thus reserving the occlusion surgical correction and/or orthodontics to the cases in which they represent an advantage.

Even if the literature does not describe the real cost (in terms of life risks) involved with pre-surgical orthodontic treatment, it is the authors' opinion that the correction of malocclusions should be reserved only for those cases wherein it represents unquestionable advantages. Therefore, we believe that occlusion correction should be excluded for all patients presenting Class I occlusions or I degree occlusal discrepancies that do not significantly and unfavorably interfere with the repositioning of the maxillary skeletal bases.

Logically, when a patient wishes to optimize both apneic and occlusal components, in the postoperative period, all the different orthodontic and prosthetic therapies will be taken into account according to each individual case. Furthermore, postponing these kinds of procedures to approximately six months from the intervention allows for the optimization and solving of possible occlusal discrepancies that occur in the postoperative period due to skeletal and/or condylar adjustments.

Unfavorable occlusal modifications

The surgical treatment of MMA in Class II patients may be correlated with unfavorable occlusal modifications including:

- predisposition to posterior crossbite due to the mandibular advancement
- reduction of the overjet.

The risk of a *transversal discrepancy rarely* limits the entity of the mandibular advancement.

If the patient is in agreement to optimize the occlusion, it is possible to execute a surgical expansion of the maxillary (during the main intervention) or, in cases of mild entity, to proceed to the postoperative orthodontic correction.

When facing the risk of a *sagittal discrepancy* in a hyperdivergent patient with an increased gonial angle, it is advisable to extract the first lower premolars and then retract and impact the lower front-canine sector through an anterior segmental subapical osteotomy from element 33 to element 43. In this way, the maxilla-mandibular sagittal relation is corrected, and it is then possible to proceed to advancements of different entities of the two bone bases (the mandible advances much more than the maxilla).

The result can be optimized by pre-operatively preparing more splints based on plaster models simulating different degrees of dentoalveolar repositioning and, thus, different degrees of maxillary advancement. This does not mean that it is necessary to use such a maneuver. In the surgery room, after achieving the pre-set mandibular advancement, the Le Fort I is then executed. The maxillary is put in occlusion with the mandible, and the aesthetic impact is evaluated (ascribable to the more consistent advancement). In the case of an anti-aesthetic result, a mandibular dentoalveolar (retraction) dissection is executed. Such a procedure is planned with consequent maxillary advancement of minor entity.

In *hypodivergent patients with a reduced gonial angle and deep bite*, a surgical mandibular advancement is executed to create a tripod occlusion, i.e., the achievement of a relation with front teeth, bilateral lateral open bite, and exclusive posterior contact in the premolar teeth area. The lateral open bite can be corrected later with an orthodontic extrusion of premolar teeth or through occlusal premolar and molar bite raising.

In patients falling in the *II Class – II Division*, it is possible to avoid preoperative orthodontics by planning a mandibular advancement with an occlusal anterior crossbite that can be successively corrected with postoperative orthodontic treatment. In these cases, the orthodontic/surgical planning plays a particularly important role in the achievement of an adequate and stable intermaxillary relation. An alternative to this treatment plan is to execute a subapical dentoalveolar segmental osteotomy to modify the inclination of the superior and inferior incisors.

If it is necessary to *expand the intercanine diameter*, it is possible to proceed with a Wunderer-type osteotomy associated with the classic Le Fort I.

In the presence of a *normal profile*, it is possible to proceed with therapeutic advancements to retract both the upper and lower dentoalveolar segments from canine to canine (with the extraction of four premolar teeth), creating an initial bi-retrusion that will be corrected with the maxillary advancement.

Postoperative course

As of yet, there are no specific studies on the postoperative course of patients subjected to MMA for OSAS. A 2003 meta-analysis led by Bays and collaborators on 688 patients who underwent orthognathic surgery reported the following results::

- recovery time of nutrition per os: immediate
- mean hospitalization time: 3.2 days
- mean time to return to work: 17.4 days
- mean time to complete recovery of mastication: 38.2 days
- percentage of patient satisfaction: 93%.

We should not forget that for patients with OSAS, the surgery involves immediate improvement, if not complete resolution of the pathology. During initial days after the intervention, the patients do not need CPAP support anymore and show a drastic decrease of AHI.

Therefore, compared with dysmorphic patients, patients with OSAS show a clearly elevated percentage of satisfaction and increased degree of compliance in dealing with certain problems related to the immediate postoperative period such as edema, need for a liquid diet, and alterations of sensitivity, among others.

REFERENCES

ABRAMNSON Z, SUSARLA S, AUGUST M. Three-dimensional computed tomographic analysis of airway anatomy in patients with obstructive sleep apnea. *J Oral Maxillofac Surg.* 2010;68:354-362.

BARKDULL CG, KHOL CA, PATEL M. Computed tomography imaging of patients with obstructive sleep apnea. *Laryngoscope.* 2008;118:1486-1492.

BAYS RA, BOULOUX GF. Complications of orthognatic surgery. *Oral Maxillofac Surg Clin N Am.* 2003;15:229-242.

BETTEGA G, PEPIN JL, VEALE D. Obstructive sleep apnea syndrome: Fifty-one consecutive patients treated by maxillofacial surgery. *Am J Respir Crit Care Med.* 2000;16:641-649.

BREVI BC, TOMA L, MAGRI AS, SESENNA E. Use of the mandibular distraction technique to treat obstructive sleep apnea syndrome. *J Oral Maxillofac Surg.* 2011 Feb;69(2):566-71.

BREVI BC, TOMA L, PAU M, SESENNA E. Counterclockwise rotation of the occlusal plane in the treatment of obstructive sleep apnea syndrome. *J Oral Maxillofac Surg.* 2011 Mar;69(3):917-923.

BRUNO CARLO B, MAURO P, SILVIA B, ENRICO S. Modified genioplasty and bimaxillary advancement for treating obstructive sleep apnea syndrome. *J Oral Maxillofac Surg.* 2008 Sep;66(9):1971-1974.

BRUSATI R, SESENNA E. Chirurgia delle deformità mascellari, Elsevier, Milano, 1988.

CODIVILLA A. On the means of lengthening in the lower limbs, the muscles and tissues which are shortened through deformity. *Am J Orthop Surg.* 1905;2:353-369.

COSTELLO BJ, POSNICK JC. The role of maxillofacial osteotomies in the treatment of obstructive sleep apnea. *Curr Opin Otolaryngol Head Neck Surg.* 2003;11:267-274.

DELAIRE J. Architectural and structural craniofacial analysis (lateral view). Theoretical principles. Some example of its use in maxillofacial surgery (translation). *Rev Stomatol Chir Maxillofac.* 1978;79(1):1-33.

DELAIRE J. Architectural and structural teleradiographic analysis of the face. *Orthod Fr.* 1971;42:411-427.

DELAIRE J, SCHENDEL SA, TULASNE JF. An architectural and structural craniofacial analysis: a new lateral cephalometric analysis.*Oral Surg Oral Med Oral Pathol.* 1981 Sep;52(3):226-238.

FAIRBURN SC, WAITE PD, VILOS G. Three-dimensional changes in upper airway of patients with obstructive sleep apnea following maxillomandibular advancement. *J Oral MaxilloFacial Surg.* 2007;65:6-12.

GOODDAY R. Diagnosis, Treatment Planning, and Surgical Correction of Obstructive Sleep Apnea. *J Oral Maxillofac Surg.* 2009;67:2183-2196.

GOTTE P. Sulla terapia chirurgica del progenismo. Esperienze e risultati ottenuti mediante una modificazione del metodo intraorale di Obwegeser. *Minerva Stomatol.* 1966;1:12.

HOCHBAN W, CONRADT R, BRANDENBURG U, ET AL. Surgical maxillofacial treatment of obstructive sleep apnea. *Plast Reconstr Surg.* 1997;99:619-626.

LEE NR, GIVENS CD, WILSON J, ET AL. Staged surgical treatment of obstructive sleep apnea syndrome: a review of 35 patients. *J Oral Maxillofac Surg.* 1999;57:382-385.

LOWE AA, FLEETHAM JA, ADACHI S. Cephalometric and computed tomographic predictors of obstructive sleep apnea severity. *Am J Orthod Dentofac Orthop.* 1995;107:589-595.

MCCARTHY JG, SCHRIEBER J, KARP N, THORNE CH, GRAYSON BH. Lengthening the human mandible by gradual distraction. *Plast Reconstr Surg.* 1992;1:89.

MCCARTHY JG. Mandibular bone lengthening. *Oper Tech Plast Reconstr Surg.* 1994b;1:99.

MCCARTHY JG. The role of distraction osteogenesis in the reconstruction of the mandible in unilateral facial microsomia. *Clin Tech Plast Surg.* 1994a;1:105.

PRINSELL JR. Maxillomandibular advancement surgery for obstructive sleep apnea syndrome. *JADA.* 2002;133:1489-1497.

PRINSELL JR. Maxillomandibular advancement surgery in a site specific treatment approach for obstructive sleep apnea in 50 consecutive patients. *Chest.* 1999;116:1519-1529.

RANDERATH WJ, VERBRAECKEN J, ANDREAS S, ET AL. (EUROPEAN RESPIRATORY SOCIETY TASK FORCE ON NON-CPAP THERAPIES IN SLEEP APNOEA). Non-CPAP therapies in obstructive sleep apnoea. *Eur Respir J.* 2011 May;37(5):1000-1028.

RILEY RW, POWELL NB, GUILLEMINAULT C. Current surgical concepts for treating obstructive sleep apnea syndrome. *J Oral Maxillofac Surg.* 1987;45:149.

RILEY RW, POWELL NB, GUILLEMINAULT C. Obstructive sleep apnea syndrome: a review of 306 consecutively treated surgical patients. *Otolaryngol Head Neck Surg.* 1993;108:117-125.

RONCHI P, NOVELLI G, COLOMBO L, VALSECCHI S, OLDANI A, ZUCCONI M, PADDEU A. Effectiveness of maxillo-mandibular advancement in obstructive sleep apnea patients with and without skeletal anomalies. *Int J Oral Maxillofac Surg.* 2010 Jun;39(6):541-547.

SAMCHUKOV ML, COPE JB, CHERKASHIN AM. *Craniofacial Distraction Osteogenesis.* Ed. Mosby; 2001.

SCHENDEL SA, POWELL NB. Surgical Orthognathic Management of Sleep Apnea. *J Craniofacial Surg.* 2007;18(4):902-911.

STEINER CC. Cephalometrics for you and me. *Am Jour Orthod.* 1953;39(10):729-755.

STEINER CC. The use of cephalometrics as an aid to planning and assessing orthodontic treatment. *Am Jour Orthod.* 1960;46(10):721-754.

TINER BD. Surgical management of obstructive sleep apnea. *J Oral Maxillofac Surg.* 1996 Sep;54(9):1109-14.

VICINI C, DALLAN I, CAMPANINI A, ET AL. Surgery vs ventilation in adult severe obstrctive sleep apnea syndrome. *Am J Otolaryngol.* 2010 Jan-Feb;31(1): 4-20.

VOS W, DE BECKER J, DEVOLDER A. Correlation between severity of sleep apnea and upper airway morphology based on advanced anatomical and functional imaging. *J Biomech.* 2007;40:2207-2213.

WAITE RW PD, WOOTEN V, LACHNER J. Maxillo-mandibular advancement surgery in 23 patients with obstructive sleep apnea syndrome. *J Oral Maxillofac Surg.* 1989;47:1256-1261.

YUCEL A, UNLU M. Evaluation of upper airway cross-sectional area changes in different degrees of severity of obstructive sleep apnea syndrome: cephalometric and dynamic CT study. *Am J Neurorad.* 2005;26:2624-2629.

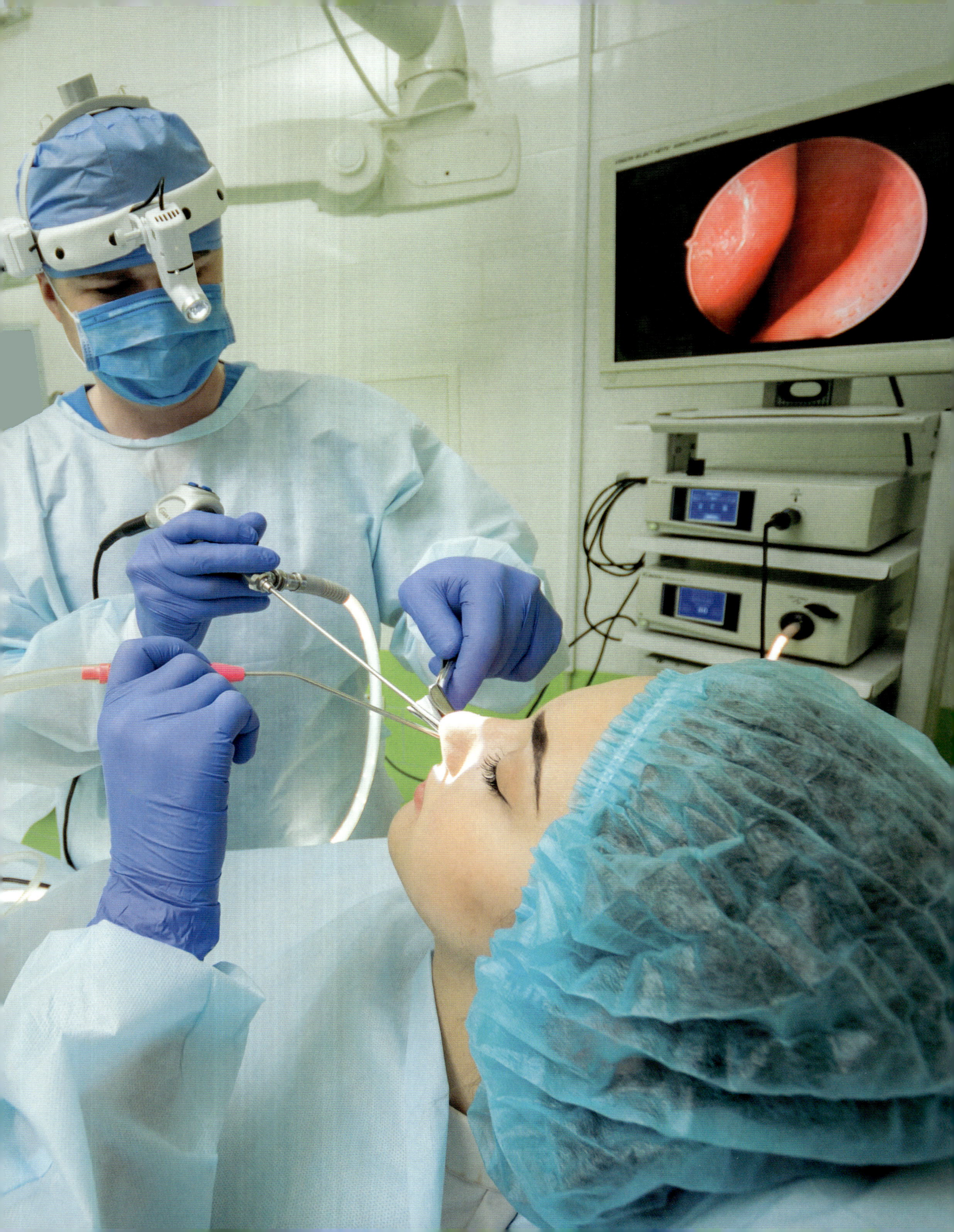

Surgical ENT therapy

Claudio Vicini ▪ Filippo Montevecchi ▪
Andrea De Vito ▪ Giuseppe Meccariello ▪
Giannicola Iannella

Objectives

- Identifying the patients eligible for ENT surgery
- Understanding the various ENT surgical techniques for patients with OSAS

Introduction

Surgical treatment for snoring and OSAS (also known as ronchopathy surgery) aims to reduce or, if possible, eliminate pathological snoring and clinical manifestations associated with obstructive apnea. In this regard, ronchopathy surgery supplements and integrates all the other conventional therapeutic approach modalities, such as dietary therapy and ventilatory therapy with CPAP, as well as more recent therapies such as the use of oral devices, by augmenting the supply of all possible solutions to the problem (American Sleep Disorders Association 1996; Bäck *et al.* 2009).

Table 8.1 briefly summarizes the essential chronological stages in the history of ronchopathy surgery.

In the past, many interventions originally developed for other purposes, such as for septoplasty, adenoidectomy, and tonsillectomy, were able to contribute to the resolution of nocturnal apneas in certain patients (Bäck *et al.* 2009, Bourolias *et al.* 2008).

The **targets of surgical** corrective **treatment** are the following areas:

- Nose and nasopharynx
- Oropharynx (soft palate and palatine tonsils)
- Hypopharynx
- Trachea.

With all these areas under the scope of otolaryngology, most surgeons who perform ronchopathy surgery belong to an ENT background. However, some solutions for managing the posteroinferior respiratory and retrolingual spaces involve the facial skeleton and are therefore under the scope of maxillofacial surgeons.

Additionally, plastic surgeons or stomatologists occasionally venture into this branch of surgery. Regardless of the surgeon's area of expertise, there are general rules that must be followed (8.2 e 8.3).

8.1 Chronological stages in the history of ronchopathy surgery.

1960-1970	Tracheostomia
1970-1980	UvuloPalatoPharyngoPlasty (UPPP)
1980-1990	Laser Assisted Uvulo Palatoplasty (LAUP) Upper Airway Reconstruction (UAR)
1990-2000	Mini Invasive Procedures Radio Frequency Volume Reduction (RFVR) Lingual Stabilization
2000-2018	Expansion sphincter pharyngoplasty (ESP) Barbed reposition pharyngoplasty (BRP) Transoral Robotic Surgery (TORS) Hypoglossus Nerve Stimulation

8.2 Surgical therapy for OSAS: preliminary conditions, alternative therapies, indications, and contra-indications.

• A potential surgical treatment requires a preliminary diagnosis of certainty, with grading and topodiagnosis
• CPAP remains the cornerstone of the therapy that precedes, possibly in all cases, surgical treatment
• Surgical treatment is only applied to cases of specific dysmorphism(s) that can be surgically corrected
• Surgical therapy is indicated if: – the noninvasive treatment is not sufficient – the noninvasive treatment is rejected – the patient expressly asks for it – the patient does not present surgical contra-indications

Source: American Sleep Disorders Association 1996

8.3 Surgical therapy of OSAS: Stanford Protocol.

• The treatment aims to cure the patient
• The management of the single case is related to the situation of the case itself (tailored)
• The treatment may consist of a combination of various procedures (multi-level surgery) or may be planned in two or more stages (multi-stage surgery)
• The patient receives accurate and complete counseling
• Follow-up is an integral part of the treatment
• The objectives of the treatment are the normalization of the clinical and instrumental symptoms of the • patient

Source: Riley et al. 1995

Table 8.4 lists the different surgical modalities currently available that must be accurately selected by choosing the most adequate one for every single patient. It is possible to perform a combination of two or more interventions to simultaneously or sequentially correct all the obstructive sites involved in the pathology (American Sleep Disorders Association 1996; Cahali 2003; Canzi *et al.* 2013).

8.4 Surgical modalities employed in the treatment of snoring or nocturnal apneas.

Surgical site	Purpose of the intervention	Typology of intervention
Nose and nasopharynx	Reduction of nasal resistances, reduction of the negative endopharyngeal pressure	Septoplasty, valvuloplasty, inferior turbinoplasty, adenoidectomy, surgery of paranasal sinuses
Oropharynx and soft palate	Enlarging the oropharyngeal lumen	Tonsillectomy, classic and modified UPPP, and ESP-BRP
	Shortening, lessening, and stiffening	Classic and modified LAUP, uvulopalatal flap surgery, and radiofrequency volume reduction
Hypopharynx, lingual tonsil, base of the tongue	Enlarging the hypopharyngeal lumen, reduction of the BS volume, anterior positioning, and reduction of hypopharyngeal compliance	Lingual tonsillectomy, subglossectomy with CO2 laser, transoral robotic surgery, coblation tonsillectomy, radiofrequency volume reduction, genioglossal advancement, hyoid suspension, lingual suspension, and maxillomandibular advancement
Trachea	Shunt of the collapsible area	Tracheostomy

The subjective and more specifically, the objective (instrumental polysomnographic) results of this modern snoring surgery appear to be extremely interesting also because of the reduced and minimal risks of major complications.

Classification of ronchopathy surgery procedures

The surgical procedures developed over decades and daily employed in snoring surgery fall someway in one of the operative mechanisms listed in Table 8.1, inspired by Ptosic (American Sleep Disorders Association 1996; Frapier *et al.* 2011):

- Bypass of the nocturnal respiratory obstruction;
- Tissue ablation;
- Tissue stiffening;
- Reduction of nasal resistances;
- Nonablative volume reduction;
- Suspension suture;
- Re-tensioning of the pharyngeal muscles with repositioning of the muscular insertions;
- Pace-making of dilatory musculature.

Nasal surgery

The common denominator of these procedures is reducing the nasal and/or nasopharyngeal resistances with a double impact on the snoring pathology (Choi *et al.* 2011a and b). It involves:

- increasing the negative inspiratory pressure of the collapsible segments and reducing the risk to exceed the critical closing pressure (apnea);
- discouraging mouth breathing and thus reducing the phenomenon of retraction of the genioglossus insertion due to the open-mouth posture.

The implemented intervention type depends directly on the pathology to be treated, the settings (ambulatory or surgery room, local or general anesthesia, etc.) where the surgery is performed, and the available technology (laser, radiofrequency, debridger, etc.). In snoring surgery, the nasal factor plays an indisputable role. Even by considering some publications with different views, it seems unlikely that an isolated nasal or nasopharyngeal intervention can really solve simple snoring or OSAS problems in the majority of the cases. On the contrary, the reduction of the resistances in the first segment seems to be a required complementary intervention that is also extremely useful for a majority of patients affected with oro- and hypopharyngeal problems, whether the nasal intervention is executed simultaneously with a palatal or hypopharyngeal surgery or at a postponed time. Compared to the palatal time, the resulting pain or simple discomfort seems modest (Choi *et al.* 2011a; Choi *et al.* 2011b).

According to the experience of the authors, the most commonly adopted procedures in adult patients are listed below:

1. **Inferior turbinoplasty:** It can be executed with all the techniques currently available. The number of choices is restricted by the requirements of ronchopathy surgery (need to avoid tampons for potential immediate use of CPAP, preference for minimally invasive ambulatory procedures executed with local anesthesia, or contrarily, combined interventions, and the possibility to employ technologies also used for the palate):
   - bipolar cautery with forceps: simple, fast, cost-effective, does not require final tamponing replaced by the application of a simple silastic sheet for a few days. This is the preferred technique by the authors in the majority of cases, in association with palatal surgery under narcosis, with the patient in the Rose position;
   - volumetric reduction with CO_2 laser or diode laser: It is relatively easy but requires more effort. It appears interesting when it is associated with the palatal intervention on the same patient and for its absolute efficacy with no tamponing requirement.
   - radiofrequency volume reduction: Per the experience of the authors, its results are very encouraging. The last version with a probe and computer-aided algorithm proved to be extremely interesting when combined with the corresponding palatal use.
2. **Septoplasty:** Through the removal of deviated cartilage parts of the nasal septum and/or septum bone spurs, this surgical technique allows us to increase the space from the nasal cavity to the nocturnal airflow. Independent of the execution or experience and preference of the operator, this technique requires systems of medication different from tamponing to avoid dangerous apneas and also, to enable the use of CPAP during the postoperative nights (unless it is executed on an autonomous intervention). Per the authors' experience, the employment of Doyle-type medical-grade silicone splints and/or continuous septal sutures proved to be the height of the task.
3. **Surgery of the paranasal sinuses (FESS):** It may require the removal of nasal polyps, a middle antrostomy, and an ethmoidectomy. Nowadays, this surgery is executed using surgical optics and a microdebridger, which enhances its minimally invasive characteristics.
4. **Valvuloplasty:** A rarer but not exceptional surgery-type. To avoid a possible nocturnal valvular collapse, the authors conducted it using spreading grafts and/or alar grafts and obtained good results.
5. **Adenoidectomy:** It is also rare but not exceptional. It is required in cases of residual adenoid stenotic tissues. Technically it is not difficult, in the

majority of the cases, it is executed with cold curettes. Its execution may present a problem when it has to be performed simultaneously with palatal surgery due to the consistent risk of unpredictable and uncontrollable stenosis. The authors' practice is to perform the two procedures separately and chronologically.

Oropharyngeal surgery

The chapter on oropharyngeal surgery is certainly the most detailed. However, it is sometimes unjustly absolutized in all snoring surgeries that should not be regarded as mesopharyngeal and even less, as palate surgery. The surgical treatments of the mesopharynx have the following different objectives (Gallina *et al.* 2009; Olszewska *et al.* 2012):

- **Ablation or volumetric reduction of hypertrophic or protruding** tonsils that are responsible for sub-stenosis or obstruction;
- **Remodeling of excessive, falling and/or thickened velum-uvula** that is vibrating abnormally and/or pathologically obstructing the rear space. Generally, the different techniques reduce or eliminate uvula and shorten or thin out the soft palate (only UPF thickens it);
- **Stiffening of the soft palate** to limit the entity of vibrations with the airflow;
- **Lateral enlargement** of the oropharyngeal space.

Almost all simple snorers and the great majority of apneic subjects require one intervention on the palate.

Many snorers can be treated with an isolated palate intervention whereas the vast majority of apneic subjects need an additional nasal or hypopharyngeal procedure, if not both. Usually, palate surgery entails a painful postoperative period (even for several days) since it is performed on an organ that is richly innervated, in continuous movement (swallowing, speech), and has an unfavorable environment (saliva, bacteria).

Permanent invalidating consequences (velopharyngeal insufficiency) were relatively frequent in the past, nowadays, they represent an exception. On the contrary, mild but extended over time disorders, like retropalatal paresthesia (foreign body sensation due to the scar) and minor dysphagia disorders (difficulty in swallowing, major incidences of accidentally inhaling food), remain quite common.

For better clarity, the oropharyngeal procedures are distinguished in:

- Minor procedures, or procedures that can also be executed with local anesthesia;
- Major procedures that require general anesthesia.

In general, but not as a rule, the former addresses simple snoring whereas the second mainly targets cases of UARS or real OSAS.

MINOR OROPHARYNGEAL PROCEDURES

1. **Uvulectomy and single-stage snare dissection UPP (SUPP)** with tonsil snare: the dissection of the uvular base with a tonsil snare is certainly a fast, cost-effective, and simple procedure. It is particularly implemented and appreciated among English-speaking professionals (Herford *et al.*; Weingarten 1995) and it is limited to the snoring. It can also be described as a simple dissection with scissors after an extended clamping (Gallina *et al.* 2009; Lundkvist *et al.* 2009; Olszewska *et al.* 2018).
2. **Injections of sclerotherapy agents (snoreplasty)** Injections of chemical substances promoting sclerosis phenomenon with consequent stiffening of the palate. This procedure is not very common. It is an interesting technique in cases of snorer subjects who have already been treated with non-satisfying results.
3. **Interstitial laser therapy** It is mainly executed with diode laser applied several times at different points of the palate (Gallina *et al.* 2009; Huang *et al.*2012) which aims to remove a series of submucosal linear scars with hardening of the palate. It is easy and well-tolerated but costly. It certainly deserves more attention among the minor approaches to palatal snoring (Yaremchuck *et al.* 2016).
4. **Ambulatory uvulopalatopharyngoplasty**, single-stage: It is executed using an electro-scalpel to perform a sort of minimal UPPP by dissecting the uvula and a variable trait of the free border of the palate, and later sutured with four to five absorbable stitches. However, it is not easy to perform in local anesthetic and ambulatory settings. A very similar procedure, named the modified UPPP, is thus adopted by the Stanford group (Gallina *et al.* 2009; Rashwan *et al.* 2018).
5. **Palatal radiofrequency volume reduction (RFVR), submucosal radiofrequency UPP (SUPP)**: it requires the use of a needle-probe adequately shaped and adapted to the morphology of the single soft palate. During one or more sessions, this probe is inserted in the median and lateral palatal space with the aim of producing coagulative necrosis at low temperatures through the extremely selective radiofrequency-mediated space opening. After a few weeks, this results in a volumetric reduction of approximately a third of the initial volume due to a scarring sclerosis retraction (Boudewyns and Van De Heyning 2000; Coleman *et al.* 2000). This technique is currently out of its experimental phase and has been approved by the FDA for the almost complete lack of pain, absence of effective risks of velopharyngeal insufficiency, and optimal efficacy on snoring in patients with thick palates and enlarged-brachial uvula, in the absence of contracted pharynx and tonsillar hypertrophy. However, it is necessary to mention its elevated cost. Other authors have proposed less expensive devices with the same objectives (Taliaferro 2001; Fibbi *et al.* 2009; Olszewska *et al.* 2012).

❻ **Tonsillar radiofrequency volume reduction (RFVR)** this uses the same generator (appropriately updated) and a two-needle radiofrequency probe (Nelson *et al.* 2000). The same observations can be made as for the above-described technique (Fibbi *et al.* 2009).

❼ **Classic LAUP with variations** it is the most commonly used surgical procedure worldwide, spreading almost exponentially (Camacho *et al.* 2017 and Götkas *et al.* 2014). Extremely easy technically, it is characterized by the application of a CO_2 laser (less frequently with diode laser or YAG) on two parasagittal sections of the soft palate, followed by a variable degree of reduction of the uvula (by a modest debulking of a subtotal section). The sections must be executed in consecutive sessions by applying incisions vertically higher until the patients are not able to reproduce the snoring on purpose anymore, and they have actually stopped snoring during sleep. It is certainly easy, fast, and effective when the palates are not thick, the uvula is not excessively enlarged, and especially, in the absence of a contracted oropharynx (for instance grade 2 giant tonsillolith/giant tonsillar hypertrophy grade 2. Due to the graduality of the approach in more sessions, the risk of permanent velopharyngeal insufficiency is insignificant. Contrastingly, it is necessary to consider the cost of laser use, the intense postoperative pain (it is not true at all that laser performs pain-free incisions!) on a tissue that is exposed and not sutured (and this needs to be multiplied by the three to five sessions, the necessary average), the high incidence of postoperative paresthesia, and especially, the growing doubts on the after scarring/cicatrization result (which is unpredictable), with a high risk of developing a stenosis later (Milczuk *et al.* 2012; Randerath *et al.* 2011).

❽ **Laser Assisted Serial Tonsillectomy (LAST)**: it was proposed by Kamamy for chronic scleroatrophic caseous cryptic tonsillitis. Occasionally, it is also indicated in the debulking of hypertrophic tonsils. It is not a difficult procedure to perform surgically and is certainly very painful for the patient (Pang and Woodson 2007; Randerath *et al.* 2011).

❾ **Microdebridger-assisted UPP (MAUPP)**: this requires an ambulatory setting, local anesthesia, and a microdebridger. It would be easy to recommend due to its easy execution, minor edema, less intense pain (compared to LAUP), and minor total cost at purchase. However, the data on its efficacy and follow-up results remain insufficient. It is required for knowledge and consideration purposes in case of laser unavailability (Fibbi *et al.* 2009; Milczuk 2012; Olszewska *et al.* 2012).

❿ **Cold-steel UPP (CUPP)**: it represents a further ambulatory revision (Casiano and Sheth 1996) with a different technological approach than LAUP. Here, the cutting tool is the backbiting forceps employed in endoscopic ethmoid surgery. It is certainly a genial procedure with low costs. However, it has not provided convincing clinical records yet. As above, it is to be considered in the case of laser unavailability (Fibbi *et al.* 2009; Milczuk *et al.* 2012; Olszewska *et al.* 2012).

11. **Cautery-assisted UPP (CAUPP):** another variation of LAUP which replaces the use of electro-scalpel (Zinder and Postma 1995; Gnuechtel *et al.* 1997). Also, this multi-session procedure should be considered in all cases of laser unavailability. However, further data concerning its efficacy and follow-up is required (Fibbi *et al.* 2009; Milczuk *et al.* 2012; Olszewska *et al.* 2012).
12. **Cautery-assisted palatal stiffening operation:** Differs from LAUP and similar procedures and is closer to the classic UPPP (Hoolsema 1999; Mair and Day 2000; Wassmuth *et al.* 2000). It is an ambulatory procedure performed by removing a 2cm strip of oral palatal mucosa with an electro-scalpel and allowing the wound to heal by natural cicatrization. It has been proposed for OSAS with an RDI mainly below 20; even after applying the "success" criterion of AHI reduction of >50%, it does not exceed the 40% score. Mair and Day achieved more significant positive outcomes on snoring of 99% immediately after the surgery, and 77% after one year (Fibbi *et al.* 2009; Milczuk *et al.* 2012; Olszewska *et al.* 2012).

MAJOR OROPHARYNGEAL PROCEDURES

Procedures performed on the oropharynx under general anesthesia include a wide range of interventions, which are classified in the most commonly employed categories. The procedures used by the authors are listed below (American Sleep Disorders Association 1996; Cahali 2003; Choi *et al.* 2011b; Lundkvist *et al.* 2009; Randerath *et al.* 2001):

1. UPP;
2. ESP;
3. UPF;
4. BRP;
5. Classic LAUP (see above);
6. Modified LAUP;
7. Tonsillectomy.

UPPP (Uvulopalatopharyngoplasty): The logical basic principle is to increase all the oropharyngeal diameters with simultaneous stiffening of the palatal edge as opposed to the collapsibility of the tissues in the oropharyngeal area typical in snoring/apneic patients.

To avoid ablation or dissection that may result in velopharyngeal insufficiency (VPI), it is necessary to recognize the surgical reference points intra-operatively.

- **Transition point:** It marks the passage between the hard and soft palate, representing the most cranial level of the soft palate. It is the zero in the metric estimation of the palatal section;
- **Metric point:** For the avoidance of VPI, it is a good rule to perform the palatal dissection at 2,5 cm caudally to the transition point;

- **Contact point:** This is the most cranial contact point of the palate with the posterior pharyngeal wall. It is better seen by exerting pressure on the median line until it touches the prevertebral plane. The mark left by the tool is the insuperable resection limit.

It is recommendable to use a cold/cryo scalpel and bipolar cautery.

It is necessary to respect the muscular plane; in the case of combined tonsillectomy, the arch-form incision must be done once from an anterior pillar to the other. The suture must be extroverted toward the oral cavity of the posterior mucosa, and it must be performed very accurately, being extended to the pillars when a tonsillectomy is executed, by modulating the traction on the points related to the requested degree of reduction and rigidity.

The procedure can be applied to any palate with custom-tailored maneuvers.

The entity of the resection does not influence the final result but exposes to an acceptable degree, the increase in complications (velopharyngeal insufficiency) (American Sleep Disorders Association 1996; Cahali 2003; Choi *et al.* 2011b; Lundkvist *et al.* 2009).

ESP (Expansion sphincter pharyngoplasty): It is based on the more difficult and aggressive technique of lateral pharyngoplasty described by Cahali. It has met increasing consensus and widespread application after Pang and Tucker-Woodson's description (2007) of the technique.

It can be combined with tonsillectomy. This technique is based on the isolation of a muscular rotation string (palatopharyngeus muscle) that is transected and cranially rotated to be fixed near the pterygoid hamulus.

Based on the experience of the authors, this technique proved to be superior to UPPP both in terms of the retrovelopharyngeal space (endoscopically detected) and, especially, objective parameters of the sleep study.

Unlike the techniques described above in literature, the authors do not execute the dissection of anterior mucosa of the soft palate, and the string is fixed not only near the pterygoid hamulus (guaranteeing a tri-directional traction, namely superior-lateral and anterior), but also laterally to the pterygomaxillary raphe (increasing lateral traction) (Milczuk 2012; Pang and Woodson 2007).

Barbed reposition pharyngoplasty. This technique has been recently introduced in palatal surgery. It requires specific surgical sutures (self-anchoring bidirectional barbed suture).

The patented technique used by the authors is a type of reposition pharyngoplasty and requires the isolation of the palatopharyngeal muscle, as well as, its anterolateral repositioning. Through the employment of the barbed sutures, the palatopharyngeal muscle is anchored to the pterygomandibular raphe in a way to increase the transversal oropharyngeal and retropalatal spaces (📷 8.1). The cicatrization due to the reabsorption of the thread additionally determines a stiffening of the palate that reduces its vibration and collapse

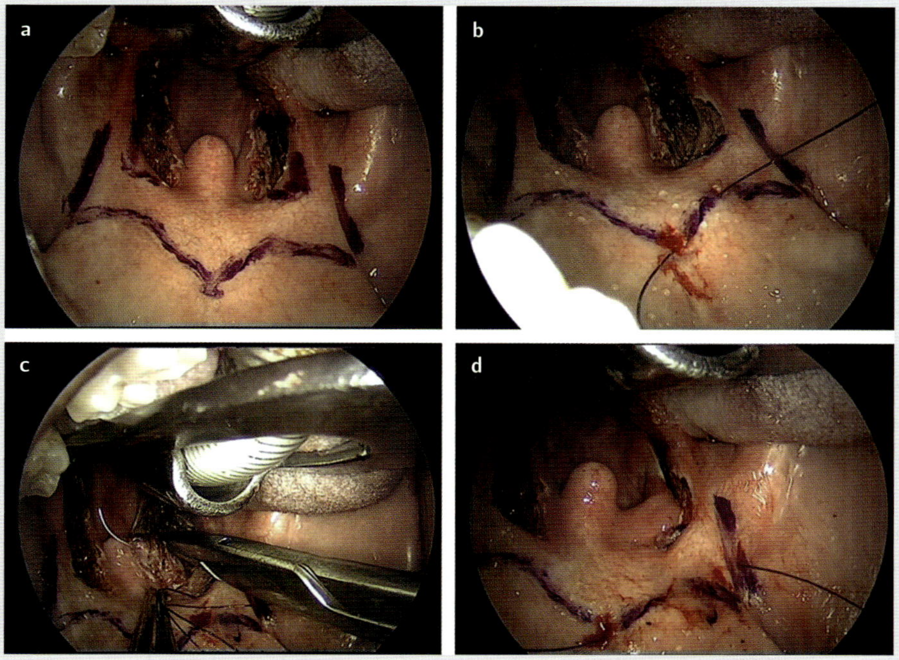

8.1 **a.** Identification of the anatomical reference points (posterior nasal spine, pterygomandibular raphe, and palatopharyngeal muscle); **b.** The bidirectional barbed suture is inserted in the posterior nasal spine and, after passing through a median transition point, is taken to the pterygomandibular raphe area; **c.** Successively, the suture is brought to the tonsillar lodge in a way to anchor the palatopharyngeal muscle; **d.** The suture is brought back to the pterygomandibular raphe to increase the oropharyngeal space with the anterolateral repositioning of the palatopharyngeal muscle.

Compared to ESP, BRP seems to offer major stability in the lateral repositioning of the palatopharyngeal muscle.

Furthermore, this surgical technique can be combined with a UPF (see below) in the case of a thinned palate and an elongated uvula.

This kind of surgery presents almost a non-existent risk of major complications (velopharyngeal insufficiency and scar stenosis) (Powell 2009; Vicini *et al.* 2014).

Uvulopalatal flap (UPF). It requires a careful selection of patients based on palatal anatomy. This surgery is exclusively indicated in the presence of a very thin palate and elongated (but not hypertrophic) uvula. Not respecting this condition leads to functional failure with a bothersome sensation of the foreign body due to the unnatural leaning of two structures (palate and uvula) that are already hypertrophic to each other. The key points of this technique are the perfect removal of excessive mucosa in the right palatal area related to the uvula margins/boundaries, the capital point (so defined because it ensures the correct leaning of the uvula to the palate without excessive traction), and the correct placement of lateral sutures to load the muscle on both sides without strangling the axial vascular pedicle.

In the case of suture dehiscence, the functional result is lost and repeating the uvula resection becomes unavoidable.

However, the real reversibility of the procedure that, per the authors, does not guarantee a lower postoperative pain than what is experienced with UPPP, remains debatable.

In contrast, there is a high risk of uvular prominence with bothersome paresthesia; this can only be partially solved with an RFVR or laser-debulking of the neo-uvula (Huang *et al.* 2011; Milczuk 2012).

Modified LAUP. It aims to broaden the indications of classic LAUP in the case of a thicker palate with ptosis and an enlarged and elongated uvula (mega-dolico uvula). Its performance requires a high-quality experience on laser-mediated snoring surgery. The technique uses oblique and lateral incisions that are extended ≥2 cm, a potential maneuver of thinning the palatal submucosa (delivered with vaporization of the adipose and muscular tissue) and subsequent suture of the edges. Normally, a CO2 laser with a back-stop, lateral mirror, and scanner, in focused continuous mode at 20–25 W, is used.

Postoperative pain is remarkable, as well as, more consistent risks of velopharyngeal insufficiency (Milczuk 2012; Randerath *et al.* 2011).

Tonsillectomy. It is executed in the classic extracapsular way and extended as best as possible to the lymphatic tissue of the lingual base focusing on the mucosa of the pillars, at least the posterior tonsillar pillars.

For pediatric patients, the focus gradually shifted to intracapsular techniques of reductive tonsillectomy with the purpose of preserving the capsule protecting vessels and nerves to avoid major bleedings and reduce postoperative pain. Based on the authors' experience with the different technologies, a dominant role is played by the microdebridger, which complies with the recommendations of the Health Department for the superiority of a cold/cryosurgical equipment concerning the risk of developing post-tonsillectomy hemorrhage.

Hypopharyngeal surgery

The extremely heterogeneous adopted surgical procedures aim to (Fibbi *et al.* 2009; Goodday and Bourque 2012; Jaspers *et al.* 2013; Randerath *et al.* 2011; Vicini *et al.* 2014):

1. perform a complete shunt of the collapsible segment through a tracheostomy;
2. generate a vector of longitudinal tension in the lateral (hyoid tension) or anteroposterior (bimaxillary advancement) wall that reduces the collapse of the same wall;
3. realize anterior vectors of enlargement or support toward the mandibular symphysis (genioglossus advancement, lingual suspension, and, partially, hyoid suspension and bimaxillary advancement);
4. remove the excessive lymphatic and/or muscular tissue at the base of the tongue (lingual tonsillectomy, median glossectomy) or reduce the mass by gradual scarring (RFVR).

The main techniques are listed below:

- **Tracheostomy:** It is the most effective procedure (nominally 100% response in 100% of cases) but the least appreciated by patients; and therefore, it is the last resort for extreme cases. The principal indication is very severe dysmorphisms of the upper air-digestive tract that cannot be resolved even with more extreme alternative techniques, especially in pathologically obese individuals or patients with associated cardiological, vascular, or neurological alterations. The surgical key of the procedure is to create a complete epithelization of the stoma, a skin-lined tracheotomy, with two (cutaneous and tracheal) flaps. This adjustment makes tracheostomy permanent with a minimal tendency to produce granulated tissues and higher compliance for the patient, who is instructed to open the cannula only when sleeping. In optimal cases, during the daytime, the cannula can be replaced by a silicone obturator/ valve in (Powell 2009; Randerath *et al.* 2011).
- **Hyoid suspension.** In the most recent version innovated by the Stanford group, this involves fixing the hyoid bone to the anterosuperior edge of the thyroidal cartilage with four suture stitches; the dissection of the stylohyoid ligament is optional. This cervicotomy surgery is very easy, fast, and cost-effective for every ENT surgeon with minimal laryngology experience. It is also acceptable to the patient due to the negligible pain, minimal scar, and the modest incidence of complications (seroma, hematoma, and keloid). The efficacy in guaranteeing the retrolingual segment patency is very high due to the combined effect of an essential action of increased longitudinal tension of the lateral walls, advancement of the insertions in the genius-hyoid muscle, a further anterior vector generated by the catenary functions of the convergence of the laryngeal insertions and superior and sub-thyroid muscles, and for the possible weakening of the stylohyoid ligament-connected posterior vector. Per the experience of the authors, this seems to be the first choice hypopharyngeal procedure for hypopharyngeal reduction with a transversal pattern of collapse and/or airspace reduction in more inferior retrolingual segments (Canzi *et al.* 2013; Tunçel *et al.* 2012; Vicini *et al.* 2014).
- **Lingual stabilization.** It is a genial transference of an originally urologic-gynecologic technique (bladder and womb suspension) into bronchopathy surgery. It involves the suspension of the superior lingual bases to the mandibular symphysis via a non-absorbable suture anchored to the mandibular cortex using a titanium screw. This end-oral technique (conditioned by the opening of the mouth) is not immediately comfortable, especially for the posterior suture. The instrument kit (anchor suture passer, tongue depressor retractor) is conceived to reduce surgery time, and it includes a costly single-use bone anchor inserter. Patients' compliance is variable, depen-

ding on the postoperative pain and dysphagia associated with the procedure to the degree of tension applied to the suture, which must be kept within certain levels. According to the Authors, this technique proved to be resolutive even over time, in cases with a high lingual tightening where the bend supports and stabilizes the lingual body while lying down. It is remarkable that, when performed with normal care, it lacks significant complications; in case of intolerance, the procedure is reversible and the suture can be removed in ambulatory settings. The cost can be minimized by adopting a slightly more invasive intervention by incising a hole with a micro-cutter and passing the suture around the mandibular body below the hole, as performed by the Authors in some cases. Finally, it is possible to implement this intervention with a more complex basilingual procedure that includes the hyoid suspension (Powell 2009; Randerath *et al.* 2011; Tunçel *et al.* 2012).

- **Genioglossus advancement.** It is another excellent development conceived by the Stanford group. Its recent version involves an anterior transfer of the genial tubercle with the insertion of the same muscle of > 1 cm. This is obtained by making (by means of an oscillating micro-saw) a rectangular parasymphyseal mandibular osteotomy. This rectangular piece of bone is advanced and stabilized with a screw. No retrolingual space is gained with this intervention, however, there is a beneficial muscular pre-tensioning that reduces the falling back of the tongue during sleep in a supine position. This intervention is not easy to perform for an inexperienced surgeon as it often presents controllable (hematoma and/or abscess of the oral floor) and sometimes, major complications (mandibular fracture). The occurrence of edema or temporary lingual hematomas that require temporary osteotomy is always possible. The Stanford clinical records report optimal functional results, where the advancement is mainly associated with the hyoid suspension and can precede a phase 2 bimaxillary advancement (Powell 2009; Randerath *et al.* 2011; Tunçel *et al.* 2012).
- **Bimaxillary osteotomy.** It is the keystone of phase 2 of the therapeutic algorithm devised by Riley, Powell, and collaborators after a potential failure of phase 1. In functional result terms, it represents one of the most effective procedures. It is mainly based on the application of bimaxillary osteotomy in ronchopathy surgery. The simultaneous liberation of the mandible and maxilla allows a new fixing with osteosynthesis in a clearly more advanced position, up to 2 cm, from the original position, with remarkable enlargement of the retrolingual space and good anteroposterior tensioning of the lateral pharyngeal walls. It is the most effective conservative intervention, providing control of apneas in > 90% of the treated cases. It requires reasonable competence in the maxilla-facial field, and it is a long and complex procedure for a surgeon. Patient compliance remains low, and it presents complications of a different character, sometimes affecting the mandibular

nerve and its occlusion considerably. Not all agree on the evidence indicating that the best efficacy is obtained after phase 1 of nasal, oropharyngeal reconstruction, and genioglossus advancement with hyoid suspension (Goodday and Bourque 2012; Jaspers *et al.* 2013; Ronchi *et al.* 2010).

- **Median subglossectomy and lingual tonsillectomy.** These are two different kinds of intervention; the first is ablative on the excessive basilingual muscle, whereas the second acts on the hyperplasia of the lingual lymphatic tissue. However, they share common aspects: they are performed in a few centers (laser availability), and they are arduous and extremely painful for the surgeon and patient, respectively. The data in literature shows a good functional efficacy when used selectively for important basilingual apneas; however, its use is outweighed by the limits represented by the need to realize a temporary tracheotomy, as well as, the several and important risks of hemorrhage and permanent dysphagia complications (Babademez *et al.* 2010; Powell 2009; Randerath *et al.* 2011; Tunçel *et al.* 2012).
- **Chabolle-TBRTHP.** The intervention conceived by Chabolle differs radically from all the other conservative techniques with a transoral approach normally proposed for the treatment of retrolingual obstruction (laser midline glossectomy, lingualplasty, surgery with radiofrequency, lingual suspension, and genioglossus advancement). This technique, performed via a pharyngotomic approach over the median hyoid bone, allows obtaining a large and full reduction of the tongue base and significant remodeling of the hyoid-glossus-epiglottic area with an enlargement of the retrolingual air space. The intervention requires a preliminary tracheostomy followed by a median cutaneous incision just above the hyoid bone with an accurate exposition of the suprahyoid musculature. These muscular structures are then incised and shortened by 1 cm to favor (with their scarring phase) the upper stabilization of the hyoid bone and the horizontalization of the mouth floor. The mylohyoid and geniohyoid muscles are first sectioned, then the lingual vessels and hypoglossal nerves are identified before cutting the hyoglossus muscle. The most delicate stage of the intervention involves the dissection of these structures, which are traced to their entry point into the lingual body. While keeping the neurovascular bundles under constant observation, the sectioning of the tongue musculature proceeds in depth following a perfectly perpendicular plane to the x neck axis until the pharynx adjacent to the glossoepiglottic valleculae. At this point, the surgery continues with a large resectioning of the tongue base until it touches the circumvallate papillae, extending laterally if required. After accurate hemostasis, the intervention proceeds with the closure of the pharyngotomy breach with a Hyo-epiglottoplasty with five Vicryl stitches. The operation ends by performing the hyoid suspension after retrospectively making two openings close to the inferior border of the mandible. The hyoid bone is raised and two large absorbable stitches are passed under its body (Powell *et al.* 2011; Randerath *et al.* 2011; Tunçel *et al.* 2012).

- **TORS**. This innovative surgical procedure was first described by the team of Authors and is now common worldwide. It utilizes the technology of the Da Vinci surgical robot and is a relatively minimally invasive surgery that can be executed transorally. It allows the introduction of a tri-dimensional endoscope in the oral cavity and two robotic arms for manipulating and resecting the excessive lingual tissue and the resectioning and remodeling of the suprahyoid epiglottis (8.2). It can be inserted in a multicenter surgery with robotic and non-robotic interventions at the lingual base and palatal level, respectively. Within 40 min, the procedure allows the removal of a significant volume of lymphatic and/or muscular tissue, with mean sizes of 14 cm3 and in extreme cases, up to 50 cm3, in the tongue base region. After preliminary tests for feasibility and safety, this technique has been shown to be effective, as confirmed by several international papers. The strength of this method lies on the possibility to execute rapidly and safely, large resections of hypopharyngeal tissues with a high percentage of success (estimated at approximately 70%-80%). It is however limited by the high console cost. Postoperative complications are scarce in terms of dysphagia and dysgeusia; long-term lymphatic re-growths are virtually absent (Vicini et al 2010; Vicini *et al.* 2014).

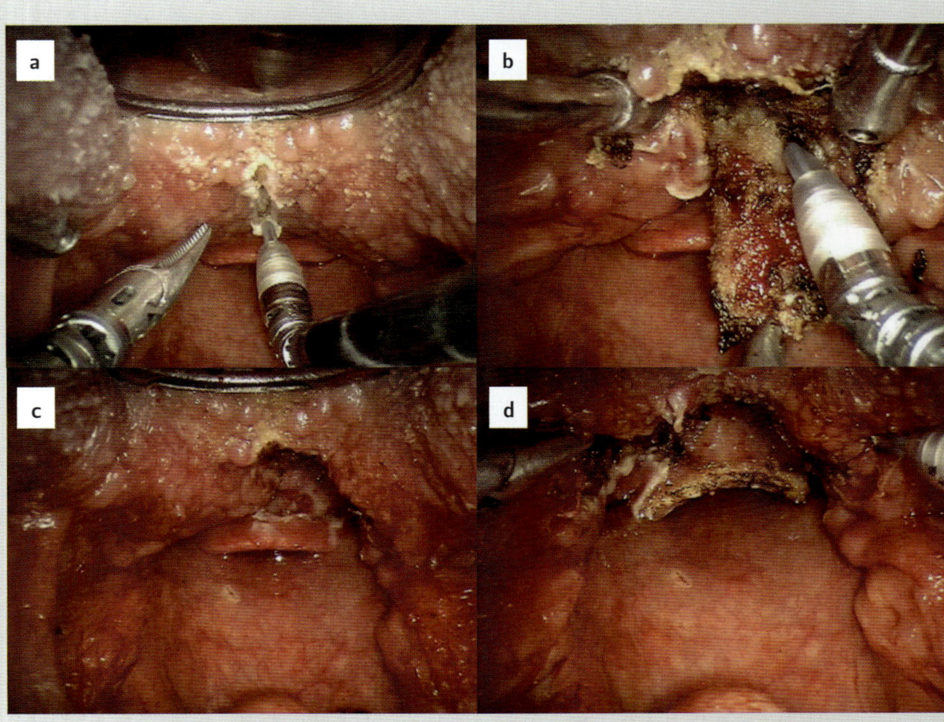

8.2 TORS Image. With a 30° view, it is possible to visualize the base of the tongue region and remove the excess tissue with the two robotic arms: a. Paramedian initial incision; b. the tissue at the base of the tongue is pulled and removed with the use of a robotic electric scalpel; c. Image after the removal of the right tongue hemibase; d. Final image after the removal of the entire excessive tissue and the free border of the epiglottis (epiglottoplasty).

- **RFVR of the lingual base**. Ambulatory intervention with local anesthesia. Although this method utilizes the radiofrequency device employed for the palate, it differs in that it uses a probe adequate for the lingual base. Through the emission of radio frequencies in several points behind the lingual V, a gradual and painless reduction of the tissues without complications is achieved. Generally, the procedure requires more sessions. The obstacle is its currently remarkable cost; however, this is not unsurmountable. It deserves, however, a prominent role in operating the base of the tongue in ronchopathy surgery (Babademez *et al.* 2010; Powell 2009).
- **Hypoglossal nerve stimulation**. It is the last procedure among the surgical solutions and involves the implantation of a pulse generator in the chest area. This device stimulates the hypoglossal nerve during sleep by means of a subcutaneous lead insert under the nerve. This technique is not completely new. After an initial experimental phase, electrical stimulation devices have then been described in literature for many years. In the last couple of years, three companies have focused more systemically on this technique, manufacturing three devices that differ in concept and functionality. The main differences among the options available on the market depend on the presence or not of a respiration sensing lead that synchronously triggers the stimulation with the respiratory cycles, on the configuration of the electrodes and the modality and chronology of the stimulation (in-full, selective or super-selective). After the experimental phase, the hypoglossal nerve stimulators are achieving a strong consensus within several authorized centers worldwide and their preliminary results arouse great interest (Powell 2009; Randerath *et al.* 2011).

Postoperative aspects

Regardless of this kind of intervention, it is always necessary to follow a control program agreed with the ENT specialist. Generally, a **postoperative short-term control** (for instance 2 weeks after the intervention) and another control after 3-6 months, which includes a fiber endoscopy of the upper aerodigestive ways, is required.

The scarring evolution, especially in the palatal area, occurs over a long times, and result analysis must be performed at ≥6 months, with a sleep study (polysomnography) that compares the preoperative condition (American Sleep Disorders Association 1996; Lundkvist *et al.* 2009, Powell 2009; Randerath *et al.* 2011; Vicini *et al.* 2014).

Acknowledgements

Special thanks are due to the following doctors: Giovanni D'Agostino, Chiara Bellini; Riccardo Gobbi, Elisabetta Firinu, Giovanni Cammaroto, Francesco Stomeo, and Bruno Brevi, who participated in writing this chapter.

REFERENCES

American Sleep Disorders Association. Practice Parameters for the Treatment of Obstructive Sleep Apnea in Adults: The Efficacy of Surgical Modifications of the Upper Airway. *Sleep*. 1996;19(2):152-155.

Babademez MA, Ciftci B, Acar B, et al. Low-temperature bipolar radiofrequency ablation (coblation) of the tongue base for supine-position-associated obstructive sleep apnea. *ORL J Otorhinolaryngol Relat Spec*. 2010;72(1):51-55.

Bäck LJ, Liukko T, Rantanen I, et al. Radiofrequency surgery of the soft palate in the treatment of mild obstructive sleep apnea is not effective as a single-stage procedure: A randomized single-blinded placebo-controlled trial. *Laryngoscope*. 2009 Aug;119(8):1621-1627.

Boudewyns A, Van De Heyning P. Temperature-controlled radiofrequency tissue volume reduction of the soft palate (somnoplasty) in the treatment of habitual snoring: results of a European multicenter trial. *Acta Otolaryngol*. 2000;120:981-5.

Bourolias C, Hajiioannou J, Sobol E, Velegrakis G, Helidonis E. Epiglottis reshaping using CO_2 laser: a minimally invasive technique and its potent applications. *Head Face Med*. 2008 Jul 25;4:15.

Cahali MB. Lateral pharyngoplasty: a new treatment for obstructive sleep apnea hypopnea syndrome. *Laryngoscope*. 2003 Nov;113(11):1961-1968.

Camacho M, Nesbitt NB, Lambert E et al. Laser-Assisted Uvulopalatoplasty for Obstructive Sleep Apnea: A Systematic Review and Meta-Analysis. *Sleep*. 2017;1:40.

Canzi P, Berardi A, Tinelli C, et al. Thirteen Years of Hyoid Suspension Experience in Multilevel OSAHS Surgery: The Short-Term Results of a Bicentric Study. *Int J Otolaryngol*. 2013;2013:263043.

Casiano RR, Sheth S. Efficacy of cold-steel uvulopalatoplasty. *Otolaryngol Head Neck Surg*. 1996;115:471-3.

Choi JH, Kim EJ, Cho WS, et al. Efficacy of single-staged modified uvulopalatopharyngoplasty with nasal surgery in adults with obstructive sleep apnea syndrome. *Otolaryngol Head Neck Surg*. 2011b Jun;144(6):994-999.

Choi JH, Kim EJ, Kim YS, et al. Effectiveness of nasal surgery alone on sleep quality, architecture, position, and sleep-disordered breathing in obstructive sleep apnea syndrome with nasal obstruction. *Am J Rhinol Allergy*. 2011a Sep-Oct;25(5):338-341.

Coleman SC, Smith TL. Midline radiofrequency tissue reduction of the palate for bothersome snoring and sleep-disordered breathing: A clinical trial. *Otolaryngol Head Neck Surg*. 2000;122:387-94.

Fibbi A, Ameli F, Brocchetti F, Mignosi S, Cabano ME, Semino L. Tongue base suspension and radiofrequency volume reduction: a comparison between 2 techniques for the treatment of sleep-disordered breathing. *Am J Otolaryngol*. 2009 Nov-Dec;30(6):401-406.

Frapier L, Picot MC, Gonzales J, et al. Ventilatory disorders and facial growth: benefits of early genioplasty. *Int Orthod*. 2011 Mar;9(1):20-41.

Gallina S, Dispenza F, Kulamarva G, Ballacchino A, Speciale R. Uvulopalatopharyngoplasty with tonsillectomy in the treatment of severe OSAS. *B-ENT*. 2009;5(4):245-250.

Gnuechtel MM, Keyser JS, Greinwald JH Jr, Postma GN. lectrocautery versus carbon dioxide laser for uvulopalatoplasty in the treatment of snoring. *Laryngoscope*. 1997;107:848-54.

Göktas Ö, Solmaz M, Göktas G, Olze H. Long-term results in obstructive sleep apnea syndrome (OSAS) after laser-assisted uvulopalatoplasty (LAUP). *PLoS One*. 2014; 30:9.

Goodday R, Bourque S. Subjective outcomes of maxillomandibular advancement surgery for treatment of obstructive sleep apnea syndrome. *J Oral Maxillofac Surg*. 2012 Feb;70(2):417-420.

Herford AS, Finn R. Single-stage CO2 laser assisted uvuloplasty for treatment of snoring and mild obstructive sleep apnoea. *J Craniomaxillofac Surg*. 2000;28:213-6.

Hoolsema EM. Cautery-assisted palatal stiffening operation and nasalance of speech. *Ann Otol Rhinol Laryngol*. 1999;108(7 Pt 1):705-7.

Huang TW, Cheng PW, Fang KM. Concurrent palatal implants and uvulopalatal flap: safe and effective office-based procedure for selected patients with snoring and obstructive sleep apnea syndrome. *Laryngoscope*. 2011 Sep;121(9):2038-2042.

Jaspers GW, Booij A, de Graaf J, de Lange J. Long-term results of maxillomandibular advancement surgery in patients with obstructive sleep apnoea syndrome. *Br J Oral Maxillofac Surg*. 2013 Apr;51(3):e37-e39.

Loube D. Radiofrequency ablation for sleep-disordered breathing. *Chest*. 1998;113:1151-2.

Lundkvist K, Januszkiewicz A, Friberg D. Uvulopalatopharyngoplasty in 158 OSAS patients failing non-surgical treatment. *Acta Otolaryngol*. 2009 Nov;129(11):1280-1286.

Mair EA, Day RH. Cautery-assisted palatal stiffening operation. *Otolaryngol Head Neck Surg*. 2000;122:547-56.

Milczuk HA. Effects of oropharyngeal surgery on velopharyngeal competence. *Curr Opin Otolaryngol Head Neck Surg*. 2012 Dec;20(6):522-526.

Nelson LM. Radiofrequency treatment for obstructive tonsillar hypertrophy. *Arch Otolaryngol Head Neck Surg*. 2000;126:736-40.

Olszewska E, Rutkowska J, Czajkowska A, Rogowski M. Selected surgical managements in snoring and obstructive sleep apnea patients. *Med Sci Monit*. 2012 Jan;18(1):CR13-CR18.

Pang KP, Woodson BT. Expansion sphincter pharyngoplasty: a new technique for the treatment of obstructive sleep apnea. *Otolaryngol Head Neck Surg*. 2007 Jul;137(1):110-114.

Powell NB. Contemporary surgery for obstructive sleep apnea syndrome. *Clin Exp Otorhinolaryngol*. 2009 Sep;2(3):107-114.

Randerath WJ, Verbraecken J, Andreas S, et al. European Respiratory Society task force on non-CPAP therapies in sleep apnoea. Non-CPAP therapies in obstructive sleep apnoea. *Eur Respir J*. 2011 May;37(5):1000-1028.

Rashwan MS, Montevecchi F, Cammaroto G et al. Evolution of soft palate surgery techniques for obstructive sleep apnea patients: A comparative study for single-level palatal surgeries. *Clin Otolaryngol.* 2018;43:584-590.

Richard W, Timmer F, van Tinteren H, de Vries N. Complications of hyoid suspension in the treatment of obstructive sleep apnea syndrome. *Eur Arch Otorhinolaryngol.* 2011 Apr;268(4):631-635.

Riley RW, Powell NB, Guilleminault C, Clerk A, Troell R. Obstructive sleep apnea. Trends in therapy. *West J Med.* 1995;162:143-8.

Ronchi P, Novelli G, Colombo L, et al. Effectiveness of maxillo-mandibular advancement in obstructive sleep apnea patients with and without skeletal anomalies. *Int J Oral Maxillofac Surg.* 2010 Jun;39(6):541-547.

Sufioğlu M, Ozmen OA, Kasapoglu F, et al. The efficacy of nasal surgery in obstructive sleep apnea syndrome: a prospective clinical study. *Eur Arch Otorhinolaryngol.* 2012 Feb;269(2):487-494.

Taliaferro C. Submucosal radiosurgical uvulopalatoplasty for the treatment of snoring: Is the monitoring of tissue impedance and temperature necessary? *Otolaryngol Head Neck Surg.* 2001;124:46-50.

Tunçel U, Inançli HM, Kürkçüoğlu SS, Enoz M. A comparison of unilevel and multilevel surgery in obstructive sleep apnea syndrome. *Ear Nose Throat J.* 2012 Aug;91(8):E13-E18.

Vicini C, Dallan I, Canzi P, et al. Transoral robotic surgery of the tongue base in obstructive sleep Apnea-Hypopnea syndrome: anatomic considerations and clinical experience. *Head Neck.* 2012 Jan;34(1):15-22.

Vicini C, Dallan I, Canzi P, Frassineti S, La Pietra MG, Montevecchi F. Transoral robotic tongue base resection in obstructive sleep apnoea-hypopnoea syndrome: a preliminary report. *ORL J Otorhinolaryngol Relat Spec.* 2010;72(1):22-27.

Vicini C, Frassineti S, La Pietra MG, De Vito A, Dallan I, Canzi P. Tongue Base Reduction with Thyro-Hyoido-Pexy (TBRTHP) vs. Tongue Base Reduction with Hyo-Epiglottoplasty (TBRHE) in mild-severe OSAHS adult treatment. Preliminary findings from a prospective randomised trial. *Acta Otorhinolaryngol Ital.* 2010 Jun;30(3):144-148.

Vicini C, Montevecchi F, Pang K, B et al. Combined transoral robotic tongue base surgery and palate surgery in obstructive sleep apnea-hypopnea syndrome: expansion sphincter pharyngoplasty versus uvulopalatopharyngoplasty. *Head Neck.* 2014 Jan;36(1):77-83.

Wassmuth Z, Mair E, Loube D, Leonard D. Cautery-assisted palatal stiffening operation for the treatment of obstructive sleep apnea syndrome. *Otolaryngol Head Neck Surg.* 2000;123(1 Pt 1):55-60.

Yaremchuk K. Palatal Procedures for Obstructive Sleep Apnea. *Otolaryngol Clin North Am.* 2016;49:1383-1397.

Zinder DJ, Postma GN. Outpatient cautery-assisted uvulopalatoplasty. *Laryngoscope.* 1995;105:1256-7.

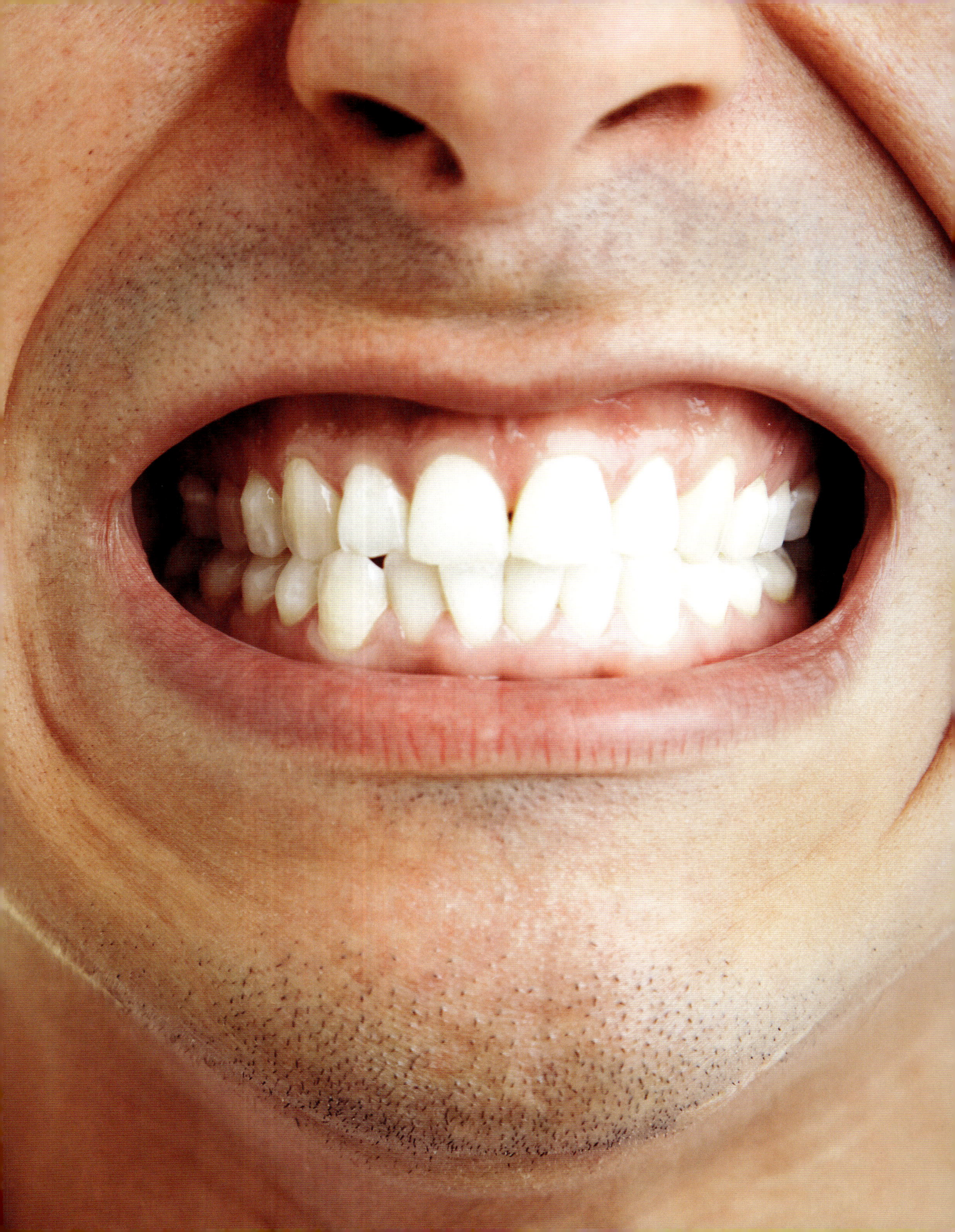

Sleep bruxism

Massimiliano Di Giosia ▪ Steven Bender
Tommaso Castroflorio ▪ Andrea Bargellini

Bruxism is defined as a repetitive jaw muscle activity that is characterized by clenching or grinding of the teeth and/or by bracing or thrusting of the mandible. It has two distinct circadian manifestations: it can occur during sleep (sleep bruxism [SB]) or during wakefulness (awake bruxism [AW]) (Lobbezoo *et al.*, 2013).

It is difficult to determine the prevalence of SB in the general population, and most data are from studies with several limitations. Indeed, the vast majority of available data are from epidemiological surveys based on self-reporting. According to the available literature, the prevalence of SB is approximately 14%–20% in the younger population, 8% in the adult population, and 3% in the elderly population (Ohayon *et al.*, 2001; Manfredini *et al.*, 2013; Castroflorio *et al.*, 2017).

Etiology and patophysiology

Traditionally, researchers in dentistry have considered SB to primarily result from peripheral morphologic etiologies. However, a more recent published study suggests a shift from peripheral-based paradigms to a more centrally regulated behavior (Lobbezoo and Naeijue, 2001). Indeed, most data suggest that SB likely involves multiple mechanisms, including genetic and environmental factors. Therefore, SB should be viewed as a behavior that probably differs from individual to individual without a single etiologic mechanism and one that is potentially related to various underlying factors. This section will focus on the more commonly suggested factors for the genesis of SB, such as morphologic, genetic, and environmental influences; psychosocial factors; and arousal-related mechanisms, such as those observed in sleep-related breathing disorders.

Occlusal Factors

In 1955, Bober observed that the prevalence of SB was higher in subjects who had what was described as "malocclusions" than in those who had occlusions that were deemed to be "normal." This work undoubtedly contributed to the morphologic philosophies that then developed over time.

However, more recent studies suggest that peripheral factors, such as dental occlusion, and other morphological factors play no significant role in the initiation or maintenance of SB activity. In a recent double-blinded randomized crossover trial, subjects had either active or dummy interferences placed on the occluding or buccal surfaces, respectively.

Interestingly, the active interference group displayed a significant reduction in the number per hour and amplitude of SB events during the experimental period. It was also observed that none of the study subjects developed signs and/or symptoms of temporomandibular disorders (TMDs) throughout the study (Michelotti *et al.*, 2005). In addition, it has been shown that the elimination of so-called "occlusal interferences" does not significantly influence jaw muscle activity during sleep. A recent review confirmed these findings by concluding that there is currently no evidence for any causal relationship between bruxism and occlusal factors (Lobbezoo *et al.*, 2012). Therefore, based on the current evidence, the idea that SB results from peripheral factors should no longer be considered valid because there is ever increasing evidence that other factors are more relevant.

Genetic and Environmental Factors

Many people, including clinicians, feel that SB is a hereditable behavior. In a recent systematic review of 10 publications dealing with heredity and bruxism, 4 studies examined the prevalence of bruxism within families, 5 were related to twins, and 1 reported on data from a previously unpublished study in which the characteristics of the subjects were not available. Based on the authors' systematic analysis, they concluded that SB is at least partially genetically determined (Lobbezoo *et al.*, 2014). In a recent polysomnography-based study investigating familial aggregation in individuals with SB, 37% of individuals with SB indicated that they had at least one first-degree relative with SB (Khoury *et al.*, 2016). As evidence, SB is a characteristic finding in individuals with Rett syndrome, Prader-Willi syndrome, and Angelman syndrome, all neurodevelopmental disorders caused by alterations in epigenetic gene expression (Carotenuto *et al.*, 2013; Maas *et al.*, 2010; Bruni *et al.*, 2004).

Ultimately, the role of genetics in SB remains to be fully elucidated, with consideration to environmental variables and epigenetic mechanisms. For example, caffeine is a known central nervous system (CNS) stimulant and has been shown to increase the risk of SB by 1.5 times. Ethyl alcohol, if particularly before sleep, may have a negative impact on sleep architecture and can affect serotonin and dopamine levels in the CNS. This potentially contributes to the initiation or worsening of SB activity. It has also been reported that smokers have a twofold greater risk of SB than non-smokers, which may be due to the influence of tobacco on the dopamine system.

Some drugs, such as selective serotonin reuptake inhibitors and amphetamines, as well as illegal substances, such as 3,4 methylenedioxymethamphetamine and cocaine, are also known to induce or enhance SB behavior. In a recent systematic review, duloxetine, paroxetine, venlafaxine, barbiturates, and methylphenidate were reported to be potentially associated with an increase in the odds for SB occurrence (Melo *et al.*, 2018). However, the authors warn that the results should be viewed with caution because the quality of the current evidence is low.

Psychosocial Factors

Although evidence on the role of psychosocial factors in SB is limited, a study has suggested that traits such as anxiety and stress are frequently associated with SB (Manfredini and Lobbezoo, 2009).

In fact, children and adults who report self-awareness of tooth grinding tend to be more anxious, aggressive, and hyperactive than those who do not have SB. In addition, it has been demonstrated that individuals with SB tend to experience more nervousness, competitive behaviors, emotional lability, and poor coping mechanisms (Bayar *et al.*, 2012).

A recent study by Seraidarian *et al.* (2009) found higher levels of urinary catecholamines in pediatric and adult subjects with SB than in control subjects. Based on animal studies, it has been postulated that the forebrain nuclei, which are related to autonomic control and stress responses, such as the lateral hypothalamus and the amygdala, may influence the activity of trigeminal motor neurons and be at least partially responsible for the genesis of SB (Mascaro *et al.*, 2009). Obviously, this work will need to be replicated in a human model. Watanabe *et al.* (2003) and van Selms *et al.* (2004) have provided contradictory evidence regarding the role of psychosocial stressors in individuals with SB. These two studies failed to find relationships between daily activity, sleep quality, and stress (anticipated and experienced) and SB. Ultimately, definitive conclusions concerning the role of psychosocial factors in SB should be viewed with caution as more work is needed in this area.

Arousal-related Mechanisms

SB has been described as a sleep-related motor activity occurring secondary to sleep arousal (Huynh *et al.*, 2006). Sleep arousal is defined as a brief awakening from sleep characterized by increased electroencephalographic, autonomic, cardiac, and muscle activity without a complete return to consciousness (Iber, 2007).

Periodic arousals during sleep are considered to be a normal response of the brain to environmental and internal physiologic stimuli. In normal sleepers, arousals occur between 6 and 14 times per hour.

A previous study has demonstrated that SB occurs in association with an increase in sympathetic tone occurring approximately 4–8 minutes prior to the SB event (Lavigne *et al.*, 2007). Another work has demonstrated that SB can be initiated by experimentally induced arousals in individuals with SB (Carra *et al.*, 2011). Approximately 80% of non-rapid eye movement (NREM) SB episodes occur in association with what is known as "cyclic alternating patterns (CAPs)." CAPS are structured and repetitive arousals that tend to occur every 20–60 seconds in NREM sleep periods and consist of the activation of electroencephalogram and electrocardiogram (ECG) patterns. These events appear to be a mechanism for preserving a degree of vigilance in the environment during sleep to maintain body homeostasis and protection during this time. Variability to normal CAP sequencing, time, and rate suggest sleep fragmentation and arousal instability (Terzano and Parrino, 2000). Although it may be tempting to suggest that sleep arousal is the initiator or triggering event for SB, it is probably more likely that the arousal period provides a "permissive window" in which SB tends to occur, similar to what is noted in other rhythmic movements observed during sleep (Carra *et al.*, 2010).

SB has been shown to frequently occur in people with sleep disordered breathing (SDB) (Hosoya *et al.*, 2014). It has been suggested that SB may play a protective role in restoring normal airway patency and respiration after a respiratory event (Manfredini *et al.*, 2015). The proponents of this theory point to reports of a significant reduction in SB in patients treated for SDB with adenotonsillectomy (Eftekharian *et al.*, 2008), mandibular advancement devices (Landry-Schonbeck *et al.*, 2009), or continuous positive airway pressure machines (Oksenberg and Arons, 2002). However, the association between SB and SDB appears to be primarily related to the occurrence of arousals that result from SDB (Hosoya *et al.*, 2014). In fact, in individuals with concomitant SDB and SB, 54% of events occurred within 0-10 seconds following the respiratory event, 25.5% occurred before the event, and 19.5% occurred without any temporal relationship with a respiratory event (Saito *et al.*, 2016, 2014). This lack of consistently observed rhythmic masticatory muscle activity (RMMA) in close approximation to abnormal respiratory events suggests that other factors are responsible for the genesis of SB. In most instances, contractions of the masticatory muscles in association with a respiratory event during sleep appear to be nonspecific, i.e., not RMMA, and are more dependent on the duration of the arousal rather than on the occurrence of the respiratory event itself (Kato *et al.*, 2013). Although it may be possible that some SB events do in fact result from respiratory events, further studies are needed to clarify the nature of this apparent link.

Effects of sleep bruxism

There is sufficient literature regarding the effects of SB. However, most studies are observational and have not been scientifically validated. Certainly, the potential damage to the dentition or dental prosthesis that can occur with this behavior is the primary concern of the dentist. Although there is conflicting evidence regarding the nature of the relationships, it is widely accepted that SB plays a significant role in the genesis and maintenance of musculoskeletal pain of the stomatognathic system. This section will focus on some of the more commonly reported signs and symptoms of SB.

Musculoskeletal Pain

A long-held perception in dental literature and clinical practice is that bruxism, particularly SB, is the primary causative factor of pain in the stomatognathic system. It has been suggested that SB produces a load on the structures exceeding the adaptive capacity of the host, thereby initiating nociception and eventual pain; the more an individual bruxes, the more pain they will experience. Many patients experiencing musculoskeletal pain of the stomatognathic structures are also convinced that their symptoms are due to bruxism.

However, most of the time, the patient's beliefs have been influenced by what they are told by their dental or medical clinician.

However, a recent systematic review concluded that when established objective criteria are used for the diagnosis of SB, there is no significant correlation between the two entities in adult subjects (Baad-Hansen *et al.*, 2019). This review arrived to the same conclusions when reviewing studies involving children. It is apparent that most of the positive correlation studies of SB and musculoskeletal pain have relied on self-reported SB and other subjective means and not on validated objective measures. These findings reinforce the need for the use of validated means for assessing SB in future studies. As evidence, a recent study found that conclusions from investigations based on self-report of SB should be viewed with caution due to significant inconsistencies between what is believed by the patient and what is observed with more objective measures (Raphael *et al.*, 2015).

Although experimental studies involving various tasks, such as tooth clenching or grinding, have observed masticatory muscle fatigue and pain, no study has shown that these tasks result in the long-lasting pain observed by most individuals with TMDs. In fact, one study demonstrated that when the experimental clenching tasks were repeated for 5 days in succession, fewer symptoms were reported on day 5 than on day 1, suggesting an adaptation mechanism in these otherwise healthy subjects (Svensson and Arendt-Nielsen, 1996). In addition, other studies have found that patients with SB without pain have higher electromyography (EMG) activity during sleep than those with SB with pain (Arima *et al.*, 2001). Patients with SB with low-frequency EMG activity during sleep are more at risk of developing craniofacial pain (Rompre *et al.*, 2007). A laboratory-based PSG study reported that most patients with painful myofascial TMDs did not exhibit any measurable SB.

One caveat to consider in this discussion is that it has been demonstrated that pain itself may play a role in decreasing SB events (Arima *et al.*, 2001). In a recent laboratory video and PSG study involving 77 subjects (56 women and 21 men) aged 18–63 years, it was found that the distribution of TMDs, which included musculoskeletal pain, between patients with and without SB was similar (Wieckiewicz *et al.*, 2020). From this, the authors concluded that SB was not a risk factor of painful TMDs. In summary, the objective measurement of SB in sleep laboratories with validated protocols has led to the conclusion that there is no consistent, reliable association between SB and musculoskeletal pain of the stomatognathic system.

Tooth Wear

The etiology of tooth wear is considered to be multifactorial via mostly mechanical and/or chemical means. A previous study in individuals with seemingly excessive tooth wear reported that erosion was the main causative factor and that bruxism appeared to be the second-most common factor (Smith and

Knight, 1984). In dentistry, tooth wear has long been primarily attributed to bruxism activity, during both AW and SB. However, a recent study seems to dispute these previous findings (Casett *et al.*, 2017). This discrepancy could potentially be explained by the methods used to diagnose SB. For example, previous studies utilizing self-report or other subjective methods for SB diagnosis often demonstrated a positive correlation of tooth wear with stomatognathic musculoskeletal pain, while studies based on more quantitative and objective methods for SB diagnosis tended to show a much lower association with musculoskeletal pain symptoms (Manfredini *et al.*, 2010). While tooth wear does in fact indicate a loss of structure due to mechanical and/or chemical mechanisms, it cannot be used to determine the timing of the events. Thus, based on the available evidence, the presence of tooth wear cannot realistically be used to determine whether SB is a current, ongoing behavior or whether it shows the severity of any previous activity.

Masticatory Muscle Hypertrophy

Early descriptions of the enlargement of the masticatory muscles include studies by Dencer (1961) and Franks (1965). Both authors suggest the pathophysiology of masticatory muscle hypertrophy may at least in part be related to bruxism or teeth clenching. However, Dencer casts doubt on the theory of etiology due to the paucity of evidence. Other studies have also concluded that the parafunctional behaviors of the stomatognathic system cannot be verified in all instances of masticatory muscle hypertrophy. Riefkohl *et al.* (1984), after reviewing case reports, indicated that only 10% of patients presenting with masticatory muscle hypertrophy elicited a history of bruxism. Ultimately, the etiology of masticatory muscle hypertrophy appears to be mostly unknown but could, in some cases, be associated with parafunctional behaviors, such as jaw clenching or SB.

Torus and Exostosis

Tori and exostoses are benign asymptomatic nodular protuberances of mature compact and cancellous bone. The terminology used for these structures depends on their anatomic location.

In general, tori are located on the lingual surface of the mandible and the midline area of the palate. On the other hand, exostoses are located on the buccal or palatal surfaces of the maxilla and the buccal surfaces of the mandible. The etiology of the formation of these structures is mostly unknown; however, it is thought to be a combination of genetic and environmental variables.

It has been suggested that increased occlusal load is responsible for the pathogenesis of these entities (Pechenkina and Benfer, 2002). Frost (1994) suggested that the Wolf's law, i.e., as the loading on a bone increases, the bone will remodel over time to become stronger, may play a role in the formation of exostoses and tori. However, in a recent systematic review, Bertazzo-Silveira *et al.* (2017) concluded that while tori do seem to be associated with the presence of abnormal tooth wear, there is currently no sufficient high-quality evidence to fully support the hypothesis that teeth grinding and/or clenching are associated with tori. In their conclusions, the authors emphasized that significant limitations in the studies reviewed were the identification of parafunctional behaviors primarily based on self-report and also that a consistent definition of these behaviors was not utilized. Therefore, better quality studies with standardized definitions of parafunctional behaviors could certainly influence future conclusions.

Tongue Indentations and Buccal Mucosa Ridging

Previous reports have suggested that buccal mucosa ridging, sometimes referred to as "linea alba," and tongue indentations are suggestive of bruxism (Kampe *et al.*, 1997). Interestingly, in a study by Yadav (2011), it was observed that tongue scalloping was more common with minimal tooth attrition, suggesting that the two cannot be reliably correlated. Findings from Yanagisawa *et al.* (2007) suggest that tongue width at rest may play a more significant role in the formation of indentations than the pressure of the tongue applied to the lingual surface of the teeth during rest, clenching, or swallowing.

Certainly, disorders that can cause tongue enlargement or macroglossia, such as hypothyroidism, sarcoidosis, amyloidosis, should be considered when indentations of the tongue borders are observed. In a study of 244 randomly selected dentulous adults aged 20–59 years, 51.2% were found to have tongue indentations, 61.5% had buccal mucosa ridging, and only 10.7% reported awareness of clenching or grinding (Piquero and Sakurai, 1999). While tongue indentations and buccal mucosa ridging may be found in some individuals suspected with a bruxism behavior, more evidence is needed to establish any causative relationship as well as to differentiate between any relevance of awake or sleep-related activity.

Headache

Headache is considered to be a near universal experience, with approximately 90% of adults reportedly having experienced headache at some point in their lifetime. A previous study has suggested that SB may be at least partially responsible for daytime headaches in both adults and children (Carra *et al.*, 2012). A recent systematic review concluded that while there may be a relationship between adults with SB and headache, there is currently not enough evidence to either support or dispute the association in children (De Luca Canto *et al.*, 2014).

In a study assessing the association between bruxism (both AW and SB) and anxiety symptoms among military personnel with frequent tension-type headaches and TMDs (painful and not painful), anxiety and AW were found to be independent risk factors of the development of frequent tension-type headaches and painful TMDs, whereas only AW was a risk factor o frequent tension-type headaches with non-painful TMDs (Wagner and Moreira Filho, 2018). Therefore, SB does not seem to play a role in painful TMDs or headaches. As with many studies concerning SB, the means by which SB is assessed can prove to be a limiting factor in these findings.

Evidence from sleep laboratory studies has shown that most headaches that patients with sleep disorders experience at awakening are not usually a consequence of SB but are more related to other sleep disorders, such as such as insomnia, SDB, and leg movement disorders (Smith *et al.*, 2009; Rompre *et al.*, 2007). Based on these and other findings, when the clinician encounters a patient who reports frequent morning headaches, other causative factors should be investigated before assuming the role that SB may play in the presentation.

Diagnosis

When we talk about bruxism and more circumstantially about SB, the first things that we think about are the altered dental shape, caused by tooth wear, and the teeth grinding noise. These views result from considering these signs as pathognomonic for SB, but are they really?

Based on actual scientific evidence, it can be stated that tooth wear facets are not just caused by parafunctional activity because there are many risk factors related to dental tissue loss (such as the degree of enamel mineralization, saliva pH, malocclusions, eating habits and disorders, drugs, and systemic diseases).

Furthermore, it must be stated that dental tissue loss is irreversible. This means that if a 50-year-old patient shows various tooth wear facets, it does not mean that they are an actual bruxer: their facets could be the effect of parafunctional activity of 20 years ago. Thus, the degree of tooth wear is not suggestive of the severity of parafunctional activity.

Instead, the teeth grinding noise with a frequency of at least twice per week is a scientifically validated sign when reported by a bedpartner. Sensibility and specificity of teeth grinding noise in a PSG examination were 78% and 98%, respectively (Lavigne *et al.*, 1996). Clinical examination is always the first and irreplaceable diagnostic approach; however, it is often insufficient to provide a definite diagnosis of SB.

Lobbezoo *et al.* (2013) has described three possible scenarios for SB diagnoses:

- Possible bruxism: based on questionnaires and history (Fig 1)
- Probable bruxism: based on questionnaires and clinical examination. In this regard, the use of the clinical diagnostic criteria for SB proposed by the American Academy of Sleep Medicine (AASM) is strongly recommended (American Academy of Sleep Medicine, 2005).
- Definite bruxism: based on questionnaires, clinical examination, and polysomonographic recordings. This means the use of PSG examination with

9.1 Questionnaire example.

Item	Yes	No	I don't know
Do you grind your teeth while sleeping?			
Has anyone told you that you grind your teeth while sleeping?			
Do you wake up with clenched teeth?			
Do you wake up with jaw pain ?			
Do you wake up with toothache?			
Do you wake up with headache in the frontal region?			
Do you feel like your jaw is stuck when you wake up?			
Have you ever noticed that you clench your teeth during daytime?			
Have you ever noticed that you grind your teeth during daytime?			

audio-video (A/V) recording or the use of validated portable devices specifically designed for SB diagnosis.

This chapter will only focus on the different instrumental quantitative approaches for SB diagnosis.

The term "diagnosis" is derived from the Greek word διάγνωσις (diágnōsis), which means "understand." Diagnosis is the identification of the nature and/or the cause of a medical condition. Talking about a patient "probably" having bruxism is not the same as talking about a diagnosis because the cause of observed signs and symptoms has not been identified with certainty. Questionnaires and various diagnostic clinical criteria are very important to identify patients at risk of SB; however, definite diagnosis of SB will only result after an instrumental evaluation.

Polysomnography (PSG)

PSG with A/V recording comprises the recording of different physiological parameters in dedicated sleep laboratories with trained technicians assisting the patients during the night of recording. See Chapter 2 for a detailed description of PSG.

A/V recording is useful to document tooth grinding/clenching and to distinguish RMMA, namely the motor model for bruxism, from other motor activities, such as deglutition or head movements. There are well-codified criteria for PSG recognition of SB. These PSG diagnostic criteria for SB show sensibility and specificity of 72% and 94%, respectively (Lavigne *et al.*, 1996). On the basis of these criteria, a subject can be classified as "non-SB" when the number of episodes per hour of sleep (RMMA index) ranges between ≥0 and <2, "slight SB" when the RMMA index ranges between ≥2 and <4, and "moderate-severe SB" when the RMMA index is >4.

However, it must be kept in mind that the PSG diagnostic criteria for SB have been validated only for research protocols to determine whether subjects are bruxers or non-bruxers and have not yet been validated from a clinical point of view. Indeed, SB does not represent any pathology per se because it manifests together with different kinds of muscular activations, some of them even with physiological meaning (e.g., probable protective reflex against sleep apnea). Therefore, it can be postulated that the SB diagnostic criteria should help in discerning non-physiologic SB, with possible negative consequences on the health of the patient, from physiologic SB.

PSG is expensive and not a routine examination for patients with SB in dental clinical practice. PSG examination must be requested when individuals show signs and symptoms of SB other than those associated with sleep disturbances (such as restless leg syndrome or obstructive apnea). In these cases, dental practitioners must refer the patient to a sleep specialist.

EMG Portable Devices

Over the past few years, to overcome the limits and costs of PSG examination in sleep laboratories, interesting devices have been developed for PSG recordings. These recordings are more or less complete according to the number of parameters effectively recorded in a home environment. Such devices have been validated via comparative studies with laboratory PSGs in terms of their recording precision and accuracy and are now used in high-level studies in various medical fields (Ng *et al.*, 2010).

The PSG criteria for SB diagnosis are based on EMG signals recorded from the masseter muscle. AASM has stated that the single criterion needed for SB diagnosis is a simple increase in EMG masticatory muscle activity (masseter and/or temporalis) (American Academy of Sleep Medicine, 2005). Over time, these guidelines have strengthened the idea that SB diagnosis in daily practice can be made by simply recording EMG masseter/temporalis activity during sleep. Subsequently, different portable devices have been developed to "diagnose" SB based on EMG activity recording.

The first portable device for SB diagnosis was introduced in the 1970s (Solberg *et al.*, 1975). The main innovation following the introduction of such EMG portable devices has made it possible to record night parafunctional activity for as many nights as desired in the patient's natural environment with a lower cost than that using PSG (Gallo *et al.*, 1999).

With this in mind, some case reports that have in some ways changed the history of dentistry have greatly contributed; for example, reinforcing the idea that "bruxism" activity increases during stressful events (e.g., university exams, quarrels with partners, and job troubles) (Rugh, 1981).

All devices described in the literature require a pre-recording titration to allow the identification of an individual's threshold and to exclude all EMG physiological signals (such as deglutition and cough.). Such a threshold can be represented by the percentage of the maximum voluntary clenching or by a certain number of standard deviations of the rest EMG activity, depending on the device used.

It is important to emphasize how the use of rest EMG activity represents an important methodological limit per se. Several researchers have studied the reliability of the rest EMG activity and have found that it is difficult to distinguish it from electric noise as they are both a measure of the order of a few microvolts (μV) (Castroflorio *et al.*, 2008). Moreover, EMG signal amplitude is extremely susceptible to electrode orientation with respect to the muscle, and because the patient must position the electrodes themselves, the quality of the recorded signal could be altered, making it even more difficult to recognize signals above the rest threshold. Therefore, devices using rest EMG activity should be avoided.

Recently, different interesting portable devices have appeared in the market, and according to some with the literature, some of them are able to provide consistent results. These systems can quantify the muscular activity in terms of the duration and number of muscular activations. Ikeda *et al.* (1996) have suggested some diagnostic criteria for SB using portable EMG devices; however, to date, there is no proof of their validity using representative samples of the population. Moreover, the same authors of the proposal have underlined an important fact: ECG recording must be associated with EMG signal.

Bitestrip (SLP, Israel) is a miniaturized wireless EMG device including two electrodes, an amplifier, a microprocessor for data gathering and analysis, an electrochemical permanent display, and a lithium battery. The entire system is integrated in a plastic container that can be attached to the skin at the height of the masseter muscle.

Bitestrip has been tested in two different scientific studies. The first study by Shochat *et al.* (2007) compared the device with an EMG recording and obtained sensitivity of 72% and a positive predictive value of 75%.

The second study by Mainieri *et al.* (2012) compared Bitestrip with PSG in a sample of bruxers and obtained a sensitivity of 84% and a positive predictive value of 100%. Both studies confirmed that Bitestrips could identify subjects with bruxism. However, none of the cited studies reported specific data. Therefore, Bitestrip cannot distinguish between bruxers and non-bruxers because it is impossible for the device to discern RMMA activity from other muscular activities. This observation is very important considering that almost

30% of masticatory muscle activity during sleep in bruxers is not related to SB (Dutra *et al.*, 2009).

Grindcare (Medotech A/S, Denmark) was unveiled in 2007 as a device that can play the dual role of diagnosing and treating SB. The device records an EMG surface signal (sEMG) from the anterior temporalis and is equipped with a biofeedback system (subthreshold electrical stimulation) activated by muscle contraction. The manufacturers claim that the biofeedback system of the device can reduce parafunctional activity.

A study by Jadidi *et al.* (2008) demonstrated the ability of the Grindcare biofeedback system to reduce the EMG activity of the temporalis during sleep for a period of 3 weeks. A similar result was reported in a previous study by Needham and Davies (2013) during an observation period of 5 weeks. In a more complete prospective study, Raphael *et al.* (2013) showed that Grindcare reduces the EMG activity of the temporalis during the period of use; however, they even demonstrated that EMG activity returned to its initial activity once treatment ended. EMG reduction is not followed by a reduction in pain in the masticatory muscle area. The same results have been reported in a randomized controlled trial pilot study by Jadidi *et al.* (2013).

Considering the aforementioned percentage of nonspecific contractions found in patients with SB, the biofeedback system could determine any "over-treatment"; therefore, there is a need to improve the system to identify certain RMMA activity and to separate it from other oromotor activities.

The Bruxoff device (OT Bioelettronica, Torino, Italy) was developed to integrate the information obtained with only EMG recording. It is the only device that can simultaneously record EMG signals from both masseters and ECG. EMG signals are recorded with innovative concentric electrodes made of AgCl (CoDe Spes Medica, Battipaglia, Italy) that not influenced by the orientation above muscular fibers, thereby reducing electric noise resulting from nearby muscles (Farina and Cescon, 2001).

The device is equipped with a software (Bruxmeter; OT Bioelttronica) that can automatically score an increase in the frequency of the heartbeat over 20% of the basal rhythm and can evaluate whether this increase is immediately followed (within 5 seconds) by a contraction of the masseter muscle, with an increase of at least 10% of the maximum voluntary clenching (recorded while awake). Literature has demonstrated that an SB episode can only be identified by an increase in the frequency of the heartbeat followed by a sudden contraction of the masseter muscle. The Bruxmeter software can determine RMMA index, supporting clinical diagnosis.

Compared with PSG recordings, the Bruxoff device shows sensibility and specificity of 92% and 91%, respectively, indicating that the software can distinguish RMMA from other oromotor activities as well as allowing clinicians to identify patients with and without SB (Castroflorio *et al.*, 2014). Moreover, in a reproducibility study during an observation period of 3 weeks, the device showed high affordability (Deregibus *et al.*, 2014). Comparing clinical diagnosis based on the diagnostic criteria proposed by AASM with the Bruxoff results revealed that only EMG evaluation results in a clinical error greater than 20% when compared with a joint evaluation of EMG and ECG, confirming the risk of an overestimation of bruxism episodes when relying only on EMG evaluation (Castroflorio *et al.*, 2013).

The additional equipment needed to perform EMG recordings of both masseter muscles makes the Bruxoff device more bulky when compared to the other devices. Nevertheless, in light of a study by Castroflorio *et al.* (2013) that showed asymmetric muscular activation during sleep, this set-up is necessary.

Among the latest generation of EMG portable devices, those associated with the EMG of masticatory muscles and heartbeat frequency seem to be the most promising in terms of diagnostic validity (screening between bruxers and non-bruxers), reliability (measurement reproducibility), and simple data interpretation at a reduced cost for patients showing signs and symptoms of SB without other underlying neurological and/or breathing disturbances.

However, clinical and anamnestic examinations are the first and irreplaceable steps to take, even if they are not sufficient to provide a definite diagnosis of SB. In light of the pathophysiology of SB, RMMAs follow the activation of the autonomic nervous system, and A/V PSG recording remains the gold standard for SB diagnosis if the patient's SB is related to other sleep disturbances, such as obstructive sleep apnea syndrome or restless leg syndrome. A good generic anamnestic questionnaire as well as other more specific tools, such as the Epworth Sleepiness Scale or the snoring, tiredness, observed apnea, high blood pressure, body mass index, age, neck circumference, and gender (STOP-BANG) questionnaire can be very helpful for detecting patients at a risk of respiratory diseases in the dental population. In daily practice, collaboration between dental practitioners and sleep medical experts is desirable.

Management

Considering its multifactorial and mainly central etiology, SB cannot be "fixed" but can be managed. Managing SB should be directed toward the possible negative effects that SB can have on dentition, prosthetic reconstructions, implants, masticatory muscles, and temporomandibular joints.

There are different approaches to manage bruxism, and the clinician should always evaluate the patient and start with more conservative management options (Beddis *et al.*, 2018).

Irreversible occlusal adjustments have no basis in evidence in the management of bruxism.

Management options can include:

- Behavioral techniques
- Oral appliances
- Pharmacological treatment

Behavioral Techniques

It is very important to educate the patient to avoid all probable triggers and risk factors of SB, such as caffeine, alcohol, and use of some drugs (Kuhn and Türp, 2018). Relaxation techniques, biofeedback, sleep hygiene, and cognitive behavioral therapy have been used to manage SB. Considering the conservative and reversible nature of these approaches, they should always be considered in the management of SB even if evidence for SB diagnosis is inadequate (Carra *et al.*, 2012).

Oral Appliances

Oral appliances are probably the most common treatment approach for the management of the effects of SB. The use of an oral appliance does not eliminate bruxism activity. In few patients, there is RMMA activity only for a short period of time. Oral appliances are mainly used to protect the teeth from excessive wear and to manage muscle and joint pain (Macedo *et al.*, 2007; Matsumoto *et al.*, 2015).

Oral appliances should have some basic features:

- They should be made of hard acrylic (soft appliances are difficult to adjust and can sometimes increase the parafunctional activity) (Okeson, 1987)
- They should provide full occlusal coverage to prevent possible occlusal changes, such as teeth extrusion
- They should allow simultaneous contact of all opposing teeth

There are some data in the literature that have reported that upper oral appliances can exacerbate obstructive sleep apnea (Gagnon *et al.*, 2004; Nikolopoulou *et al.*, 2013). An alternative approach could be the use of a mandibular appliance or a mandibular advancement device (Solanki *et al.*, 2017).

Pharmacological Treatment

Although current evidence is scarce, some medications could have a role as a short-term therapy in the clinical management of patients with severe symptoms of SB.

According to recent studies, clonazepam (a benzodiazepine) reduces SB activity (Saletu *et al.*, 2005, 2010). However, benzodiazepines have a lot of potential side effects, such as tolerance, dependence, drowsiness, unsteadiness (particularly in older people with increased risk of falls and injury), and sleepiness.

Recent studies have reported that clonidine, an alpha-2 adrenergic agonist, reduces the episodes of bruxism by 60%; however, its clinical use for the management of SB is still controversial owing to side effects, such as severe morning hypotension and sleepiness (Carra and Macaluso, 2010; Sakai *et al.*, 2017).

Botulinum toxin has been proposed as a potential treatment for SB. However, according to one study, there were no differences between placebo and botulinum toxin in the relief of jaw stiffness (Lee *et al.*, 2010). Another study showed only a slight difference between placebo and botulinum toxin (Ondo *et al.*, 2018).

The effects of botulinum toxin last only for a few months, and it has to be administered at regular intervals. A recent study showed mandibular bone changes (a significant cortical thinning at the condylar area) in adult patients who received botulinum toxin in the masticatory muscles (Kahn *et al.*, 2020).

REFERENCES

American Academy of Sleep Medicine (AASM), editor. International classification of sleep disorders. Diagnosis and coding manual. (ICSD-2). Section on sleep related bruxism. 2nd edition. Westchester (IL): *American Academy of Sleep Medicine*; 2005. pp. 189-92

ARIMA T, ARENDT-NIELSEN L, SVENSSON P. Effect of jaw muscle pain and soreness evoked by capsaicin before sleep on orofacial motor activity during sleep. *J Orofac Pain* 2001;15(3):245-56.

BAAD-HANSEN L, THYMI M, LOBBEZOO F, SVENSSON P. To what extent is bruxism associated with musculoskeletal signs and symptoms? A systematic review. *J Oral Rehabil* 2019;46(9):845-61.

BAYAR GR, TUTUNCU R, ACIKEL C. Psychopathological profile of patients with different forms of bruxism. *Clin Oral Investig* 2012;16(1):305-11.

BEDDIS H, PEMBERTON M, DAVIES S. Sleep bruxism: an overview for clinicians. *Br Dent J. Nature Publishing Group* 2018;225(6):497-501. doi: 10.1038/sj.bdj.2018.757.

BERTAZZO-SILVEIRA E, STUGINSKI-BARBOSA J, PORPORATTI AL, ET AL. Association between signs and symptoms of bruxism and presence of tori: a systematic review. *Clin Oral Investig* 2017;21(9):2789-99.

Bober H. Grundlagen der Therapie der hatiptformen Des (nachtlichen) zahneknirschens. *Öst Z Stomatol* 1955;52:450-3.

BRUNI O, FERRI R, D'AGOSTINO G, ET AL. Sleep disturbances in Angelman syndrome: a questionnaire study. *Brain Dev* 2004;26(4):233-40.

CAROTENUTO M, ESPOSITO M, D'ANIELLO A, ET AL. Polysomnographic findings in Rett syndrome: a case-control study. *Sleep Breath* 2013;17(1):93-8.

CARRA MC, HUYNH N, LAVIGNE G. Sleep bruxism: a comprehensive overview for the dental clinician interested in sleep medicine. *Dent Clin North Am* 2012;56(2):387-413.

CARRA MC, MACALUSO GM, ROMPRÉ PH, ET AL. Clonidine has a paradoxical effect on cyclic arousal and sleep bruxism during NREM sleep. *Sleep* 2010;33(12):1711-6.

CARRA MC, ROMPRÉ PH, KATO T, ET AL. Sleep bruxism and sleep arousal: an experimental challenge to assess the role of cyclic alternating pattern. *J Oral Rehabil* 2011;38(9):635-42.

CARRA MC, MACALUSO GM, ROMPRÉ PH ET AL. Clonidine has a paradoxical effect on cyclic arousal and sleep bruxism during NREM sleep. *Sleep* 2010;33(12):1711-6.

CARRA MC, HUYNH N, LAVIGNE G. Sleep bruxism: A comprehensive overview for the dental clinician interested in sleep medicine. *Dent Clin North Am* 2012;56(2):387-413. doi: 10.1016/j.cden.2012.01.003.

CASETT E, RÉUS JC, STUGINSKI-BARBOSA J, ET AL. Validity of different tools to assess sleep bruxism: a meta-analysis. *J Oral Rehabil* 2017;44(9):722-34.

Castroflorio T, Bracco P, Farina D. Surface electromyography in the assessment of jaw elevator muscles. *J Oral Rehabil* 2008;35(8):638-45.

Castroflorio T, Deregibus A, Bargellini A, Debernardi C, Manfredini D. Detection of sleep bruxism: comparison between an electromyographic and electrocardiographic portable Holter and polysomnography. *J Oral Rehabil* 2014;41(3):163-9.

Castroflorio T, Mesin L, Tartaglia GM, Sforza C, Farina D. Use of electromyographic and electrocardiographic signals to detect sleep bruxism episodes in a natural environment. *J Biomed Health Inform* 2013;17(6):994-1001.

Castroflorio T, Bargellini A, Rossini G, Cugliari G, Deregibus A. Sleep bruxism and related risk factors in adults: A systematic literature review. *Arch Oral Biol.* Elsevier Ltd 2017;83:25-32. doi: 10.1016/j.archoralbio.2017.07.002.

De Luca Canto G, Singh V, Bigal ME, Major PW, Flores-Mir C. Association between tension-type headache and migraine with sleep bruxism: a systematic review. *Headache* 2014; 54(9):1460-9.

Dencer D. Bilateral idiopathic masseteric hypertrophy. *Br J Plast Surg* 1961;14:149-52.

Deregibus A, Castroflorio T, Bargellini A, Debernardi C. Reliability of a portable device for the detection of sleep bruxism. *Clin Oral Investig* 2014;18(8):2037-43.

Dutra KMC, Pereira FJ, jr, Rompré PH et al. Oro-facial activities in sleep bruxism patients and in normal subjects: a controlled polygraphic and audio-video study. *J Oral Rehabil* 2009;36(2):86-92.

Eftekharian A, Raad N, Gholami-Ghasri N. Bruxism and adenotonsillectomy. *Int J Pediatr Otorhinolaryngol* 2008;72 (4):509-11.

Farina D, Cescon C. Concentric-ring electrode systems for noninvasive detection of single motor unit activity. *IEEE Trans Bio Med Eng* 2001;48(11):1326-34.

Franks AS. Masticatory muscle hyperactivity and temporomandibular joint dysfunction. *J Prosthet Dent* 1965;15(6) :1122-31.

Frost HM. Wolff's law and bone's structural adaptations to mechanical usage: an overview for clinicians. *Angle Orthod* 1994;64(3):175-88.

Gagnon Y, Mayer P, Morisson F, Rompré PH, Lavigne GJ. Aggravation of respiratory disturbances by the use of an occlusal splint in apneic patients: a pilot study. *Int J Prosthodont* 2004;17(4):447-53.

Gallo LM, Gross SS, Palla S. Nocturnal masseter EMG activity of healthy subjects in a natural environment. *J Dent Res* 1999;78(8):1436-44.

Hosoya H, Kitaura H, Hashimoto T, et al. Relationship between sleep bruxism and sleep respiratory events in patients with obstructive sleep apnea syndrome. *Sleep Breath* 2014;18 (4):837-44.

Huynh N, Kato T, Rompré PH, et al. Sleep bruxism is associated to micro-arousals and an increase in cardiac sympathetic activity. *J Sleep Res* 2006;15(3):339-46.

Iber C. The AASM manual for the scoring of sleep and associated events: rules. *Terminol Tech Specif* 2007.

Ikeda T, Nishigawa K, Kondo K, Takeuchi H, Clark GT. Criteria for the detection of sleep-associated bruxism in humans. *J Orofac Pain* 1996;10(3):270-82.

Jadidi F, Castrillon E, Svensson P. Effect of conditioning electrical stimuli on temporalis electromyographic activity during sleep. *J Oral Rehabil* 2008;35(3):171-83.

Jadidi F, Castrillon EE, Nielsen P, Baad-Hansen L, Svensson P. Effect of contingent electrical stimulation on jaw muscle activity during sleep: A pilot study with a randomized controlled trial design. *Acta Odontol Scand* 2013;71(5):1050-62.

Kahn A, Kün-Darbois JD, Bertin H, Corre P, Chappard D. Mandibular bone effects of botulinum toxin injections in masticatory muscles in adult. *Oral Surg Oral Med Oral Pathol Oral Rad.* Mosby Inc. 2020;129(2):100-8. doi: 10.1016/j.oooo.2019.03.007.

Kampe T, Tagdae T, Bader G, Edman G, Karlsson S. Reported symptoms and clinical findings in a group of subjects with longstanding bruxing behaviour. *J Oral Rehabil* 1997;24(8):581-7.

Kato T, Katase T, Yamashita S, et al. Responsiveness of jaw motor activation to arousals during sleep in patients with obstructive sleep apnea syndrome. *J Clin Sleep Med* 2013;9 (8):759-65.

Khoury S, Carra MC, Huynh N, Montplaisir J, Lavigne GJ. Sleep bruxism-tooth grinding prevalence, characteristics and familial aggregation: A large cross-sectional survey and polysomnographic validation. *Sleep* 2016;39(11):2049-56.

Kuhn M, Türp JC. Swiss Dent J 2018;128(2):118-24. Available at: https://pubmed.ncbi.nlm.nih.gov/29533049/ (Accessed: 26 June 2020).

Landry-Schönbeck A, de Grandmont P, Rompré PH, Lavigne GJ. Effect of an adjustable mandibular advancement appliance on sleep bruxism: a crossover sleep laboratory study. *Int J Prosthodont* 2009;22(3):251-9.

Lavigne GJ, Huynh N, Kato T, et al. Genesis of sleep bruxism: motor and autonomic-cardiac interactions. *Arch Oral Biol* 2007;52(4):381-4.

Lavigne GJ, Rompré PH, Montplaisir JY. Sleep bruxism: validity of clinical research diagnostic criteria in a controlled polysomnographic study. *J Dent Res* 1996;75(1):546-52.

Lee SJ, McCall WD, Kim YK, Chung SC, Chung JW. Effect of botulinum toxin injection on nocturnal bruxism: A randomized controlled trial. *Am J Phys Med Rehabil* 2010;89(1):16-23. doi: 10.1097/PHM.0b013e3181bc0c78.

Lobbezoo F, Ahlberg J, Glaros AG et al. Bruxism defined and graded: an international consensus. *J Oral Rehabil* 2013;40(1):2-4.

Lobbezoo F, Ahlberg J, Manfredini D, Winocur E. Are bruxism and the bite causally related? J Oral Rehabil 2012; 39(7):489-501.

Lobbezoo F, Naeije M. Bruxism is mainly regulated centrally, not peripherally. *J Oral Rehabil* 2001;28(12):1085-91.

LOBBEZOO F, VISSCHER CM, AHLBERG J, MANFREDINI D. Bruxism and genetics: a review of the literature. *J Oral Rehabil* 2014;41(9):709-14.

LOBBEZOO F, AHLBERG J, GLAROS AG ET AL. Bruxism defined and graded: an international consensus. *J Oral Rehabil* 2013; 40(1):2-4. doi: 10.1111/joor.12011.

MAAS AP, SINNEMA M, DIDDEN R, ET AL. Sleep disturbances and behavioural problems in adults with Prader-Willi syndrome. *J Intellect Disabil Res* 2010;54(10):906-17.

MACEDO CR, SILVA AB, MACHADO MA, SACONATO H, PRADO GF. Occlusal splints for treating sleep bruxism (tooth grinding). John Wiley and Sons Ltd. Cochrane Database Syst Rev 2007;(4):CD005514. doi: 10.1002/14651858.

MAINIERI VC, SAUERESSIG AC, PATTUSSI MP, FAGONDES SC, GROSSI ML. Validation of the Bitestrip versus polysomnography in the diagnosis of patients with a clinical history of sleep bruxism. *Oral Surg Oral Med Oral Pathol Oral Radiol* 2012;113(5):612-7.

MANFREDINI D, GUARDA-NARDINI L, MARCHESE-RAGONA R, LOBBEZOO F. Theories on possible temporal relationships between sleep bruxism and obstructive sleep apnea events. An expert opinion. *Sleep Breath* 2015;19(4):1459-65.

MANFREDINI D, LOBBEZOO F. Relationship between bruxism and temporomandibular disorders: a systematic review of literature from 1998 to 2008. *Oral Surg Oral Med Oral Pathol Oral Radiol Endod* 2010;109(6):e26-50.

MANFREDINI D, LOBBEZOO F. Role of psychosocial factors in the etiology of bruxism. *J Orofac Pain* 2009;23(2):153-66.

MANFREDINI D, WINOCUR E, GUARDA-NARDINI L, PAESANI D, LOBBEZOO F. Epidemiology of bruxism in adults: A systematic review of the literature. *J Orofac Pain.* Quintessence Publishing 2013;27(2):99-110. doi: 10.11607/jop.921.

MASCARO MB, PROSDÓCIMI FC, BITTENCOURT JC, ELIAS CF. Forebrain projections to brainstem nuclei involved in the control of mandibular movements in rats. *Eur J Oral Sci* 2009;117 (6):676-84.

MATSUMOTO H, TSUKIYAMA Y, KUWATSURU R, KOYANO K. The effect of intermittent use of occlusal splint devices on sleep bruxism: A 4-week observation with a portable electromyographic recording device. *J Oral Rehabil.* Blackwell Publishing Ltd 2015;42(4):251-8. doi: 10.1111/joor.12251.

MELO G, DUTRA KL, RODRIGUES FILHO R, ET AL. Association between psychotropic medications and presence of sleep bruxism: A systematic review. *J Oral Rehabil* 2018;45(7):545-54.

MICHELOTTI A, FARELLA M, GALLO LM, ET AL. Effect of occlusal interference on habitual activity of human masseter. *J Dent Res* 2005;84(7):644-8.

NEEDHAM R, DAVIES SJ. Use of the Grindcare® device in the management of nocturnal bruxism: a pilot study. *Br Dent J* 2013;215(1):E1.

NG SS, CHAN TO, TO KW ET AL. Validation of Embletta portable diagnostic system for identifying patients with suspected obstructive sleep apnoea syndrome (OSAS). *Respirology* 2010;15(2):336-42.

NIKOLOPOULOU M, AHLBERG J, VISSCHER CM ET AL. Effects of occlusal stabilization splints on obstructive sleep apnea: A randomized controlled trial. *J Orofac Pain.* Quintessence Publishing 2013;27(3):199-205. doi: 10.11607/jop.967.

OHAYON MM, LI KK, GUILLEMINAULT C. Risk factors for sleep bruxism in the general population. *Chest. American College of Chest Physicians* 2001;119(1):53-61. doi: 10.1378/chest.119.1.53.

OKESON JP. The effects of hard and soft occlusal splints on nocturnal bruxism. *J Am Dent Assoc* 1987;114(6):788-91. doi: 10.14219/jada.archive.1987.0165.

OKSENBERG A, ARONS E. Sleep bruxism related to obstructive sleep apnea: the effect of continuous positive airway pressure. *Sleep Med* 2002;3(6):513-5.

ONDO WG, SIMMONS JH, SHAHID MH ET AL. Neurology. Lippincott Williams & Wilkins 2018;90(7):e559-64. doi: 10.1212/WNL.0000000000004951.

PECHENKINA EA, BENFER RA, JR. The role of occlusal stress and gingival infection in the formation of exostoses on mandible and maxilla from Neolithic China. *Homo* 2002;53(2):112-30.

PIQUERO K, ANDO T, SAKURAI K. Buccal mucosa ridging and tongue indentation: incidence and associated factors. *Bull Tokyo Dent Coll* 1999;40(2):71-8.

RAPHAEL KG, JANAL MN, SIROIS DA, ET AL. Validity of self-reported sleep bruxism among myofascial temporomandibular disorder patients and controls. *J Oral Rehabil* 2015;42(10):751-8.

RAPHAEL KG, JANAL MN, SIROIS DA, SVENSSON P. Effect of contingent electrical stimulation on masticatory muscle activity and pain in patients with a myofascial temporomandibular disorder and sleep bruxism. *J Orofac Pain* 2013;27(1):21-31.

RIEFKOHL R, GEORGIADE GS, GEORGIADE NG. Masseter muscle hypertrophy. *Ann Plast Surg* 1984;12(6):528-32.

ROMPRÉ PH, DAIGLE-LANDRY D, GUITARD F, MONTPLAISIR JY, LAVIGNE GJ. Identification of a sleep bruxism subgroup with a higher risk of pain. *J Dent Res* 2007;86(9):837-42.

RUGH JD. Psychological stress in orofacial neuromuscular problems. *Int Dent J* 1981;31(3):202-5.

SAITO M, YAMAGUCHI T, MIKAMI S ET AL. e Temporal association between sleep apnea-hypopnea and sleep bruxism events. *J Sleep Res* 2014;23(2):196-203.

SAITO M, YAMAGUCHI T, MIKAMI S, ET AL. Weak association between sleep bruxism and obstructive sleep apnea. A sleep laboratory study. *Sleep Breath* 2016;20(2):703-9.

SAKAI T, KATO T, YOSHIZAWA S ET AL. Effect of clonazepam and clonidine on primary sleep bruxism: a double-blind, crossover, placebo-controlled trial. *J Sleep Res.* Blackwell Publishing Ltd 2017;26(1):73-83. doi: 10.1111/jsr.12442.

SALETU A, PARAPATICS S, SALETU B ET AL. On the pharmacotherapy of sleep bruxism: placebo-controlled polysomnographic and psychometric studies with clonazepam. *Neuropsychobiology* 2005;51(4):214-25. doi: 10.1159/000085917.

SALETU A, PARAPATICS S, ANDERER P, MATEJKA M, SALETU B. Controlled clinical, polysomnographic and psychometric studies on differences between sleep bruxers and controls and acute effects of clonazepam as compared with placebo. *Eur Arch Psychiatry Clin Neurosci* 2010;260(2):163-74. doi: 10.1007/s00406-009-0034-0.

Seraidarian P, Seraidarian PI, das Neves Cavalcanti B, Marchini L, Claro Neves AC. Urinary levels of catecholamines among individuals with and without sleep bruxism. *Sleep Breath* 2009;13(1):85-8.

Shochat T, Gavish A, Arons E et al. Validation of the BiteStrip screener for sleep bruxism. *Oral Surg Oral Med Oral Pathol Oral Radiol Endod* 2007;104(3):e32-9.

Smith BG, Knight JK. A comparison of patterns of tooth wear with aetiological factors. *Br Dent J* 1984;157(1):16-9.

Smith MT, Wickwire EM, Grace EG, et al. Sleep disorders and their association with laboratory pain sensitivity in temporomandibular joint disorder. *Sleep* 2009;32(6):779-90.

Solanki N, Singh BP, Chand P et al. Effect of mandibular advancement device on sleep bruxism score and sleep quality. *J Prosthet Dent*. Mosby Inc. 2017;117(1):67-72. doi: 10.1016/j.prosdent.2016.04.009.

Solberg WK, Clark GT, Rugh JD. Nocturnal electromyographic evaluation of bruxism patients undergoing short term splint therapy. *J Oral Rehabil* 1975;2(3):215-23.

Svensson P, Arendt-Nielsen L. Effects of 5 days of repeated submaximal clenching on masticatory muscle pain and tenderness: an experimental study. *J Orofac Pain* 1996;10(4):330-8.

Terzano MG, Parrino L. Origin and significance of the cyclic alternating pattern (CAP). REVIEW ARTICLE. REVIEW ARTICLE. *Sleep Med Rev* 2000;4(1):101-23.

van Selms MK, Lobbezoo F, Wicks DJ, Hamburger HL, Naeije M. Craniomandibular pain, oral parafunctions, and psychological stress in a longitudinal case study. *J Oral Rehabil* 2004;31(8):738-45.

Wagner BA, Moreira Filho PF. Painful temporomandibular disorder, sleep bruxism, anxiety symptoms and subjective sleep quality among military firefighters with frequent episodic tension-type headache. A controlled study. *Arq Neuro Psiquiatr* 2018;76(6):387-92.

Watanabe T, Ichikawa K, Clark GT. Bruxism levels and daily behaviors: 3 weeks of measurement and correlation. *J Orofac Pain* 2003;17(1):65-73.

Wieckiewicz M, Smardz J, Martynowicz H, et al. Distribution of temporomandibular disorders among sleep bruxers and non-bruxers-A polysomnographic study. *J Oral Rehabil* 2020;47(7):820-6.

Yadav S. A study on prevalence of dental attrition and its relation to factors of age, gender and to the signs of TMJ dysfunction. *J Indian Prosthodont Soc* 2011;11(2):98-105.

Yamaguchi T, Abe S, Rompré PH, Manzini C, Lavigne GJ. Comparison of ambulatory and polysomnographic recording of jaw muscle activity during sleep in normal subjects. *J Oral Rehabil* 2012;39(1):2-10.

Yanagisawa K, Takagi I, Sakurai K. Influence of tongue pressure and width on tongue indentation formation. *J Oral Rehabil* 2007;34(11):827-34.

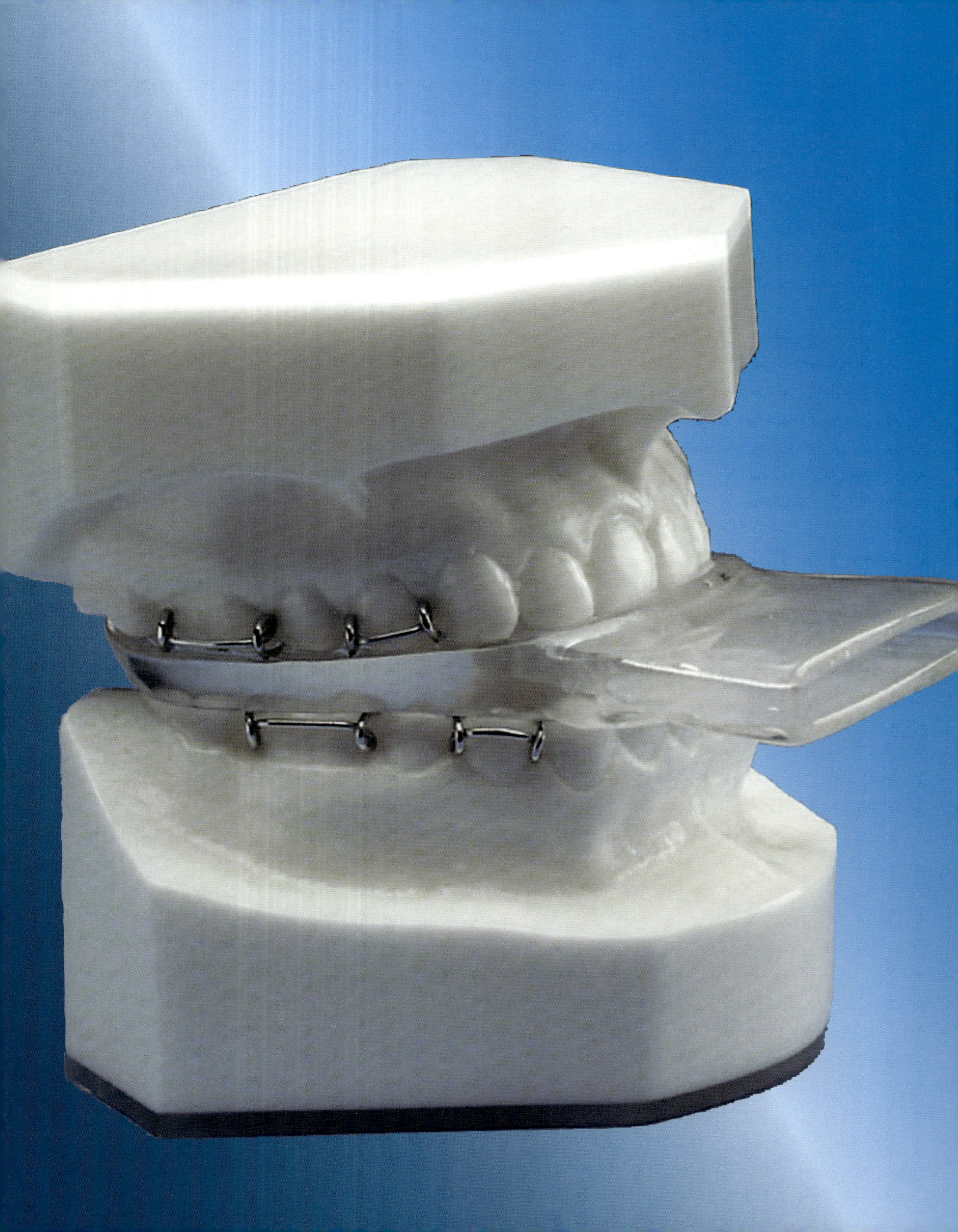

Oral devices

Francesca Milano · Antonio L. Gracco

Objectives

- Understanding the action mechanisms of oral devices (OAs)
- Understanding the available devices in the market
- Selecting the most adequate device for patients according to patient characteristics and disorders
- Understanding the titration mechanisms of the devices
- Understanding and managing the side effects of several devices

Oral appliances (OAs)

Oral appliances (OAs) are one of the conservative therapeutic choices for the treatment of obstructive sleep apnea syndrome (OSAS). They are used to stabilize the upper airways and increase their diameters.

Pierre Robin was the first who understood the close correlation among the lingual posture, mandibular position, and respiratory function. His hypothesis led to the development of a device—"monobloc"—that aimed at preventing the posterior collapse of the tongue in children with glossoptosis, mandibular hypoplasia, and mouth breathing via mandibular anterior repositioning (Robin 1902, 1934).

In the 1970s, McNamara (1979) demonstrated the effects of mandibular propulsion obtained using an OD on the airways and initiated the investigation of the effects of mouth breathing on mandibular development in subjects who were still in the growing phrase.

The forerunners of ODs for treating OSAS in adult patients were functional devices designed with a corrective purpose for deviant craniofacial development.

Tongue-retaining devices (TRDs) and mandibular advancement devices (MADs)

ODs used for treating sleep respiratory disorders are categorized as follows:

1. TRDs
2. MADs

TRDs are soft acrylic hollow bulbs that hold the tongue forward by suction due to negative pressure (📷 10.1). This *vacuum effect* on the tongue determines its protrusion during sleep and favors major tension of the pharyngeal walls (Sutherland *et al.* 2014).

TRDs were the first devices designed to reduce apnea and snoring in adult patients. The original idea was introduced by a psychologist—Charles Samelson—who aimed at treating his chronic snoring problem, which was affecting his wife who was a pianist and was concerned about losing her musical ear because of her husband's snoring.

Samelson understood that his snoring was caused by the collapse of his tongue. He collaborated with Rosalind Cartwright (Director of the Sleep Disorder Center of Rush University Medical School of Chicago) to develop a device that was able to hold the tongue in the most protruded position during sleep.

In 1982, Cartwright and Samelson reported their initial findings on 14 patients using TRDs and stated that it was possible to obtain a significant decrease in the number of nocturnal events (Cartwright and Samelson 1982).

In the literature, reports have provided limited evidence on the efficacy of TRDs because they are not well accepted or tolerated by patients. A TRD can be a treatment option for patients with insufficient dental anchorage or insufficient abili-

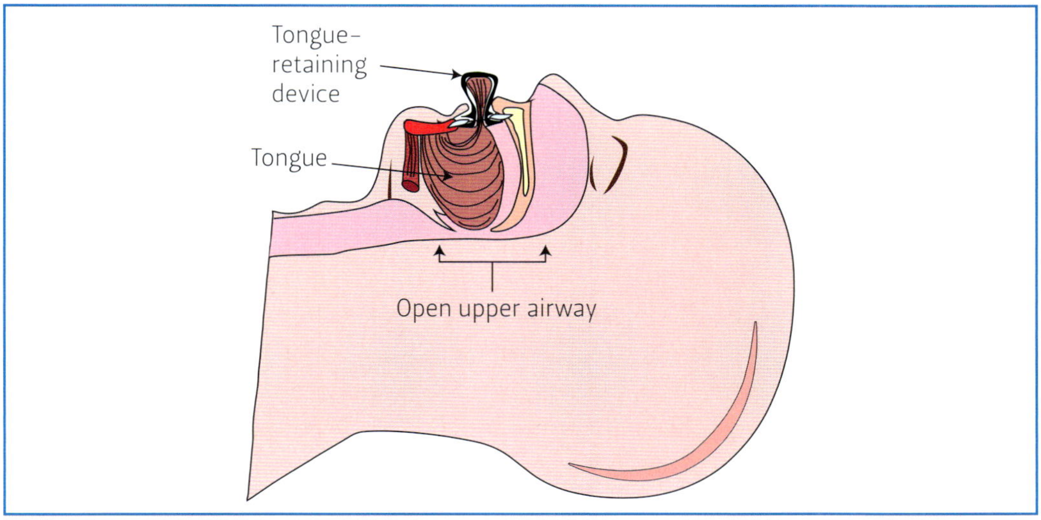

10.1 Action mechanism of a tongue-retaining device (TRD).

ty to protrude the mandible as long as there is no increase in the nasal resistance, (Deane *et al.* 2009).

MADs have different designs that allow mandibular advancement and downward distraction (10.2).

Dental anchorage guarantees control of the mandibular position.

MADs were first applied between the end of the 1980s and the beginning of the 1990s. The initial results regarding their efficacy were published in *The New England Journal of Medicine* in an article written by Peter George about an

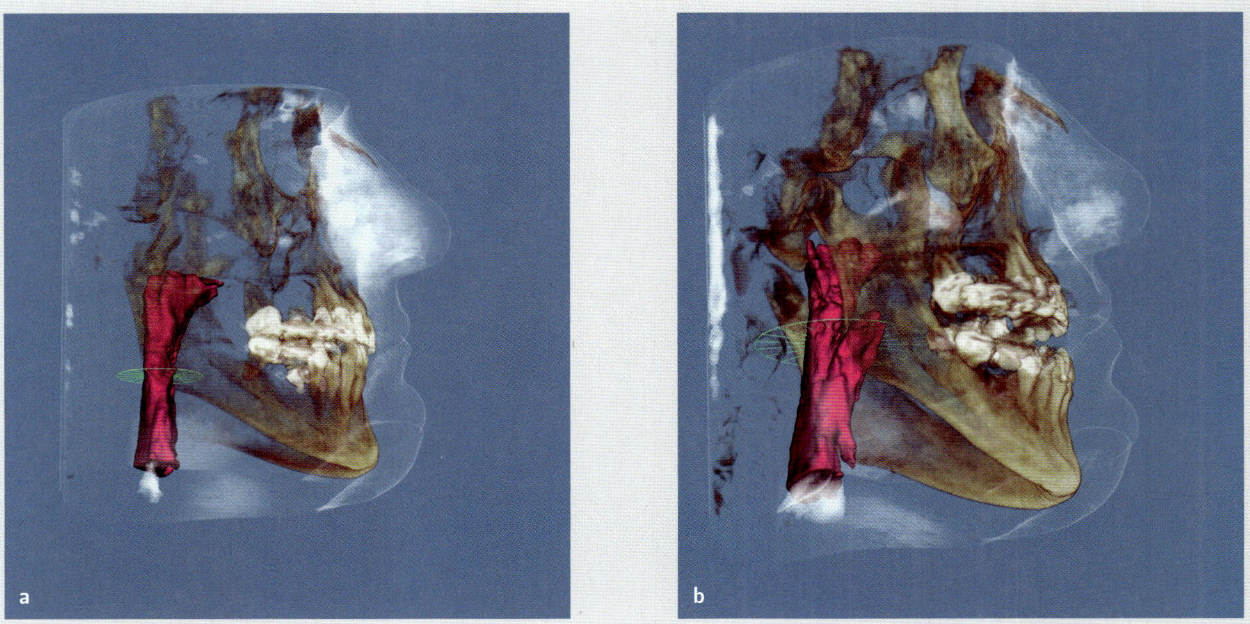

10.2 a. Mandibular morphological and volumetric cone beam computed tomography (CBCT) without a mandibular advancement device. b. Morphological and volumetric CBCT of the upper airways with a mandibular advancement device.

acrylic monobloc device with clasps for tooth grip, (Nocturnal Airway Patency Appliance NAPA; 10.3) (George and Soli 1985).

The evolution of MADs was the design of bimaxillary devices connected by a coupling mechanism that could allow to the patient to advance the mandible in a gradual manner (titration). *Titrable devices gave* the possibility to achieve a larger final advancement, reducing the risk of discomfort.

Over time, several **mechanisms of propulsion** have been proposed, assessed, and compared.

At the beginning of the 1990s, Alan Lowe (Professor and Chair, Division of Orthodontics of the University of British Columbia) proposed Klearway® (10.4), the first *titrable device*, which used a snap lock expansion screw placed at the center of the superior splint (Lowe *et al.* 1990). With increments of 0.25 mm per time, the screw allows an 11-mm range of anteroposterior movement.

The device is made of thermoactive acrylic material for easy insertion on dental arches.

A few years later, Thornton introduced the Thornton Adjustable Positioner (TAP®; Thornton and Roberts 1996), which is a device with two trays connected by a frontal hook attached to a bar or a sock in the opposite splint (10.5). The mechanism allows minimal freedom of lateral movements of the mouth (especially the version with the bar in the lower splint and dream TAP).

The research to achieve improved patient comfort with major freedom in the mandibular opening movement led to the development of MADs characterized by a propulsion system, such as HERBST (Rider 1998), with a metallic telescopic rod per side (SUAD).

In the version proposed by Dr. Hinz, i.e., the Intraoral Snoring Therapy Appliance (IST®), the length of the rod can be increased by an adjustable nut mechanism (10.6a).

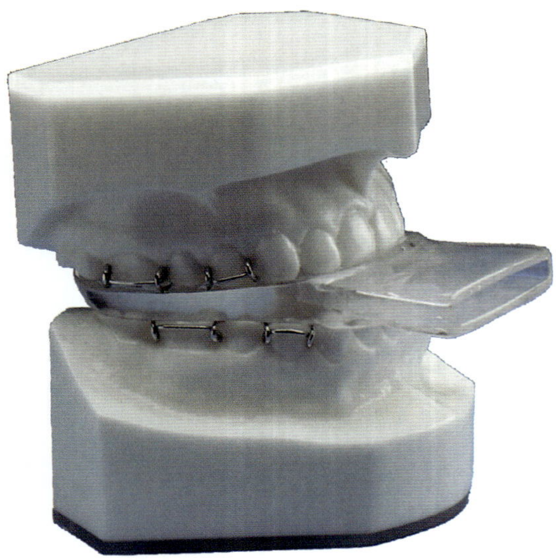

10.3 Nocturnal airway patency appliance (NAPA).

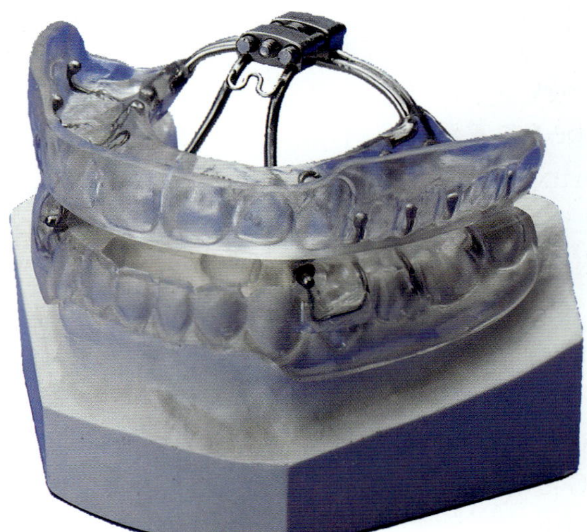

10.4 Klearway®.

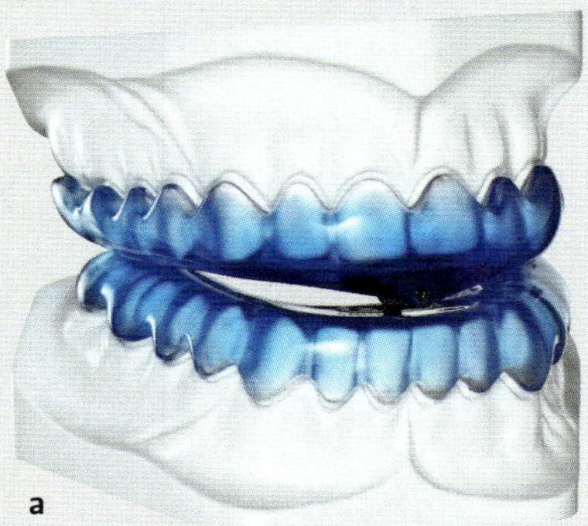

a

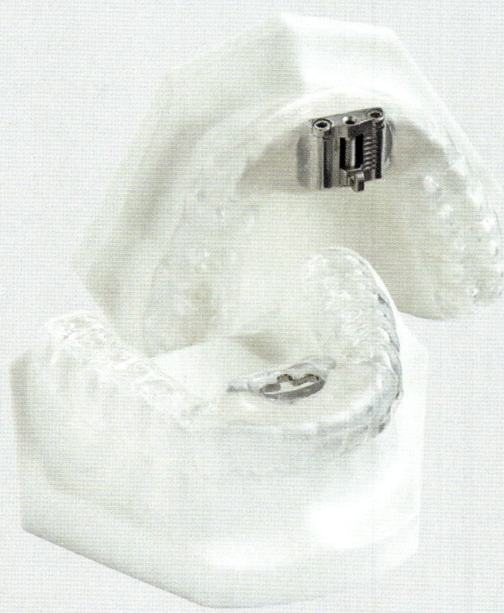

b

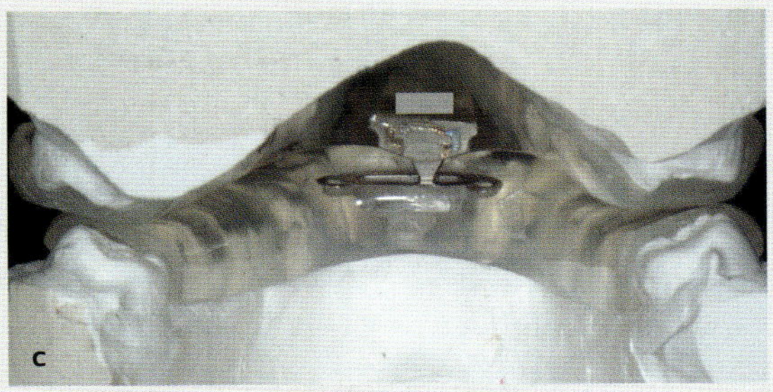

c

10.5 a. Thornton Adjustable Positioner (TAP®). b. TAP 3®, and c. posterior view of the advancement mechanism.

10.6 a. Intraoral Snoring Therapy Appliance (IST®), b. gradually advancing telescopic rod, c. presicion Herbst of ProSomnus with telescopic advancer mechanism of Leone.

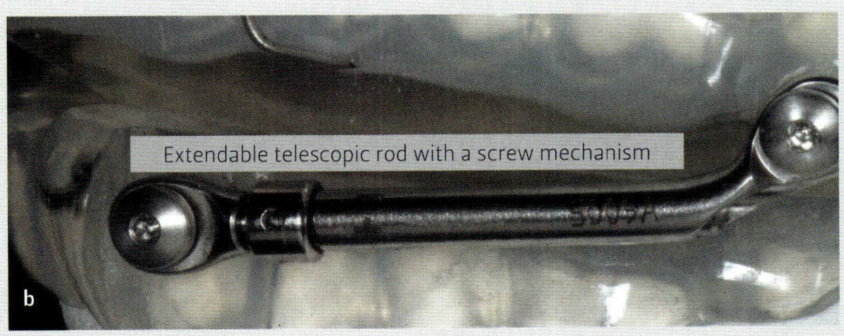

b

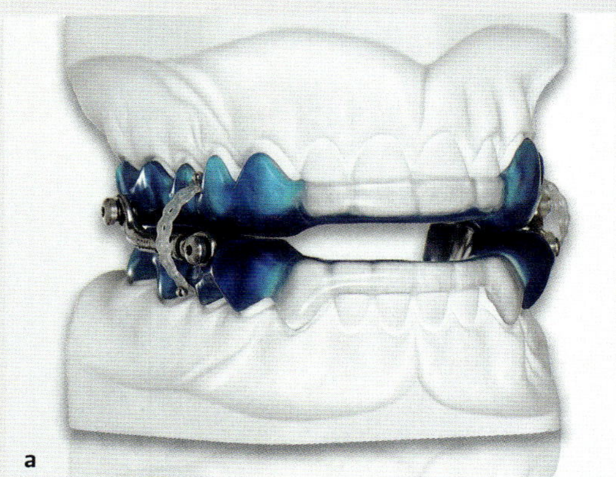

a

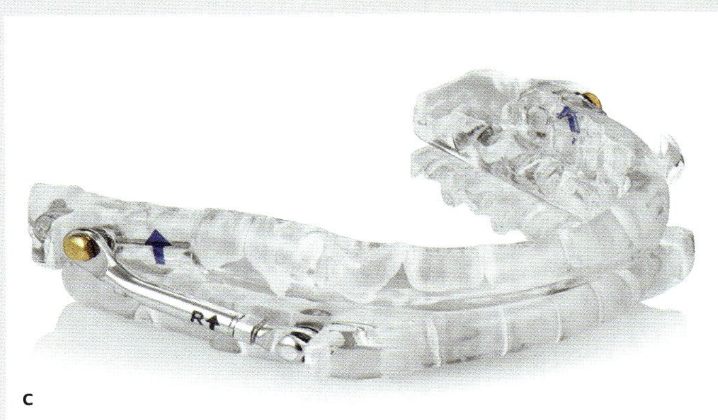

c

There is also a version in which the direction of the telescopic rod can be inverted (reverse rod) to increase mandibular protrusion if the mouth opens. The last telescopic rod wich has been developed, is the Telescopic advancer of Leone (10.6b), that can be choosen also in the Prosomnus CAD/CAM Precision Herbst version (10.6c). The device can be titrated with a wrench that tights the square head screws, elongating the rod.

Other MADs propulsion mechanisms are made by inclined ramps as Twin block appliance (Clark and Nakono 1988). The first of these mechanisms was Somnodent®, proposed by Richard Palmisano at the beginning of 2000. The device presents two vestibular fins placed on both sides of the lower splint. These fins have a 17° inclination and they are opposed to ramps placed in the upper tray that can be gradually advanced to 0.1 mm at one time by adjusting the screw embedded in the resin (10.7). In the latest version (10.8), the wings can be replaced with wings of different thicknesses to enable the possibility of a major advancement.

Due to the lack of a mechanism connecting the two splints and the improved inner soft material, this device can also be applied to patients who are completely edentulous in the upper arc (10.9).

The last fin mechanisms those have been proposed in the market are Leone Forward and Prosomnus IA (Iterative Advancement) and CA (Continuos Advancement) versions.

Leone Forward presents fins with an inclination of 30°, matching with the 70° angulated body of the upper metal screw. Each activation of the screw generates 0.1 mm of advancement (10.10a) Prosomnus CA and IA are made with computer-aided design/computer-aided manufacturing (CAD/CAM) and can be customized, designing different dual ramps angles (10.11 a-b).

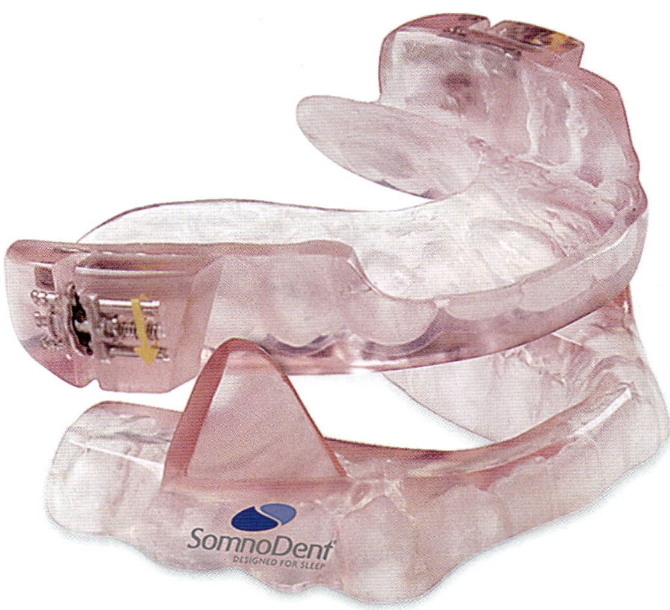

10.7 SomnoDent Flex®.

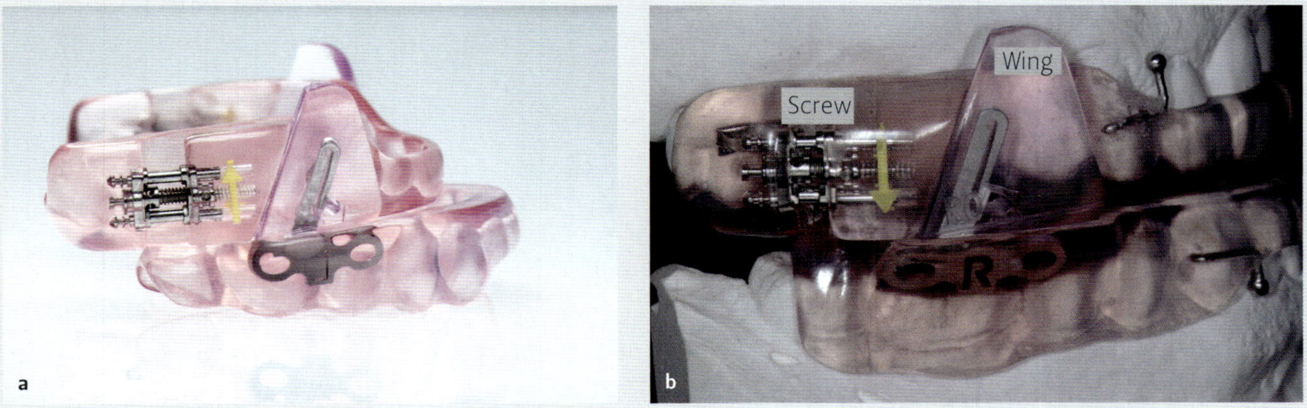

10.8 a. SomnoDent Fusion®. b. advancement mechanism: adjustment screw and interchangeable fin.

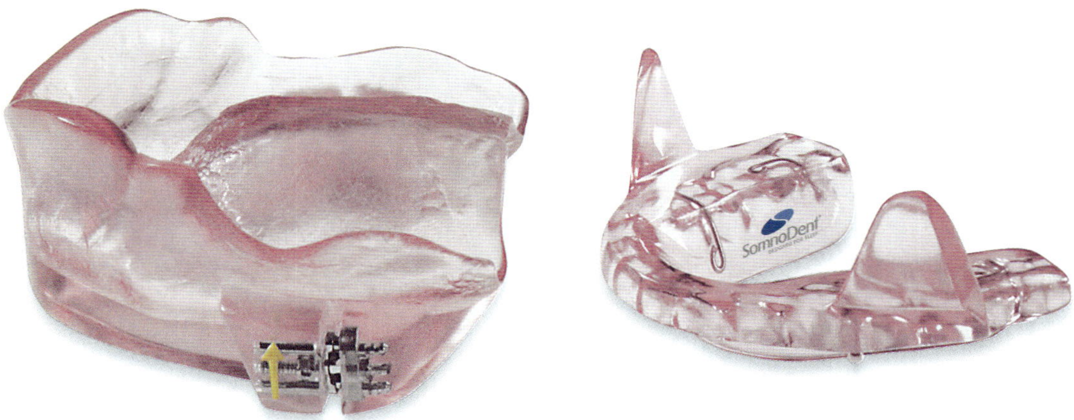

10.9 SomnoDent Edentulous®.

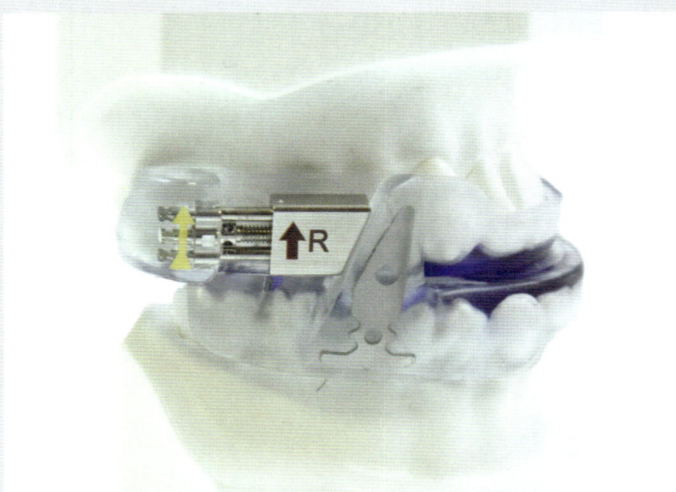

10.10 Leone Forward®

10.11 **a**. ProSomnus CA inclined ramps. **b**. ProSomnus IA straight ramps, **c**. Stepwise titration.

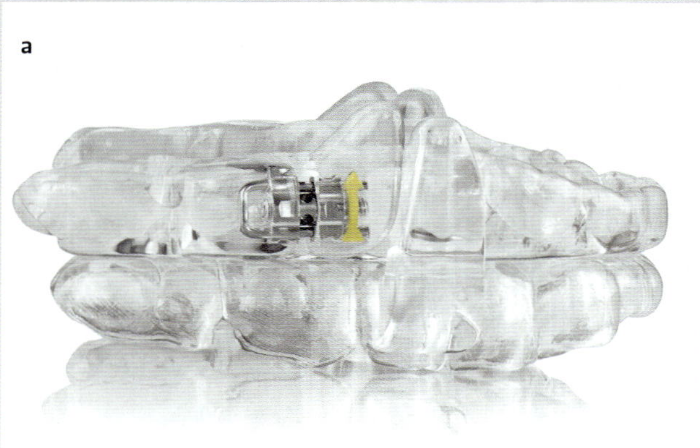

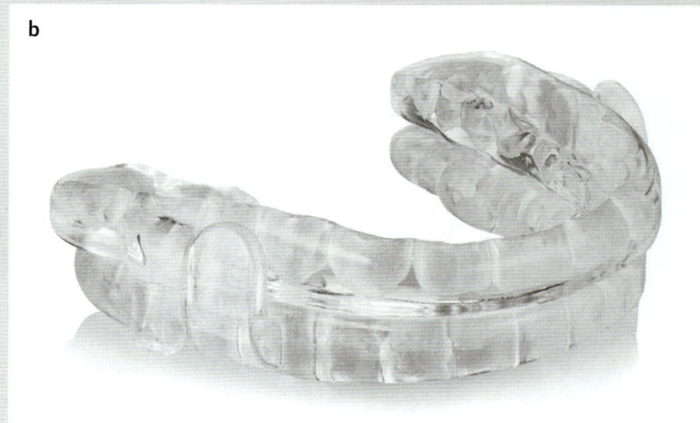

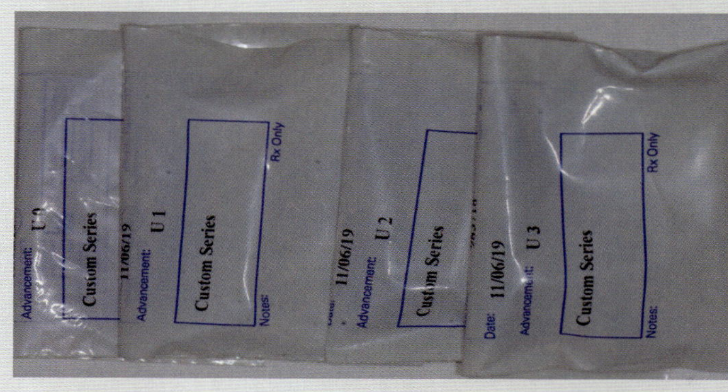

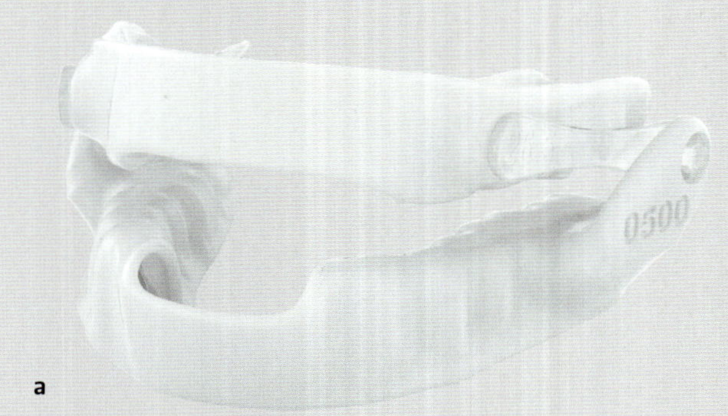

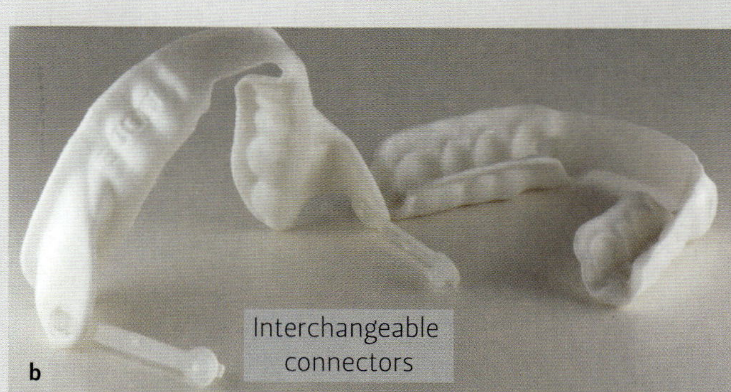

10.12 **a**. Narval® CC. **b**. Connector of the device (courtesy of Dr. Edoardo Manfredi).

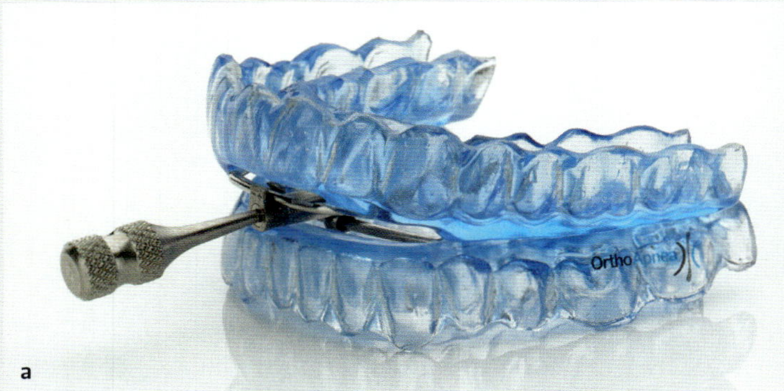
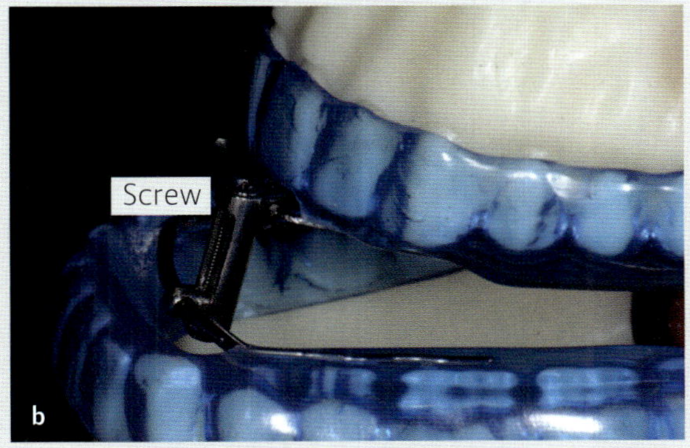

10.13 a. OrthoApnea®. b. Screw of the device.

Ramps can be inclined or straights: the second ones hinder the mandible retrusion when the patient open his mouth, during the night. In IA version the final advancement is technology achieved by a stepwise titration (with upper and lower sequential trays) and not with a screw mechanism. (10.11 c). Another device that has been introduced in 2009 is t Narval® CC (10.12a), a bimaxillary device that is fabricated with CAD/CAM technology. It has lateral straps that are provided with different lenghts and are exchangeable to obtain a gradual advancement of 0.5 mm at one time 10.12b).

Among frontal mechanism we can avail of inverted rod of OrthoApnea® that is attached to two bars, placed in the vestibular area of the upper and the lower trays (10.13a) or the frontal strap of the new Somnodent Avant® (10.14) that is attached from the posterior part of the lower tray to the frontal part of the upper tray.

The first one (10.13b) presents a screw mechanism titration (a full turn of the screw generates 0.4 mm of advancement), while the second one has a stepwise mechanism titration (different lenght straps to obtain an advancement of 1mm at one time).

Narval, Orthoapnea and Somnodent Avant push the mandible forward when the patient opens the mouth and control mouth opening in varyng degrees.

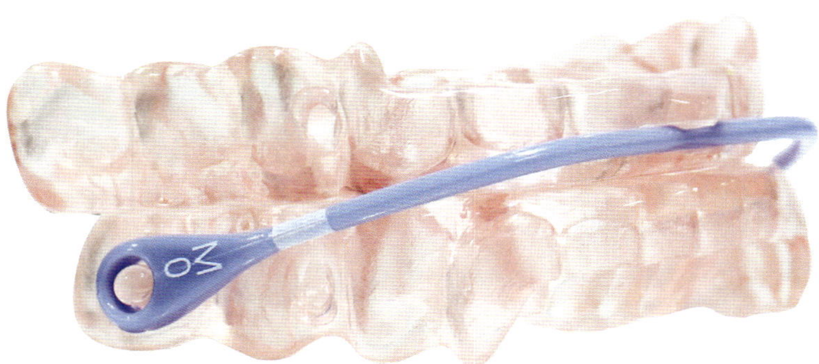

10.14 SomnoDent Flex®.

The **action mechanism** that enables MADs to increase their airway patency has not been completely elucidated to date. However, studies conducted using three dimensional (3D) imaging techniques [computed tomography (CT) and magnetic resonance (MR)] and direct vision of airways during induced sleep (sleep endoscopy) have provided important indications (Ryan *et al.* 1999; Kyung *et al.* 2005; Chan *et al.* 2010a and b; Sutherland *et al.* 2011).

Our understanding of the mechanism underlying the increase in upper airway patency must be improved to carefully select patients eligible for dental therapy.

The major difficulty in defining the effects of these devices on the upper airways lies in the differences in the pharyngeal dimension between sleep and wakefulness. A study published in 2012 on 32 patients with OSAS investigated an area of a pharyngeal section using MR to compare both wakefulness and induced sleep (with propofol) upper airways volumes in each patient. They showed a mean reduction of 75.5% during sleep (Faria *et al.* 2012).

Mandibular propulsion causes the following:

- an increase in the velopharyngeal diameter, particularly in its lateral side, for the anatomical proximity of the jaw, tongue, and tonsillar pillars (palatopharyngeal muscles and palatoglossus);
- an increase in the muscular tone at the base of the tongue that moves away from the posterior pharyngeal wall;
- protraction of the hyoid bone and stabilization of the epiglottis with a consequent increase in the hypopharyngeal diameter (Chan *et al.* 2010a).

These abovementioned effects cause an increase in the posterior air space at the retrolingual (hypopharyngeal) level and an increase in the pharyngeal diameter at the retropalatal level (velopharyngeal), particularly in the lateral direction (vedi 📷 10.4).

The hypothesis about the effects of **downward mandibular distraction** on airway patency states that such distraction influences the increase in the velopharyngeal diameter because of the traction exerted by such distraction on the pharyngeal superior constrictor and the palatoglossal muscle (George 2001).

The response of the muscular tone to protrusion is not always predictable and may lead to insufficient normalization of the caliber of the airways.

Indications

American Academy of Sleep Medicine (AASM)

The first guidelines on the use of OAs were published in 1995 by AASM.

In 2002, a task force gathered again to update the guidelines considering the advancements achieved in Sleep Dentistry and the number of published articles with high scientific rigor. This task force reviewed the available literature and selected a database with 141 publications that complied with the requirements set by them. Using this knowledge base, the indications and recommendations were updated and published in 2006. The last revised AASM guidelines were written in collaboration with the American Academy of Dental Sleep Medicine and are listed in Table 10.1.

10.1 American Academy of Dental Sleep Medicine (AADSM): Indications for using mandibular advancement devices (MADs).

Patients with simple snoring
Patients with mild, moderate, or severe OSAS preferring MADs over continuous positive airway pressure (CPAP) or those not responding to CPAP or not being eligible for it

Source: Ramar et al. 2015

European Respiratory Society (ERS)

In 2011, a task force of ERS published a report with the aim of summarizing the evidence on the efficacy of all nonCPAP therapies. The results of the ERS task force concluded that MADs are recommended for patients with mild to moderate OSAS as an alternative treatment to continuous positive airway pressure (CPAP) and for patients with severe OSAS who cannot tolerate CPAP (Randerath *et al.* 2011).

In addition to the abovementioned indications, MADs can be associated with positional therapy; ear, nose, and throat (ENT) surgical therapy; and CPAP with the purpose of obtaining the best possible outcomes for individual patients.

The combination of MAD with positional therapy aims at controlling the body position when several respiratory events occur even at the end of the therapy, particularly in the supine position.

The rationale of ENT surgery associated with MADs is to intervene at more levels when required based on the anatomy of the obstructive sites (Millman *et al.* 1998).

The correction of high nasal resistance and/or retropalatal obstruction may improve the outcomes of treatment with MADs.

ENT surgery may be indicated before dental therapy or subsequently when the obtained results were not acceptable or were considered improbable.

Finally, MADs can be combined with CPAP to reduce its pressure in patients who cannot tolerate it well (El-Sohl *et al.* 2011) and to replace the interface in cases wherein patients can barely tolerate it.

Contraindications

The major contraindications for using MADs as reported by AASM are as follows:

- inadequate number of healthy teeth
- insufficient dental health

- periodontal disease in the active phase
- severe tooth mobility
- temporomandibular (TM) joint disorder
- functional limitations of the TM joint.

The number of teeth in a dental arch must guarantee sufficient anchorage to the device. Conservative (periodontal and prosthetic) pretreatments must be performed when possible before bite registration. The patients must be instructed regarding hygiene practices. Current or regressed painful TM joint pathologies or functional limitations require careful gnathological evaluation.

Efficacy

Objective of the therapy

With **simple snoring**, the therapeutic objective is to eliminate or significantly reduce the snoring noise (a polysomnographic follow-up is not necessary), whereas for OSAS, the aim is to increase the upper airway space, resolve daytime sleepiness, reduce sleep fragmentation, improve quality of life, manage the associated comorbidities, and reduce cardiovascular risks.

Criteria to define cured OSAS

According to the criteria proposed by AASM for CPAP titration (Kushida *et al.* 2008), the polysomnographic follow-up scoring indicates excellent result when there is a residual apnea-hypopnea index (AHI) of <5 events/hour.

In severe patients a good result can be considered a residual AHI of <10 events/hour.

An acceptable result is a reduction of >75% in baseline AHI.

Polysomnographic control must be repeated during the therapy whenever the patients report aggravation of the symptoms.

Regardless of the variable used to evaluate efficacy, the sleep odontologist with the sleep physician evaluates the outcomes of the treatment. This can be performed by interpreting the context of the comorbidities associated with individual patients (e.g., daytime pressure values and reduction in possible arrhythmia episodes), the alleviation of symptoms and by analyzing the number of residual respiratory events in the supine and nonsupine positions and the quality of nocturnal oxygenation (ODI and CT of <90%).

If the obtained outcomes are insufficient or can be improved, titration can be continued according to the tolerability of the patient or the opportunity for complementary therapy should be evaluated.

As suggested previously, treatment with MADs can be associated with CPAP therapy, ENT surgical therapy and/or positional therapy.

If sleepiness persists significantly, the sleep medicine specialist must determine if a specific pharmacological treatment needs to be prescribed (Rosenberg and Doghramji 2009).

Percentage of success of MAD therapy

In 2005, a task force of AASM set the objective to investigate the efficacy of MADs.

A systematic review was published in Sleep in 2006 and it concluded that even if MADs do not achieve an efficacy similar to that of CPAP in reducing the number of nocturnal respiratory events, they can reduce AHI to <5 events/hour in 42% of the patients and AHI to <10 events/hour in 52% of the patients and obtain a response (reduction of at least 50% in AHI compared with the baseline AHI) in 65% of the patients. These results were confirmed by Hoffstein in the following year (Hoffstein 2007).

Having ascertained the reliability of MADs for treating chronic snoring and mild or moderate OSAS, AASM developed new guidelines that were published in 2006.

The indications to therapy were based on the evidence that the response is associated with the original level of severity. The response percentage is 57%–81% in patients with mild-moderate OSAS, whereas this response percentage decreases in patients with moderate-severe OSAS wherein the probability of response to the treatment with MADs is 52%. Literature reports have indicated a percentage of success between 41% and 51% for patients with severe OSAS according to the criteria used to define cured OSAS (AHI < 5 and AHI < 10, respectively) (Pancer *et al.* 1999; Rose *et al.* 2002).

The most recent update on the efficacy of MADs was published by Kate Sutherland and collaborators, and this report confirmed that considering the criteria for cured OSAS with achievements of AHI < 5 (reduced by at least 50% compared with the baseline), 48% of the patients responded to the therapy (in a group of nonselected patients with mild to severe OSAS). If the criteria for cured OSAS is the achievement of AHI <10 (reduced by at least 50% compared to the baseline), the percentage of responders is 64% of the treated patients.

Regarding the effects of MAD on snoring and daytime symptoms, the data reported in the literature indicate an improvement, particularly subjective improvements, in the snoring noise (Schmidt-Nowara *et al.* 1995; Bates and McDonald 2006; Maguire *et al.* 2010), a reduction in daytime sleepiness, and an improvement in the scores of test on quality of life (FOSQ and SF-36), which are similar to those reported for the ventilatory therapy (Engleman *et al.* 2002; Barnes *et al.* 2004; Naismith *et al.* 2005; Gagnadoux *et al.* 2009).

The data elaborated by Hoffstein allowed pinpointing the measure of the efficacy of treatment with MADS for investigating snoring and daytime sleepiness (10.2).

Furthermore, no significant differences have been reported for patients treated with MADs and CPAP in the simulated driving test after 2–3 months of treatment (Hoekema *et al.* 2007). Therefore, a revision published in the Cochrane Database (Lim *et al.* 2006) affirmed that there was no significant difference between the two therapies in improving the diurnal symptoms.

The importance of polysomnographic control has been highlighted by two randomized and controlled studies, which compared MADs and inactive OAs and reported that a high percentage of patients treated with placebo—as controls—reported subjective symptoms and wished to continue the therapy (Gotsopoulos *et al.* 2002; Johnston *et al.* 2002).

In three of the trials reviewed by Hoffstein that evaluated the control of cardiovascular comorbidities, an improvement in arterial pressure (both diastolic and systolic) of 3–5 mmHg was associated with treatment with MADs.

In 2013, Anandam and collaborators presented the results of a cohort study conducted for more than 6 years on 562 patients with severe OSAS. All the patients had been initially treated with CPAP but treatment was interrupted in 319 patients (57%) after 3 months from titration, and these patients chose to undergo treatment with MADs. The purpose of the study was to compare the risk of mortality for cardiovascular events in patients treated with MADs, those treated with CPAP, a group of severe nontreated patients, and a group of healthy patients with AHI of <5. The results confirmed an increased risk of mortality in the severe nontreated patients, and they demonstrated that patients treated with CPAP and MADs had an overlapping mortality risk, which was similar to that observed in patients who did not have OSAS. These results are in line with those reported by Phillips and collaborators on the short-term efficacy of the two therapies in terms of health benefits (Phillips *et al.* 2013) and with the conclusion reported in the revision on the cardiovascular benefits of treatment with MADs that was recently published by Van Haesendonck and collaborators (2015).

10.2 Efficacy of MADs in improving the symptoms.

Snoring
Observed patients: 529*
Percentage of improvement in symptoms: 45%
Daytime sleepiness
Observed patients: 854
Baseline Epworth sleepiness score (EES): 11.2 vs. EES with MAD: 7.8
Percentage of improvement in symptoms: 30%

* The indicators of snoring are not homogenously defined scales depending on the trial. They are available separately, but it is not possible to calculate the average.

The reason why health benefits and the resolution of symptomatology are so similar for patients treated with a MAD or CPAP despite the treatment with MADs being less efficacious in reducing AHI, probably lies in the relation between residual AHI and the degree of adherence to the therapy, which is often higher in patients treated with MADs.

Adherence to therapy

Adherence is defined as the degree of constancy of the patient to follow the prescribed therapy (Sabate 2001). It is a multidimensional phenomenon determined by the interaction of several factors. Adherence to therapy with MADs is correlated with the characteristics of the patient (severity of the symptoms, subjective perception of the therapy benefits, self-motivation, awareness of the risks associated with apnea, presence of comorbidities, awareness of the adverse effects that MAD may involve, and presence of strong nasal resistance), with environmental factors (support received, family and social background), the kind of device used (comfort, retention, gradual advancement), and with the therapist (ability to educate, motivate and encourage the patient; competence in predicting the risk of occurrence of complications, identifying and managing these complications and remote supervision) (10.15).

In the literature, the level of adherence to treatment with MADs has been reported in terms of the following:

- percentage of patients using the device at follow-up
- number of hours during which the device is used on average per night
- number of days in which the device is used on average per week

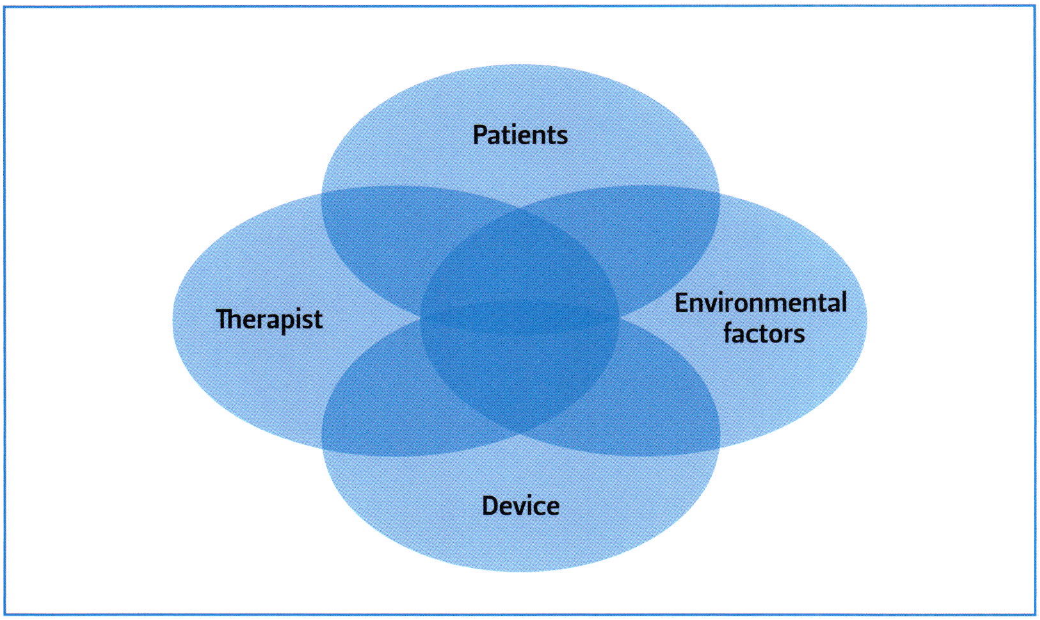

10.15 Factors affecting patient adherence to treatment with MADs

From the data of the 21 of the studies analyzed by Hoffstein, the mean data on a total of 3,107 patients indicated 56%–68% of the subjects used the device after 33 months since the beginning of the therapy, whereas the revision of AASM indicates a mean value of 77% one year after treatment with the device (Ferguson *et al.* 2006) and a mean use of 6.8 hours per night (Gotsoupoulos *et al.* 2002).

A study on 180 patients after 10 years since the beginning with treatment with MADs reported an adherence of 65% and the percentage of patients wearing it at least six nights per week was 55% (Jauhar *et al.* 2008) (■ 10.3).

■ **10.3** Therapeutic adherence reported subjectively by patients treated with MADs.

Observed patients: 3,017
Follow-up duration: 33 months
Percentage of adherence: 56%–58%

The limit for assessing adherence to treatment with MADs lies in the difficulty of evaluating the data in an objective way, similar to that in ventilatory therapy. Recently, a Belgian group led by Vanderveken and Braem published the results of a study on the use of thermosensitive microsensors integrated into a MAD to evaluate the number of hours the device was used per night. The analysis of the data after 3 months of therapy revealed that thermosensitive microsensors integrated into an OD were used for a mean duration of 6.7 ± 1.3 hours per night.

None of the patients interrupted the use of the device after 3 months, whereas 84% of the patients use this device for more than 5 days a week over more than 4 hours per night. The sensor did not cause adverse effects (Vanderveken *et al.* 2012).

In conclusion, it is worth highlighting the extent to which the outcomes of the treatment depend on the accuracy of the diagnosis and the experience of the dentist in terms of specific education in Sleep Medicine. The knowledge of the mechanics and physiologic principles underlying the action mechanisms of the device, and the clinical implications underlying the choice of a particular device are critical issues to achieve good results.

A high degree of adherence to treatment with MADs must be considered as the primary objective.

The percentage of adherence is hardly predictable because it depends on several factors and it is a dynamic process, which is susceptible to motivational support from the odontologist and the family and social context of the patient over time.

Predictive factors of MADs therapy success

Several studies have been conducted with an aim to evaluate the possibility of gaining positive prognostic factors for treatment with MADs.

The literature describes a correlation among response to the therapy; the severity of the syndrome; the prevalence of obstructive events in the supine position; the age, sex, and body mass index (BMI) of the patient; the skeletal conformation; the site and pattern of obstruction; the capacity of protrusion; and the potential weight gain or loss during the treatment (10.4).

The most conflicting data in the literature are those identifying cephalometric predictive factors as reported in the revision by Sutherland and collaborators (Sutherland *et al.* 2014).

Regarding positionality, the devices that better control the AHI in the supine position are those favoring the control of mouth opening.

The efficacy of treatment with MADs in terms of the present obstructive characteristics depends on the site and pattern of the airway collapse during sleep.

Among ENT evaluations, the negative impact exerted by high nasal resistance (frequent in patients with OSAS) on the outcomes of therapy is crucial (Zheng *et al.* 2008).

A recent study aimed at evaluating the percentage of success of MAD in patients selected according to the characteristics described by an ENT specialist in respiratory sleep disorders demonstrated it was possible to obtain an AHI <10 in 73% of 42 of the studied patients (with mild to severe pathology) and an AHI <10 in 50% of the patients affected with severe OSAS. All the patients included in the sample had low nasal resistance during wakefulness, a prevalent retrolingual obstruction and a tonsillar grading <3.

The inclusion criteria are illustrated in 10.5.

10.4 Predictive factors for efficacy.

Anthropometric and physiologic factors
Young age
Female sex
BMI and neck circumference reduced
Positional OSAS
Reduced baseline AHI
Capacity of protrusion (6 mm at least)
Cephalometric factors
Reduced thickness of the tongue
Reduced length of the soft palate
Low overjet
Normal mandibular length
Normal or hypodivergence
Anatomic factors of the upper airways
Improvement in respiratory latency during simulation of mandibular advancement on sleep endoscopy or with Müller's maneuver
Low nasal resistance
Prevalent retrolingual (hypopharyngeal) obstruction

Table 10.5 Inclusion criteria.

Mild to moderate OSAS or severe OSAS in case patients refuse CPAP or surgical treatment and they are intolerant to CPAP
Retrolingual collapse ≥ 50% and retropalatal collapse ≥ 50% during Müller's maneuver
Tonsillar grading < 3
Low nasal resistance
Presence of at least six teeth in the lower dental arch
Absence of significant dental morbidity or nontreated periodontal disease
Absence of pain in the TM joints
Capacity to protrude the jaw for more than 6 mm

Source: Milano et al. 2013b

The evaluation of success predictability may become even more sophisticated by studying the patient during drug-induced sleep endoscopy (DISE). Therefore, when the patient is already a candidate for sleep endoscopy, to complete the diagnostic procedure in view of a surgical intervention, the treatment plan should be elaborated after having simulated mandibular advancement during the induced sleep (Eichler *et al.* 2012).

Therefore, Johal and collaborators published their data on the usefulness of simulation of advancement during sleep endoscopy to predict a positive outcome with treatment with MADs in 2005 and 2007 (Johal *et al.* 2005, 2007). In the studied patients, the simulation of mandibular advancement during DISE was obtained with a pull-up maneuver that consisted of delicately advancing the jaw during induced sleep. However, the obtained protrusion was arbitrary, not quantifiable, not repeatable and did not take into account the vertical distraction produced by MAD. Hence, it is recommendable to use a more predictable technique, utilizing a custom-made simulation bite during DISE (Milano *et al.* 2013).

The University of Antwerp published results on an evaluation of the efficacy of mandibular protrusion with a simulator during DISE, confirming the validity of this method to increase the percentage of success of the treatment with MADs (Vroegop *et al.* 2013).

A study on a remotely controlled mandibular protrusion during a full night polysomnography demonstrated that it can be a good method to predict the efficacy in patients affected with severe OSAS, who refuse or cannot be a candidate for ventilatory and surgical therapy. This practice has already been established for CPAP and it could be used to select responses to therapy and the ideal advancement (📷 10.16) (Cistulli *et al.* 2007; Almeida *et al.* 2009). Another option could be low cost test devices that can be titrated before to perform the control home sleep test (📷 10.17).

Il MATRx™ (see 📷 10.16) is a diagnostic medical device. It was presented in 2011 and approved by Food and Drug Administration (FDA) in 2012. It comprises two trays (one for the higher dental arch and one for the lower arch) to be filled with a silicon putty. After recording the habitual position, the max-

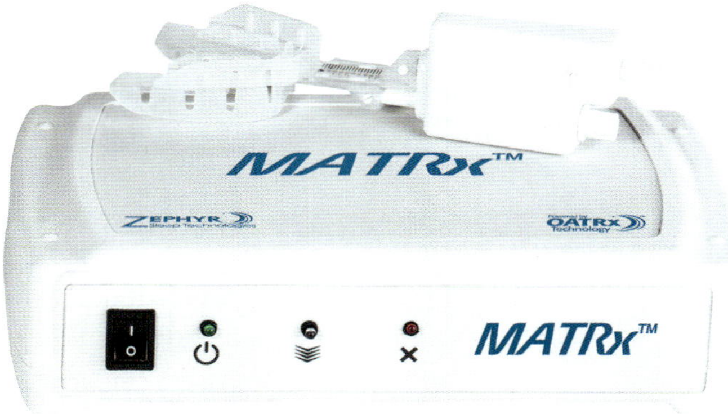

10.16 MATRx™.

imum protrusion, the initial advancement, and the maximum advancement tolerated by the patient, the odontologist reports the information to the sleep lab technician. At this point during a full night polysomnography, the technician can slide the two trays through the MATRx™ remote control to induce a gradual protrusion during sleep and identify the necessary advancement to solve the obstructive events in all the sleep phases [nonrapid eye movement (nREM) and rapid eye movement (REM)] and in all the positions (supine and nonsupine positions).

MyTAP™ (see 10.17) is a temporary appliance designed to last for a month. It comprises two trays (higher and lower) made of thermoplastic acrylic materials and is connected by a screw that allows gradual adjustment.

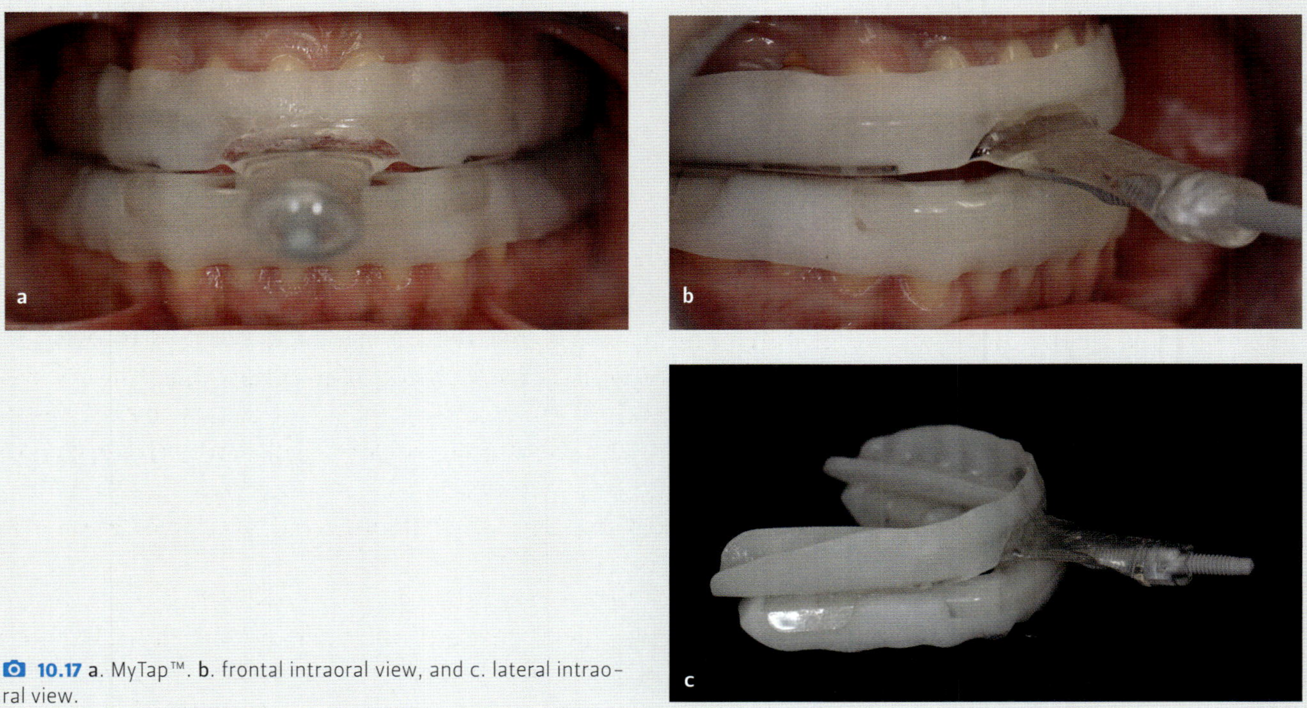

10.17 a. MyTap™. b. frontal intraoral view, and c. lateral intraoral view.

The trays are molded to the arches after being immersed in hot water and the material guarantees optimal retention. After recording the patient's habitual position and the maximum protrusion, the device can be advanced by the odontologist and then titrated (gradually advanced) by the patient during the first 3 weeks. When the final advancement is achieved, the patient can be subjected to a home sleep test to evaluate the efficacy of the appliance.

Finally, evaluation of the nonCPAP necessary pressure for resolution of the respiratory events can be considered to be a useful predictive factor for patients who use nonCPAP devices and show scarce adherence to therapy or for patients who wish to proceed to a MAD therapeutic attempt after a trial with a nonCPAP device. A nonCPAP pressure superior to 10.5 cmH2O is considered a negative prognostic factor for MAD treatment response (Tsuiki *et al.* 2010).

10.6 Side effects.

Short term
Hypersalivation or xerostomia
Dental tightness or soreness
Headache
TM joint discomfort
Occlusal alterations at awakening
Long term
Reduction of overjet and overbite
Reduction in the quantity and intensity of posterior occlusal contacts

Side effects

MADs have to be put on every night. This is why the potential adverse effects play a very important role in the selection and management of a patient and the choice of a device (10.6).

When planning a treatment, the risks and benefits must be individually evaluated for each patient considering that the time and difficulty of adaptation are correlated with the inherent comfort of the MAD and the initial therapeutic position. It is advisable to plan starting position calibrated on individual tolerability of patients during bite registration and to gradually increase the protrusion only after having allowed the patient to adapt to the initial position.

The side effects and their management are described more thoroughly in Chapter 12.

REFERENCES

Almeida FR, Lowe AA, Otsuka R, Fastlicht S, Farbood M, Tsuiki S. Long-term sequellae of oral appliance therapy in obstructive sleep apnea patients: Part 2. Study-model analysis. *Am J Orthod Dentofacial Orthop.* 2006 Feb;129(2);205-213.

Almeida FR, Lowe AA, Sung JO, Tsuiki S, Otsuka R. Long-term sequellae of oral appliance therapy in obstructive sleep apnea patients: Part 1. Cephalometric analysis. *Am J Orthod Dentofacial Orthop.* 2006 Feb; 129(2);195-204.

Almeida FR, Parker JA, Hodges JS, Lowe AA, Ferguson KA. Effect of a titration polysomnogram on treatment success with a mandibular repositioning appliance. *J Clin Sleep Med.* 2009 Jun 15; 5(3);198-204.

American Academy of Sleep Medicine. An American Academy of Sleep Medicine report. Practice parameters for the treatment of snoring and obstructive sleep apnea with oral appliances: an update for 2005. *Sleep.* 2006 Feb;29(2);240-243.

American Academy of Sleep Medicine. Practice parameters for the treatment of snoring and obstructive sleep apnea with oral appliances. *Sleep.* 1995 Jul;18(6);501-510.

Anandam A, Patil M, Akinnusi M etal. Cardiovascular mortalityin obstructive sleep apnea treated with continuous positiveairway pressure or oral appliance: an observational study. *Respirology.* 2013;18:1184-1190.

Barnes M, McEvoy RD, Banks S, Tarquinio N, et al. Efficacy of positive airway pressure and oral appliance in mild to moderate obstructive sleep apnea. *Am J Respir Crit Care Med.* 2004 Sep 15;170(6):656-664. Epub 2004 Jun 16.

Bates CJ, McDonald JP. Patients' and sleeping partners' experience of treatment for sleep-related breathing disorders with a mandibular repositioning splint. *Br Dent J* 2006;200(2):95-101.

Cartwright RD, Samelson CF. The effects of a nonsurgical treatment for obstructive sleep apnea. The tongue-retaining device. *JAMA.* 1982 Aug 13;248(6);705-709.

Chan AS, Lee RW, Srinivasan VK, et al. Nasopharingoscopic evaluation of oral appliance therapy for obstructive sleep apnoea. *Eur Resp J.* 2010b Apr;35(4);836-842.

Chan AS, Sutherland K, Schwab RJ, et al. The effect of mandibular advancement on upper airway structure in obstructive sleep apnoea. *Thorax.* 2010a Aug;65(8):726-732.

Cistulli PA, Chan AS, Lee RW. Dental appliance treatment for obstructive sleep apnea. *Chest.* 2007 Aug;132(2);693-699.

Clark GT, Nakono M. Dental appliances for the treatment of obstructive sleep apnoea. *J Am Dent Assoc.* 1989;118:611-617.

Deane SA, Cistulli PA, Ng AT, Zeng B, Petocz P, Darendeliler MA. Comparison of mandibular advancement splint and tongue stabilizing device in obstructive sleep apnea: a randomized controlled trial. *Sleep.* 2009;32(5):648-653.

Eichler C, Sommer JU, Stuck BA, Hörmann K, Maurer JT. Does drug-induced sleep endoscopy change the treatment concept of patients with snoring and obstructive sleep apnea? *Sleep Breath.* 2012 Mar;17(1);1-6.

El-Solh AA, Moitheennazima B, Akinnusi ME, Churder PM, Lafornara AM. Combined oral appliance and positive airway pressure therapy for obstructive sleep apnea: a pilot study. *Sleep Breath.* 2011 May;15(2):203-208.

Engleman HM, McDonald JP, Graham D, et al. Randomized crossover trial of two treatments for sleep apnea/hypopnea syndrome: continuous positive airway pressure and mandibular repositioning splint. *Am J Respir Crit Care Med.* 2002 Sep 15;166(6);855-859.

Faria AC, Garcia LV, dos Santos AC, Beserra Diniz PR, Ribeiro HT, de Mello-Filho FV. Comparison of the area of the pharynx during wakefulness and induced sleep in patients with Obstructive Sleep Apnea (OSA). *Braz J Otorhinolaryngol.* 2012 Feb;78(1);103-108.

Ferguson KA, Cartwright R, Rogers R, Schmidt-Nowara W. Oral appliances for snoring and obstructive sleep apnea: a review. *Sleep.* 2006 Feb;29(2);244-262.

Gagnadoux F, Fleury B, Vielle B, et al. Titrated mandibular advancement versus positive airway pressure for sleep apnoea. *Eur Respir J.* 2009 Oct;34(4):914-920.

George PT, Soli BA. Treatment of obstructive sleep apnea with a nocturnal airway patency appliance. *N Engl J Med.* 1985 Aug 8;313(6);386-387.

George PT. A Modified Functional Appliance for Treatment of Obstructive Sleep Apnea. *JCO.* 1987 Mar;21(3);171-175.

George PT. Selecting sleep-disordered-breathing appliances: Biomechanical considerations. *J Am Dent Assoc.* 2001 Mar;132(3);339-347.

Gotsopoulos H, Chen C, Qian J, Cistulli PA. Oral Appliance Therapy Improves Symptoms in Obstructive Sleep Apnea. A Randomized Controlled Trial. *Am J Respir Crit Care Med.* 2002;166(5):743-748.

Hoekema A, Stegenga B, Bakker M, et al. Simulated driving in obstructive sleep apnoea-hypopnoea; effects of oral appliances and continuous positive airway pressure. *Sleep Breath.* 2007 Sep;11(3);129-138.

Hoffstein V. Review of oral appliances for treatment of sleep-disordered breathing. *Sleep Breath.* 2007 Mar;11(1);1-22.

Jauhar S, Lyons MF, Banham SW, Cameron DA, Orchardson R. Ten-year follow-up of mandibular advancement devices for the management of snoring and sleep apnea. *J Prosthet Dent.* 2008;99(4):314-321.

Johal A, Battagel JM, Kotecha BT. Sleep nasendoscopy: a diagnostic tool for predicting treatment success with mandibular advancement splints in obstructive sleep apnoea. *Eur J Orthod.* 2005 Dec;27(6):607-614.

Johal A, Hector MP, Battagel JM, Kotecha BT. Impact of sleep nasendoscopy on the outcome of mandibular advancement splint therapy in subjects with sleep-related breathing disorders. *J Laryngol Otol.* 2007 Jul;121(7);668-675.

Johnston CD, Gleadhill C, Cinnamond M, Gabbey J, Burden DJ. Mandibular advancement appliances and obstructive sleep apnoea: a randomized clinical trial. *Eur J Orth.* 2002;24:251-262.

Kushida CA, Chediak A, Berry RB, et al. Positive Airway Pressure Titration Task Force; American Academy of Sleep Medicine Clinical guidelines for the manual titration of positive airway pressure in patients with obstructive sleep apnea. *J Clin Sleep Med.* 2008 Dec 15;4(6);157-171.

Kushida CA, Morgenthaler TI, Littner MR, et al. Practice parameters for the treatment of snoring and Obstructive Sleep Apnea with oral appliances: an update for 2005. *Sleep.* 2006 Feb;29(2):240-243.

Kyung SH, Park YC, Pae EK. Obstructive sleep apnea patients with the oral appliance experience pharyngeal size and shape changes in three dimensions. *Angle Orthod.* 2005 Jan;75(1):15-22.

Levrini L, Sacchi F, Milano F, et al. Italian recommendations on dental support in the treatment of adult obstructive sleep apnea syndrome (OSAS). *Annali di Stomatologia.* 2015;6(3-4):81-86

Lim J, Lasserson TJ, Fleetham J, Wright J. Oral appliances for obstructive sleep apnoea. *Cochrane Database Syst Rev*, 2006 Jan 25;(1).

Lowe AA, Fleetham J. Effects of a Mandibular Repositioning Appliance Used in the treatment of Obstructive Sleep Apnea on Tongue Muscle Activity. *Sleep and Respiration.* 1990;395-405; discussion 405.

Maguire J, Steele JG, Gibson GJ, Wilson JA, Steen N, McCracken GI. Randomised cross-over study of oral appliances for snoring. *Clin. Otolaryngol.* 2010 Jun;35(3),204-209.

McNamara JA, ed. *Naso-respiratory function and craniofacial growth. Center for Human Growth and Development.* The University of Michigan, Monograph number 9. Ann Arbor, MI: Michigan University Press, 1979 Feb. 23; 27-40.

Milano F, Gobbi R, Scaramuzzino G, et al. Combined Treatment of a Severe OSAS Patient Planned after a Sleep Endoscopy Performed with and without a Mandibular Protrusion Simulator. *A Case Report Journal of Sleep Disorders: Treatment & Care.* 2013b;2(4):1-4.

Milano F, Mondini S, Billi MC, Gobbi R, Gracco AL, Sorrenti G. The impact of a multidisciplinary approach on response rate of mandibular advancing device therapy in patients with obstructive sleep apnoea syndrome. *Acta Otorhinolaryngologica Italica.* 2013a;33(5):337-342.

Millman RP, Rosenberg CL, Carlisle CC, Kramer NR, Kahn DM, Bonitati AE. The efficacy of oral appliances in the treatment of persistent sleep apnea after uvulopalatopharyngoplasty. *Chest.* 1998 Apr;113(4):992-996.

Naismith SL, Winter VR, Hickie IB, Cistulli PA. Effect of oral appliance therapy on neurobehavioral functioning in obstructive sleep apnea: a randomized controlled trial. *J Clin Sleep Med.* 2005 Oct 15;1(4);374-380.

Pancer J, Al-Faifi S, Al-Faifi M, Hoffstein V. Evaluation of variable mandibular advancement appliance for treatment of snoring and sleep apnea. *Chest.* 1999 Dec;116(6);1511-1518.

Petit FX, Pépin JL, Bettega G, Sadek H, Raphaël B, Lévy P. Mandibular advancement devices: rate of contraindications in 100 consecutive obstructive sleep apnea patients. *Am J Respir Crit Care Med.* 2002 Aug 1;166(3);274-278.

Phillips CL, Grunstein RR, Darendeliler MA, et al. Health outcomes of continuous positive airway pressure versus oral appliance treatment for obstructive sleep apnea. *Am J Respir Crit Care Med.* 2013;187:879-887.

Ramar K, Dort LC, Katz SG, et al. Clinical practice guideline for the treatment of obstructive sleep apnea and snoring with oral appliance therapy: an update for 2015. *Journal of Dental Sleep Medicine.* 2015;2(3):71- 125.

Randerath WJ, Verbraecken J, Andreas S, et al. European Respiratory Society task force on non-CPAP therapies in sleep apnoea. Non-CPAP therapies in obstructive sleep apnoea. *Eur Respir J.* 2011 May;37(5);1000-1028.

Rider EA. Removable Herbst Appliance for treatment of Ostructive Sleep Apnea. *JCO.* 1988 Apr;22(4);256-257.

Robin P. Demonstration pratique sur la construction et la mise enbouche d'un Nouvelle appareil de redressement. *Revue de Stomatologie.* 1902;9:561-590.

Robin P. Glossoptosis due to atresia and hypotrophy of the mandible. *Am J of disease of children.* 1934 Sept.;48(3);541-547.

Rockville, MD. *Class II special controls guidance document: intraoral devices for snoring and/or obstructive sleep apnea: guidance for industry and FDA.* US Food and Drug Administration Center for Devices and Radiologic Health. 2002.

Rose E, Staats R, Schulte-Mönting J, Jonas IE. Treatment of obstructive sleep apnea with the Karwetzky oral appliance. *Eur J Oral Sci.* 2002 Apr;110(2);99-105.

Rosenberg R, Doghramji P. Optimal Treatment of Obstructive Sleep Apnea and Excessive Sleepiness. *Adv Ther.* 2009;26(3):295-312.

Ryan CF, Love LL, Peat D, Fleetham JA, Lowe AA. Mandibular advancement oral appliance therapy for obstructive sleep apnoea: effect on awake calibre of the velopharynx. *Thorax.* 1999 Nov;54(11):972-977.

Sabate E. *WHO Adherence Meeting Report.* Geneva: World Health Organization; 2001.

Schmidt-Nowara W, Lowe A, Wiegand L, Cartwright R, Perez-Guerra F, Menn S. Oral appliances for the treatment of snoring and obstructive sleep apnea: a review. *Sleep.* 1995 Jul;18(6);501-510.

Schwarting S, Huebers U, Heise M, Schlieper J, Hauschild A. Position paper on the use of mandibular advancement devices in adults with sleep-related breathing disorders. A position paper of the German Society of Dental Sleep Medicine (Deutsche Gesellschaft Zahnaerztliche Schlafmedizin, DGZS). *Sleep Breath.* 2007 Jun;11(2); 125-126.

Sutherland K, Deane SA, Chan AS, et al. Comparative effects of two oral appliances on upper airway structure in obstructive sleep apnea. *Sleep.* 2011 Apr 1;34(4):469-477.

Sutherland K, Vanderveken OM, Tsuda H, et al. Oral appliance treatment for obstructive sleep apnea: an update. *J Clin Sleep Med.* 2014 Feb 15;10(2):215-227.

Thorton WK, Roberts D. Nonsurgical management of the obstructive sleep apnea patient. *J Oral Maxillofac Surg.* 1996 Sep;54(9):1103-1108.

Tsuiki S, Kobayashi M, Namba K, et al. Optimal positive airway pressure predicts oral appliance response to sleep apnoea. *Eur Respir J.* 2010 May;35(5);1098-1105.

Van Haesendonck G, Dieltjens M, Kastoer C, et al. Cardiovascular benefits of oral appliance therapy in obstructive sleep apnea: a systematic review. *Journal of Dental Sleep Medicine.* 2015;2(1):9-14.

Vanderveken OM, Dieltjens M, Wouters K, De Backer WA, Van de Heyning PH, Braem MJ. Objective measurement of compliance during oral appliance therapy for sleep-disordered breathing. *Thorax.* 2012;0:1-6.

Vroegop AV, Vanderveken OM, Dieltjens M, et al. Sleep endoscopy with simulation bite for prediction of oral appliance treatment outcome. *J Sleep Res.* 2013 Jun;22(3):348-355.

Zeng B; Ng AT; Qian J; Petocz P; Darendeliler MA; Cistulli PA. Influence of nasal resistance on oral appliance treatment outcome in obstructive sleep apnea. *Sleep.* 2008;31(4):543-547.

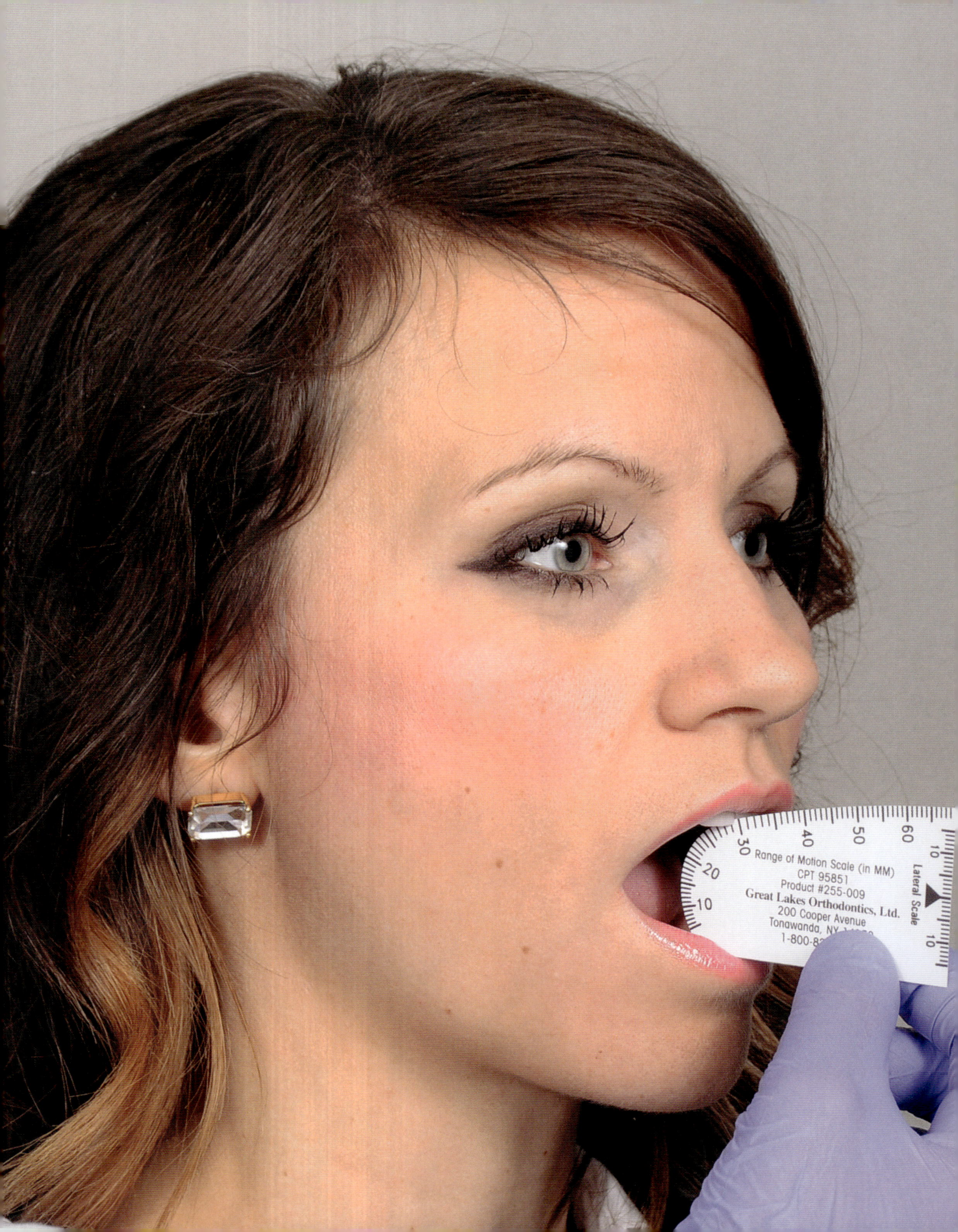
Range of Motion Scale (in MM)
CPT 95851
Product #255-009
Great Lakes Orthodontics, Ltd.
200 Cooper Avenue
Lateral Scale

Clinical dental approach

Francesca Milano ▪ Antonio L. Gracco ▪
Massimiliano Di Giosia

Objectives

- Understanding the dental diagnostic path for patients with obstructive sleep apnea syndrome (OSAS)
- Learning to define the roles of the dental sleep medicine practitioner in the multidisciplinary team
- Identifying the most appropriate mandibular advancement device (MAD) for the patient with OSAS
- Learning to titrate MADs

Introduction

As recommended by American Academy of Sleep Medicine, the dentist who treats patients affected by snoring and/or OSAS should be aware of the biological and anatomical basis underlying MADs mechanism of action, the limitations of the treatment, the required diagnostic and polysomnographic procedures, and the management of these patients over time.

The two substantial roles of the odontologist are as follows:

1. recognizing the patients that could be affected by OSAS and guiding them to the necessary diagnostic examinations;
2. treating the patients with snoring and OSAS that have already gone through the diagnostic procedures and are therefore candidates for therapy.

Because of the multiplicity of recognizable signs and symptoms shown by individuals receiving dental treatments, the first essential task includes screening.

The characteristics predisposing an individual to sleep obstructive respiratory disorders are male sex, age > 45 years, obesity (BMI > 29 kg/m^2 and neck diameter > 43 cm for men or > 41 cm for women), short or retruded jaw, narrow and high arched palate, macroglossia or reduced lingual space, redundant soft palate, and enlarged uvula. Therefore, it is important to interview subjects presenting one or more of these abovementioned traits about the quality of their sleep and the possible presence of snoring.

Total *edentulism* must be considered a risk factor due to the anatomical changes impairing the size of the upper airways (decreased posterior and retropharyngeal airspace) caused by the diminished vertical dimension (Bucca *et al.* 2006). Therefore, some authors recommend continuing the use of dentures during sleep despite the increased risk of developing candidiasis.

While investigating the presence of signs and symptoms of OSAS, particular attention should be given to patients requiring occlusal splint therapy for treating bruxism. In fact, this condition is often associated with the presence of apnea (Ohayon *et al.* 2001), and the bite can cause aggravation of the respiratory disturbance, as hypothesized and demonstrated by Lavigne in 2004 (Gagnon *et al.* 2004).

In cases of suspected OSAS, patients should be informed about the related risks and be directed to a specialist in sleep medicine (Ramar *et al.* 2015).

The second task for the odontologist is to treat the patient in collaboration with the sleep medicine physician and all the healthcare providers involved in the therapy.

The therapeutic stages include the initial examination, medical record collection, treatment plan development, clinical procedures for the fabrication of the device, delivery, follow-up, and efficacy control and monitoring.

First visit

The purpose of the first visit is to acknowledge the requests and attitudes of patients, to characterize the level of severity of the clinical situation, to ascertain the completeness of the instrumental investigations already performed (if necessary, recommending their completion), and to evaluate the main inclusion and exclusion criteria for dental therapy.

Anamnesis records

The patient's **medical anamnesis** should be investigated for the presence of possible comorbidities such as cardiovascular pathologies, diabetes, metabolic syndrome, gastroesophageal reflux and symptoms that influence life quality.

Information about cardiovascular and metabolic pathologies and the daytime symptoms is important in order to distinguish the level of severity of the pathology and evaluate the need for treatment.

The presence of *neoplasia and past chemoradiotherapy* in the head and neck area may provide indications on possible alterations on the anatomy and elasticity of the airway walls. In 2001, Friedman and collaborators reported a very high prevalence of OSAS in these patients, highlighting the importance of identifying the affected subjects and treating them to improve their quality of life (Friedman *et al.* 2001).

Pregnancy may also represent a risk factor for the onset and aggravation of respiratory sleep disorders, which are in turn associated with a risk of pregnancy-induced hypertension and gestational diabetes (Fung *et al.* 2012).

The protective effect of female hormones decreases in the *post-menopausal* period; hence, knowing the age of menopause onset is a useful part of medical history for detecting a risk of OSAS (Kapsimalis and Kryger, 2002).

The quality of *nasal breathing* influences the patient's tolerance of the oral device and affects therapeutic choices.

It is important to ask the patient about their *quality of sleep*, awakening, daytime symptoms (sleepiness, memory and concentration), possible sleepiness when driving and their sleep position, with targeted questions to evaluate the night respiratory pattern and the presence of positive or negative prognostic factors.

It is helpful if the bed partner participates in the collection of information, because patients are often not aware of their disturbed sleep and do not report any daytime symptoms. The questions should focus on the depth of sleep, the frequency of snoring and possible respiratory pauses during sleep.

If the patient reports nocturnal awakenings, it is useful to verify their number and investigate their causes.

Male patients with respiratory sleep disorders report a higher prevalence of nocturia (more than two-three time per nights in patients with severe OSAS) caused by an excessive production of natriuretic hormone. Additionally, patients with excessive nasal resistance often wake up to drink water owing to an increased tendency to oral breathing.

A reduction in these events can be a positive signal in the evaluation of the efficacy of the therapy (Kaynak *et al.* 2004).

The behavioral habits must be investigated (smoking, alcohol consumption, narcotics and sedative drugs) the patient must be instructed about the important role played by these substances in determining the night respiratory events.

The patient's height and weight, which are necessary for BMI calculation, must be reported in their medical chart. The evaluation of BMI before and after the treatment allows correct interpretation of MAD therapy outcomes.

The *occupation* of the patient may have a considerable weight in evaluating the indications and choosing the treatment. Respiratory sleep disorders can result in unsuitability for military service and daytime sleepiness is highly significant for those individuals whose occupation requires driving.

In the **anamnesis**, it is important to collect information about the presence of fixed and removable dental prostheses, nocturnal parafunctions, possible symptoms related to the temporomandibular joint and previous traumas affecting this joint, headaches, periodontal and dental health, previous orthodontic treatments, ENT surgery and sleep respiratory disease during childhood.

Information regarding nocturnal parafunctions is helpful in the choice of the device in terms of design and resistance to wear and breakage.

The following information on **previous specialist assessments** should also be collected:

- medical and/or dental examinations
- polysomnographic examinations
- radiological examinations
- prescribed therapies (CPAP, surgery, oral appliances).

Unless a sleep medicine clinician has already administered the **Epworth sleepiness scale**, the examination must be completed with this questionnaire to obtain objective data on daytime sleepiness for comparison after the initial oral device delivery date.

Clinical examination

The diagnostic evaluation must be completed with a thorough objective examination including the following:

- *face:* analysis of the shape, proportions and symmetry of the face

- *profile*: evaluation of divergence and convexity
- *dental examination*: evaluation of the dental formula, presence of tooth decay and conservative and prosthetic treatments, veneers, tooth enamel erosion, anomalies, diastema and teeth overcrowding, analysis of the curve of Spee
- *transverse diameters*: evaluation of the shape and width of palate and lower dental arch and analysis of transversal relationship
- *dental relationships*: evaluation of the dental class, overjet, overbite and of the symmetry of the median lines
- *periodontal examination*: evaluation of the patient's hygiene situation and the presence of periodontal pockets, gingival recessions and dental mobility
- *soft tissue examination*: examination of the oral mucosa, the thickness and volume of the tongue (Mallampati score), tonsillar grading

The use of MAD may be associated with some side effects, which are most often transient and reversible. In some cases, they may be a reason for discontinuing the treatment. One of the most frequent side effects is pain in the masticatory muscles and/or the temporomandibular joint.

Hence, aside from the dental and periodontal evaluation, it is also important to conduct an accurate screening of the masticatory/cervical muscles and temporomandibular joints before beginning MAD therapy to identify patients with a higher risk of side effects. If present, this disorder must be treated before starting MAD therapy.

TMDs are musculoskeletal disorders of the masticatory system. The American Academy of Orofacial Pain defines them as "different clinical problems that may arise in the masticatory musculature, temporomandibular joints and/or related structures" (de Leeuw and Klasser 2013).

The most frequent symptoms are as follows:

- pain in the muscles and/or temporomandibular joints
- joint noise (clicking sounds, crepitus etc.)
- limitation or changes in mandibular movements.

Such disorders are quite widespread in the general population and their prevalence (9%–45%) is higher than the real need for treatment (3%–9% of symptomatic patients) (de Leeuw and Klasser 2013).

A diagnosis of TMD is made after a detailed anamnesis, an accurate clinical examination and, when necessary, the use of imaging diagnostic techniques (magnetic resonance Imaging – MRI, computed tomography – CT, cone-beam computer tomography – CBCT) (Klasser 2006). Other instrumental examinations such as electromyography, kinesiographic recordings, sonography etc. are not indicated due to their low sensitivity and specificity (Suvinen *et al.* 2007; Manfredini *et al.* 2011; Al-Saleh *et al.* 2012).

The *evaluation of muscles* is performed by direct palpation (masseter, temporal, medial pterygoid muscles) and indirect or functional examination (lateral pterygoid area). Evaluation of the *temporomandibular joints* is performed by the palpation of the lateral pole of the condyle, a joint play test and auscultation of joint noises.

Evaluation of mandibular mobility is also important (range of opening and lateral motion) and the mandibular dynamic (deviation from linear gait during opening).

Listed below are some simple questions that may help the clinician in the diagnosis of dysfunctions affecting the masticatory muscles and/or temporomandibular joints (de Leeuw and Klasser 2003).

- Do you experience difficulty or pain when you open your mouth, for example, when you yawn?
- Have you ever had any episodes of mandibular block (difficulty opening the mouth completely)?
- Do you have pain when you chew or after talking for a long time?
- Do you feel sometimes that your facial muscles are tense and/or tired?
- Do you hear clicking or popping noises in the temporomandibular joint when opening and closing your mouth?
- Do you have frequent headaches, neck pain or toothache?

A positive answer to one or more of these questions should lead to the suspicion of dysfunction in the masticatory muscles and/or temporomandibular joints. This suspicion must be confirmed with anamnesis, clinical evaluation and, in some cases, appropriate instrumental investigations (MRI, CT, CBCT).

CLINICAL EVALUATION OF THE TEMPOROMANDIBULAR MUSCLES AND JOINTS

The clinical evaluation of the masticatory and cervical muscles and the temporomandibular joints consists of the following:

- muscular palpation;
- palpation and auscultation of the temporomandibular joints;
- joint play test;
- evaluation of mandibular movements.

Muscular palpation

A healthy muscle does not hurt during palpation. The purpose of palpation is to identify or exclude the presence of pain by applying a pressure of 1 kg for extra-oral sites and 0.5 kg for intraoral sites and the temporomandibular joint (Schiffman *et al.* 2014).

During palpation maneuvers, it is important to evaluate the presence of trigger points, which appear clinically as hypercontracted areas within the muscle. Trigger points can be a source of referred pain, with standardized pain maps (Simons 1999; Okeson 2013).

The *masseter muscle* must be palpated starting from the zygomatic arch until its attachment to the angle of the mandible. The deep portion of masseter muscle is very close to the temporomandibular joint, and it is therefore very important to identify it by asking the patient to contract the muscle. If there are trigger points in the masseter muscle, they can induce referred pain to the area of the temporomandibular joint or the ear and to the posterior teeth of the two arches (Dommerholt and Fernandez-de-las-Penas 2013) (📷 11.1).

The *temporalis muscle* must be palpated in its three bundles: anterior, medial and posterior, Possible trigger points may cause referred pain to the superior dental arch (Dommerholt and Fernandez-de-las-Penas 2013) (📷 11.2).

The *temporalis tendon*, which is inserted into the coronoid process, can be palpated from inside the oral cavity (📷 11.3).

The evaluation of the lateral pterygoid muscle requires a functional manipulation, asking the patient to make protrusive and lateral movements against resistance (📷 11.4).

Direct intraoral palpation, posterior to the tuber maxillae, is not reproducible (Thomas and Okeson 1987).

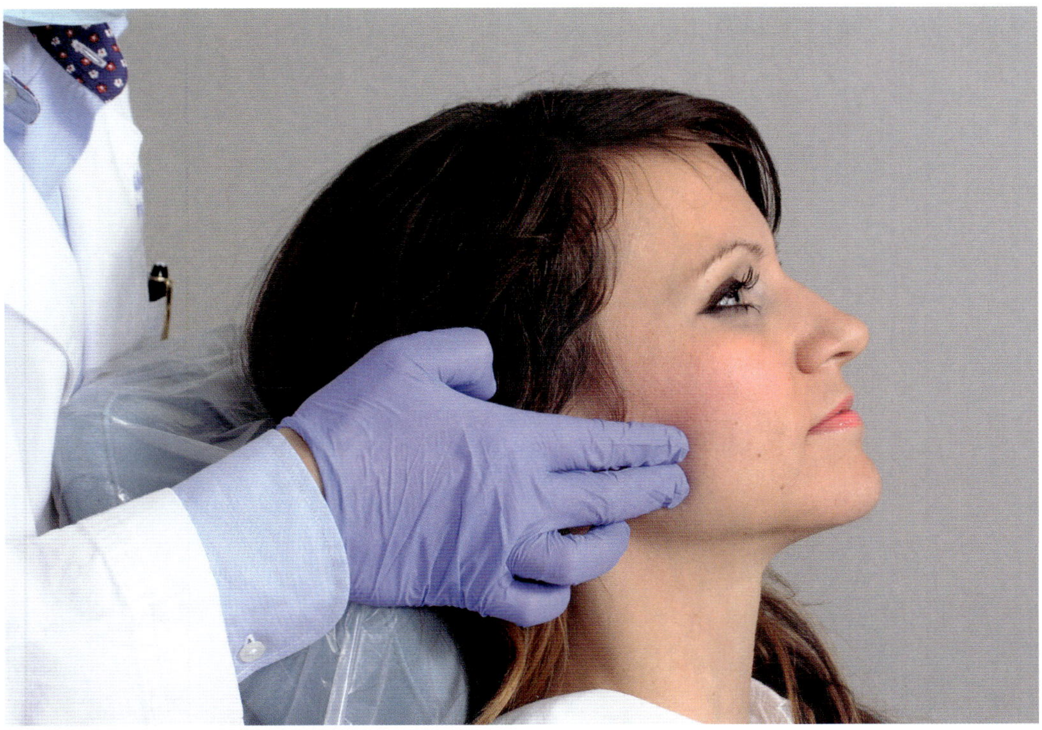

📷 **11.1** Palpation of the masseter muscle.

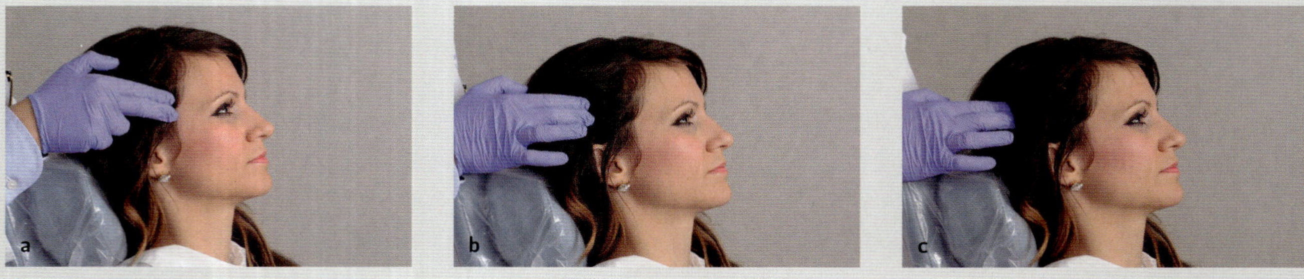

11.2 Palpation of the (**a**), anterior, (**b**) medial and (**c**) posterior bundles of the temporalis muscle.

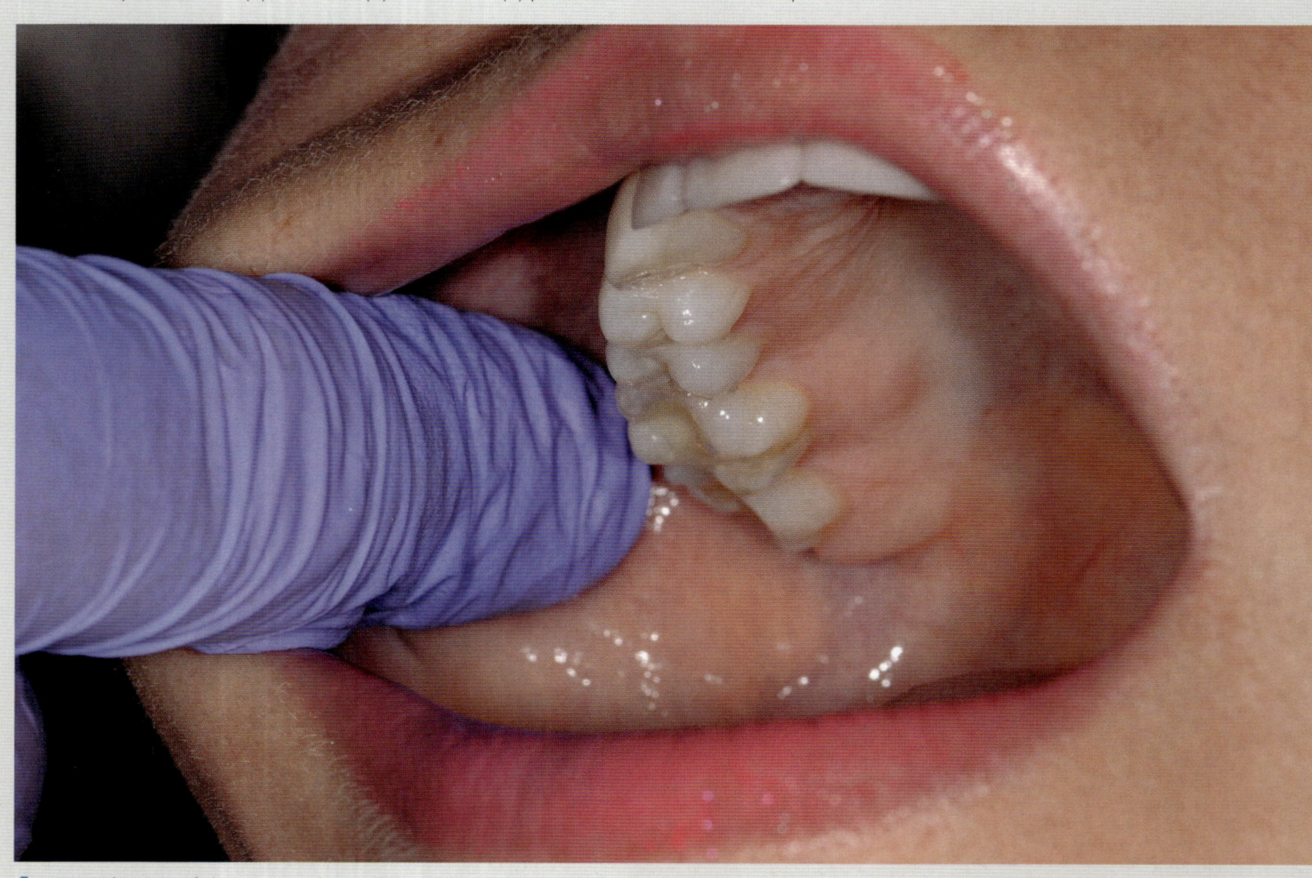

11.3 Palpation of the temporalis tendon.

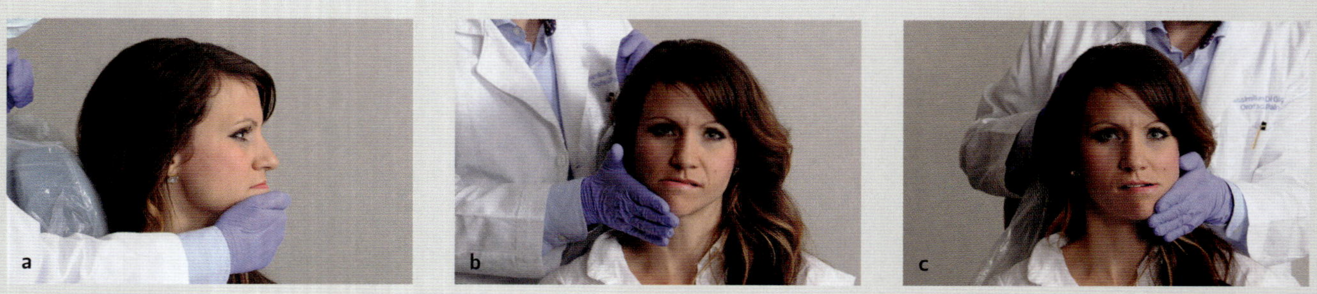

11.4 Evaluation of the pterygoid lateral muscle. **a.** Opposition to the movement of protrusion. **b.** Opposition to lateral movement toward the right. **c.** Opposition to lateral movement toward the left.

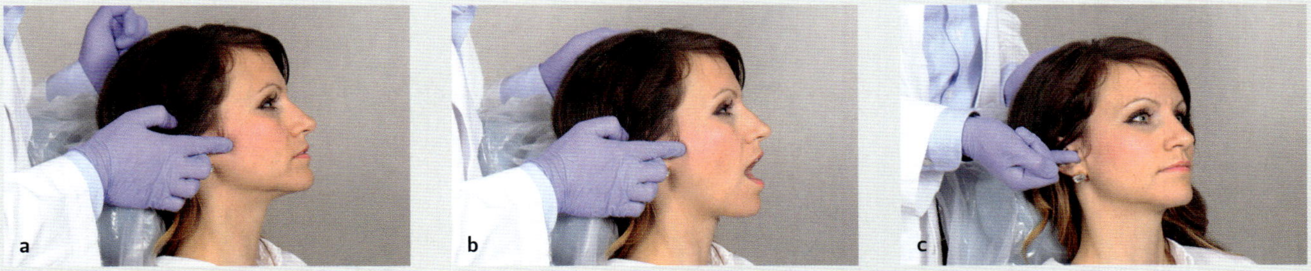

11.5 Evaluation of the temporomandibular joints. **a.** Palpation of the lateral pole of the condyle. **b.** Palpation of the dorsal pole of the condyle. **c.** Palpation in the internal auditory meatus.

Palpation and auscultation of temporomandibular joints

Clinical examination of the temporomandibular joints is needed to evaluate the presence of pain, joint noises and limited motion range.

The joint must be palpated laterally by placing the fingertips on the preauricular area corresponding to the lateral pole of the condyle and dorsally in the posterior area of the condyle with the patient keeping their mouth open. The pressure to apply is 0.5 kg.

For evaluation of the retrodiscal area, the condyle can be palpated by placing the little finger inside the acoustic meatus and applying pressure in the anterior direction with the mouth closed and with it open (Palla 2011) (11.5).

The condition of the temporomandibular joints can also be evaluated using the joint play test by executing distraction and translation movements (passive) and compression of the joint. The presence of pain indicates an inflammatory joint pathology.

To evaluate the presence of joint noises (clicking, crepitus), auscultation must be performed by gently placing the fingertips on the lateral poles of the temporomandibular joints and asking the patient to open and close the mouth.

Joint clicking should not be considered as a pathology and it is not a contraindication to treatment with a MAD. Epidemiologic data show that clicking has a prevalence varying from 18 to 30% in the general population, and it does not require any therapy if it is not associated with pain (Naje 2013).

A contraindication to treatment with a MAD could be a disc displacement without acute reduction (closed lock). In this case, it is necessary to first treat the joint problem and then begin MAD therapy.

Evaluation of mandibular movements

During the evaluation of the range of mandibular motion, in addition to the interincisal distance at maximal opening and laterality, it is also necessary to evaluate the maximal protrusion.

A limited protrusion (below 5 mm) could reduce the probability of treatment success with a MAD.

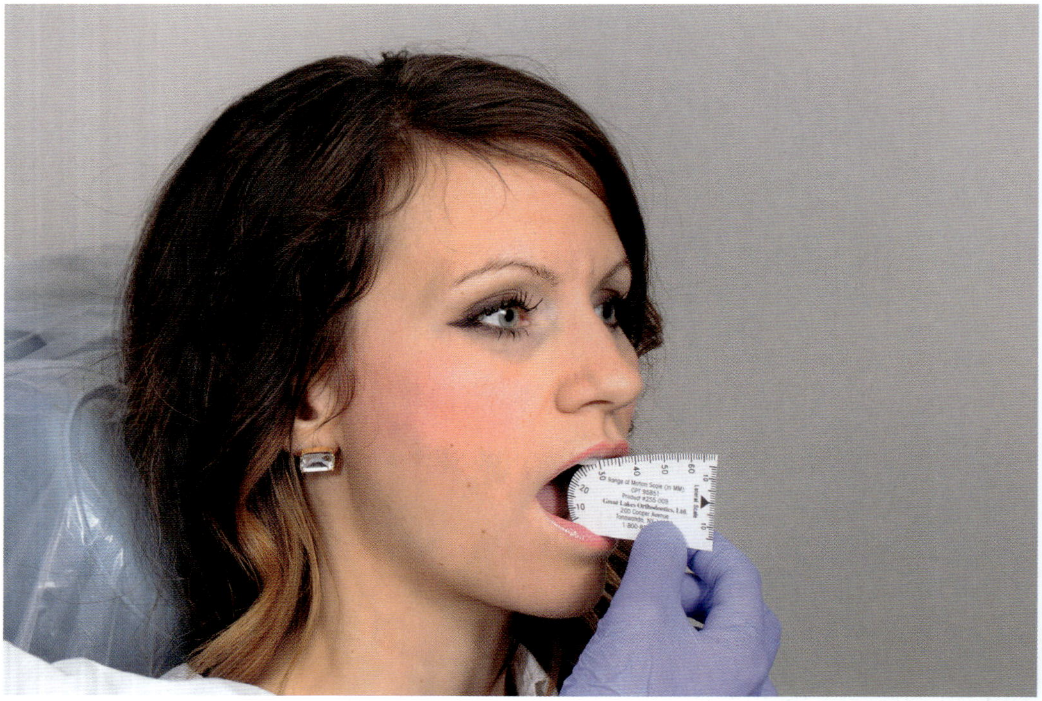

11.6 Measuring the opening.

An interincisal distance over 40 mm can be considered normal (11.6).

In cases of reduced opening, it is necessary to understand whether the limitation is caused by a muscular or a joint problem. In differential diagnosis, the end-feel evaluation test can be helpful. The patient's mouth opening is forced and followed by evaluation of the end-feel. If the end-feel is soft (in such case the patient can open the mouth much more, even if with pain) or rigid. A soft end-feel is typical of a muscular limitation whereas a hard end-feel is due to a joint limitation (11.7).

In the evaluation of the mandibular gait on the frontal plane, a deflection (a deviation without return to the center) must produce the suspicion of a disc displacement without ipsilateral reduction. In patients with disc displacement without ipsilateral reduction, the lateral movement is normal toward the side of the blockage, whereas it is reduced contralaterally.

A deviation with an "S" pattern (deviation with return to the center) may indicate a disc displacement with reduction (joint clicking noise) or anomalies of the condylar surface or fossa.

Preliminary diagnostic examinations

Before indicating and starting a therapy, it is essential for the patient to undergo polysomnography or cardiorespiratory monitoring performed by an expert sleep clinician.

In order to exclude a physical cause and increase the probability of success of the dental therapy, which is influenced by the presence of high nasal resistance

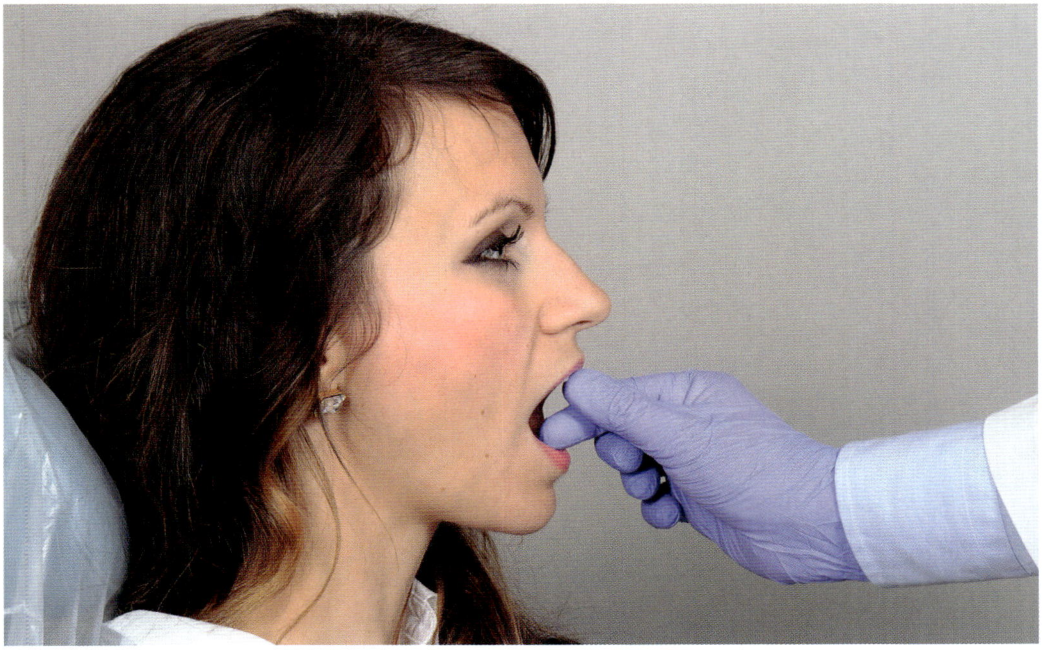

11.7 End-feel.

and the sites of the obstruction pattern, an ENT evaluation of the obstructive sites is necessary before starting therapy with a MAD (Mulla *et al.* 2011).

Record collection

The purpose of the collection of records is to be able to analyze the case and possibly discuss it with colleagues. Study **models** and **photos** are needed to document the dental and occlusal characteristics and evaluate changes over time.

Orthopantomography provides indications of dental and periodontal health, the quality of previous restorative and conservative interventions and the shape and symmetry of the condyles.

Lateral **teleradiography** of the skull allows examination of the cephalometric tracing (11.8).

Cephalometric analysis

Despite the limitations caused by the two-dimensional nature of the method and the fact that the examination is performed during wakefulness, the cephalometric analysis of teleradiography in latero-lateral projection allows the survey of (Fleisher and Kryger 2007; Santos *et al.* 2011):

- anatomy of the skull;
- profile of the soft tissues;
- skeletal class;
- skeletal divergence;

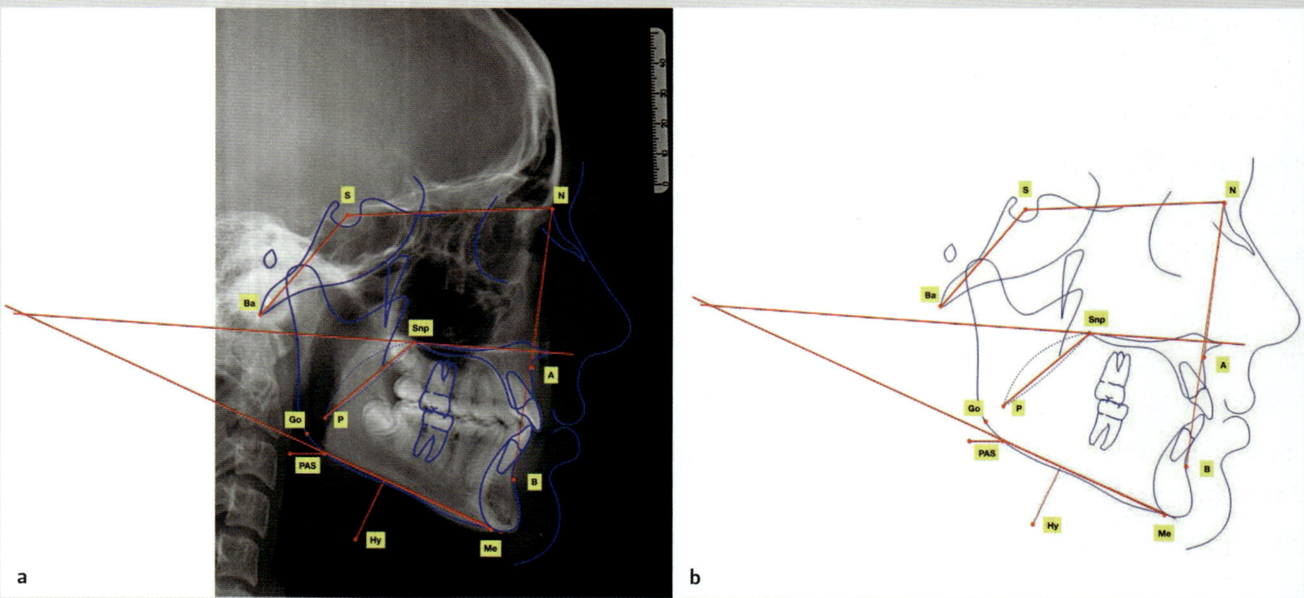

11.8 **a.** Lateral teleradiography of the skull. **b.** Cephalometric tracing. S (Sella) median point of sella turca; N (Nasion) most anterior point of the frontonasal suture; Ba (Basion posterior limit to the rim of the basal part of the occipital bone; Snp, posterior nasal spine, P, the tip of the uvula; Go (Gonion) intersection point between the posterior border of the mandible and PM; Me (Menton) lowest point of the mandibular symphysis; Hy (Hyoid) antero-superior point of hyoid bone; PM (Mandibular plane) plane passing through the points Go and Me; Hy-PM, distance from Hy to the intersection point between PM and the orthogonal projection of Hy on PM; posterior airway space (PAS), distance between the posterior pharyngeal wall and the intersection between PM and the anterior pharyngeal wall

- dentoskeletal relationships;
- morphology of the upper airways.

Literature has attempted to provide records for a better recognition of the common craniofacial characteristic among patients with OSAS, yet the data provided are conflicting.

The most frequent craniofacial characteristics appearing in the apneic patient are as follows (Lowe *et al.* 1986; Battagel *et al.* 1996; Seto *et al.* 2001; Johal and Conaghan 2004):

- mandibular retrusion (increased SNB angle);
- reduction in the anterior cranial base (diminished SN distance);
- increased length of the soft palate (Pns-P distance);
- increased mandibular plane-hyoid bone (MP-Hy);
- diminished PAS.

Latero-lateral teleradiography is useful for evaluating the possibility of maxillofacial surgery and, for the dental sleep medicine practitioner, to identify the distance between the hyoid bone and the mandibular plane (when this is highly increased, it may represent a negative predictive factor for ENT surgery). There is no real evidence in the literature about the benefits of this radiological examination in detecting patients with OSAS or to predict the outcome of MAD therapy. However, the authors believe that when the patient already has this documentation, it is useful to include these data in the medical reports:

- skeletal class (ANB: norm $2^\circ \pm 2^\circ$);
- position of the superior maxilla compared to the cranial base (SNA: norm $82^\circ \pm 2^\circ$);
- position of the inferior maxilla compared to the cranial base (SNB: norm $80^\circ \pm 2^\circ$);
- skeletal divergence (SN $\wedge$ MP: norm 36°);
- length of the soft palate (Pns–P: norm 35 mm);
- distance between the hyoid bone and the mandibular bone (MP–Hy: norm 12 mm in females and 15 mm in males);
- PAS: norm $>$ 9 mm.

Treatment plan

Briefly, the diagnostic process must be based on the expertise of a team of specialists. The accurate evaluation of the sleep disorder, daytime sleepiness and symptoms, polysomnographic examination, the evaluation of comorbidities, the clinical and instrumental examination of obstructive sites and craniofacial morphology represent the most complete approach to devise an ideal treatment plan respecting the guidelines, predictive factors for the efficacy of the potential therapeutic choice and the preferences of the patient.

During discussion of the treatment plan, it is up to the odontologist to explain MAD therapy to the patient and propose possible therapeutic alternatives according to the situation.

It is important to explain the treatment plan, the need for dental and polysomnographic follow-up and the side effects that may appear.

In summary, the following **information** must be discussed with the patient:

- mechanism of action of the MAD;
- superiority of the efficacy of ventilatory therapy according to the severity of OSAS and associate comorbidities;
- possibility of therapy failure;
- possible short- and long-term side effects;
- the need for polysomnographic follow-up;
- the need for dental follow-up.

Choice of device

The protocol of the American Academy of Dental Sleep Medicine strongly recommends knowledge of different devices for the treatment of OSAS, since no device is effective for the treatment of all patients.

There are many devices available on the market. They differ in their materials of fabrication, mechanisms of advancement, freedom of vertical and lateral mandibular movement, the possibility to be custom-made and the graduality of advancement.

The choice of the device is impacted by the following factors:

- cost;
- resistance to wear, breakage and deformation;
- difficulties involved in achieving a good retention;
- need to allow freedom for vertical and lateral movements of the jaw;
- graduality and simplicity of advancement;
- time spent in the chair at the operator's place;
- patient comfort.

Being a lifelong therapy, the durability of the device and, therefore, the material it is made from and its design are very important.

In 2010, Martinez-Gomis and coworkers observed that, during five years of MAD therapy, 36 IST-type devices (using a telescopic arm as an advancement mechanism) reported 96 cases of breakage and 54 cases needing repairs in the dental laboratory (Martinez-Gomis *et al.* 2010).

A MAD can be custom-made or preformed, monobloc or bimaxillary, adjustable or fixed.

CUSTOM-MADE OR PREFORMED?

The construction of a custom-made device involves a long fabrication time and high cost: this has led to the manufacture of preformed devices made from thermoplastic material (boil and bite devices).

In 2008, in a randomized controlled trial, Vanderveken and coworkers compared the two types of devices in a group of 35 patients. The custom-made devices proved to be effective in obtaining a response (reduced AHI by at least 50% compared to the baseline values) in 60% of the patients, whereas the preformed device achieved this objective only in 31% of patients. A total of 63% of the patients who showed compliance failure with a boil and bite device responded well to treatment with a custom-made appliance. This study is clinically very important because, aside from confirming the efficacy of custom-made devices, it eliminates the possibility of considering preformed MADs as test devices (Vanderveken *et al.* 2008).

In addition to their lower efficacy, boil and bite devices are associated with a lower adherence to therapy as they are fabricated with less accuracy and thus provide less comfort for the patient (Tsuda *et al.* 2010; Friedman *et al.* 2012).

MONOBLOC OR BIMAXILLARY?

Monobloc devices are constructed as a single piece that does not allow any mandibular movement, whereas bimaxillary devices are made from two splints connected by different mechanisms that induce mandibular advancement, allowing different degrees of freedom for vertical and lateral movement.

There have been two studies comparing monobloc and bimaxillary devices (Bloch *et al.* 2000; Rose *et al.* 2002).

Generally, no significant differences in terms of efficacy were observed between the two types of MAD; an exception is found in the study by Rose *et al.*, who reported that the Karwetzky (monobloc) device proved more effective than the Silensor® (bimaxillary) device in reducing respiratory events. The authors hypothesize that this difference may depend on the design of the devices and the materials used in their construction: the Silensor® often presents a poor retention, and the loss of the lower mask may cause the jaw to be in a more retruded position.

The other hypotesis is that monoblokc devices may be more effective because it doesn't allow mouth opening adapt to and are more likely to result in temporomandibular joint pain.

FIXED OR ADJUSTABLE ADVANCEMENT?

Fixed propulsion mechanisms are less expensive and easier to use, whereas those with gradual advancement mechanisms can be adjusted individually according to the response and tolerability for the patient in searching for the therapeutic position.

High-level performance is provided by those appliances that allow minimal advancements (circa 0.1 - 0.25 mm per activation), as they make muscular adaptation easier.

In 2011, Lettieri and coworkers published a comparison between the results obtained from 203 patients treated with a MAD with fixed advancement (60%-80% of maximum protrusion) and 602 patients treated with an adjustable device that the patient could advance by 0.5 mm per day until the subjective symptoms are resolved, according to individual tolerability (Thornton Adjustable Positioner, TAP). The devices with gradual advancement proved to be more effective in reducing AHI (74.4% reduction versus 65% with fixed devices) (Lettieri *et al.* 2011).

OCCLUSAL COVERAGE

An oral appliance should always provide a **complete occlusal coverage** (Fransson *et al.* 2002; Rose *et al.* 2002a; Hugentobler M *et al.* 2010) for the following reasons:

- guarantee homogeneous distribution of the reaction forces to the mandibular protrusion and reduce the mean pressure applied to the individual elements;
- counter the risk of occlusal changes due to the extrusion of any elements not included by the device.

Observations relating to different MADs

According to the clinical experience of the authors, the most-used MADs are: Silensor®, IST®, TAP® and SomnoDent®.

Silensor® (11.9) is a widely used device thanks to its low cost. It is a bimaxillary device whose advancement mechanism is a bilateral exchangeable plastic connector on each side, of variable length, allowing a gradual protrusion of 1 mm per time. The orientation of the connector (from the upper canine to the lower molar) induces an increase in the degree of advancement at the opening of the patient's mouth, in an attempt to counteract the negative effects of mouth opening on the airway patency. Although its efficacy has been proven (Nakano *et al.* 2013), its fragility makes it more suitable for use as a test device in patients with severe negative predictive factors.

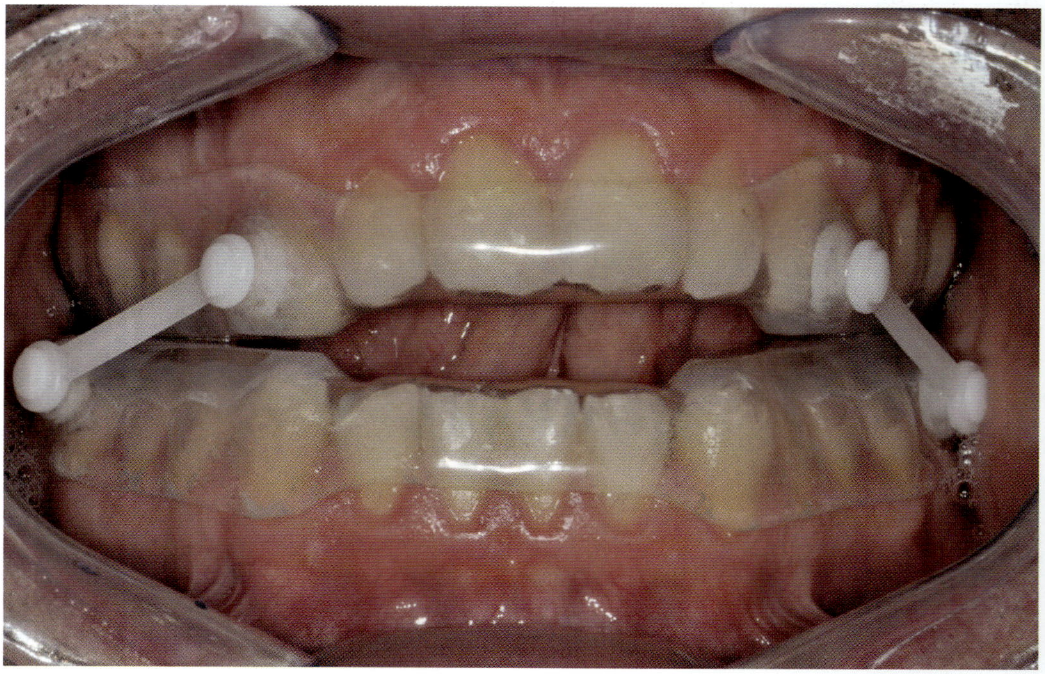

11.9 Silensor® Device..

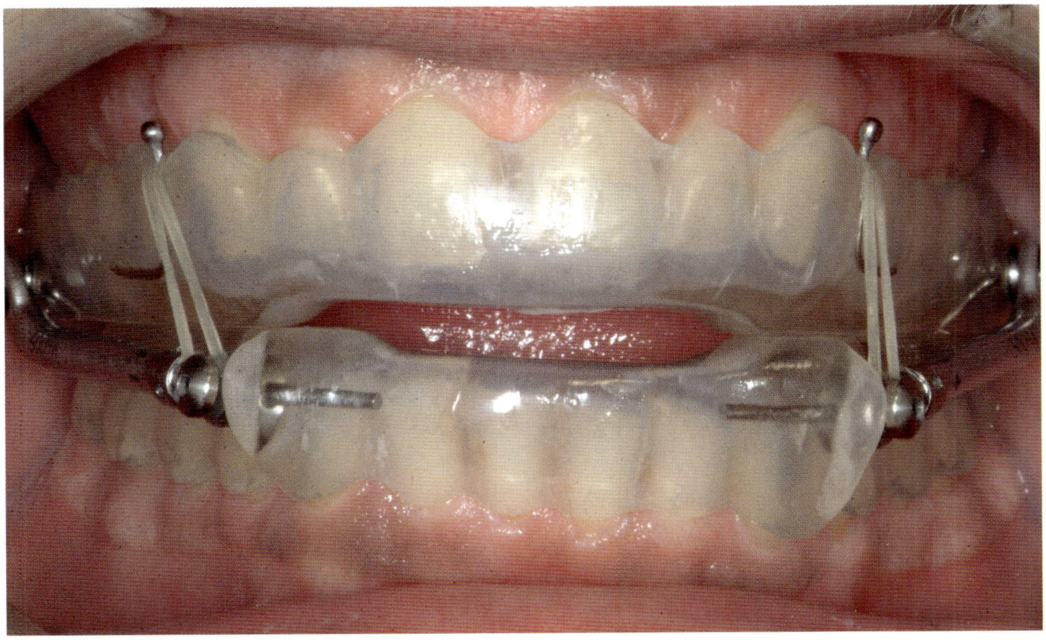

11.10 a. IST® appliance.

IST® (11.10a) Prosomnus precision Herbst and Leone Telescopic Advancer® (11.10b) a bimaxillary devices that use a telescopic rods with a screw titration mechanism, allowing a gradual protrusion of 0.016 mm (IST) or 0.1 mm (Leone and Prosomnus) per time. IST has two versions with opposite rod orientations. The IST Classic has a rod going from the first upper molar to the lower canine and is designed to guarantee freedom of vertical and lateral movement, whereas the Classic New has a telescopic arm (inverted rod) and, like Silensor®, increases the protrusion at the opening of the mouth. It is advisable to use both of them with hooks for vertical elastics, which allow the control of mouth opening. The telescopic rod devices efficacy is well documented (Lawton *et al.* 2005) and it has a good price-quality relationship. The point of attachment of the arm to the splint carries the most stress and there is a moderate risk of wear and breakage (Martinez-Gomis *et al.* 2010).

SomnoDent® (11.11a) and LEONE Forward® (11.11d) are bimaxillary MAD using inclined fins and ramps with a 17° or 30° inclination to induce and maintain the protrusion. They can be gradually advanced by 0.1 mm per time. It was introduced by Metha and Cistulli in 1998. It allows the greatest freedom for mouth opening and a moderate freedom for lateral movements. Its most important innovations are:

- the material of fabrication, SMH BFlex, providing a soft inner surface that maintains retention and can be relined
- edentulous version (11.11b), extending on the soft palate and allowing to be used in cases of complete edentulism in the upper arch as long as there are at least four teeth in the lower arch.

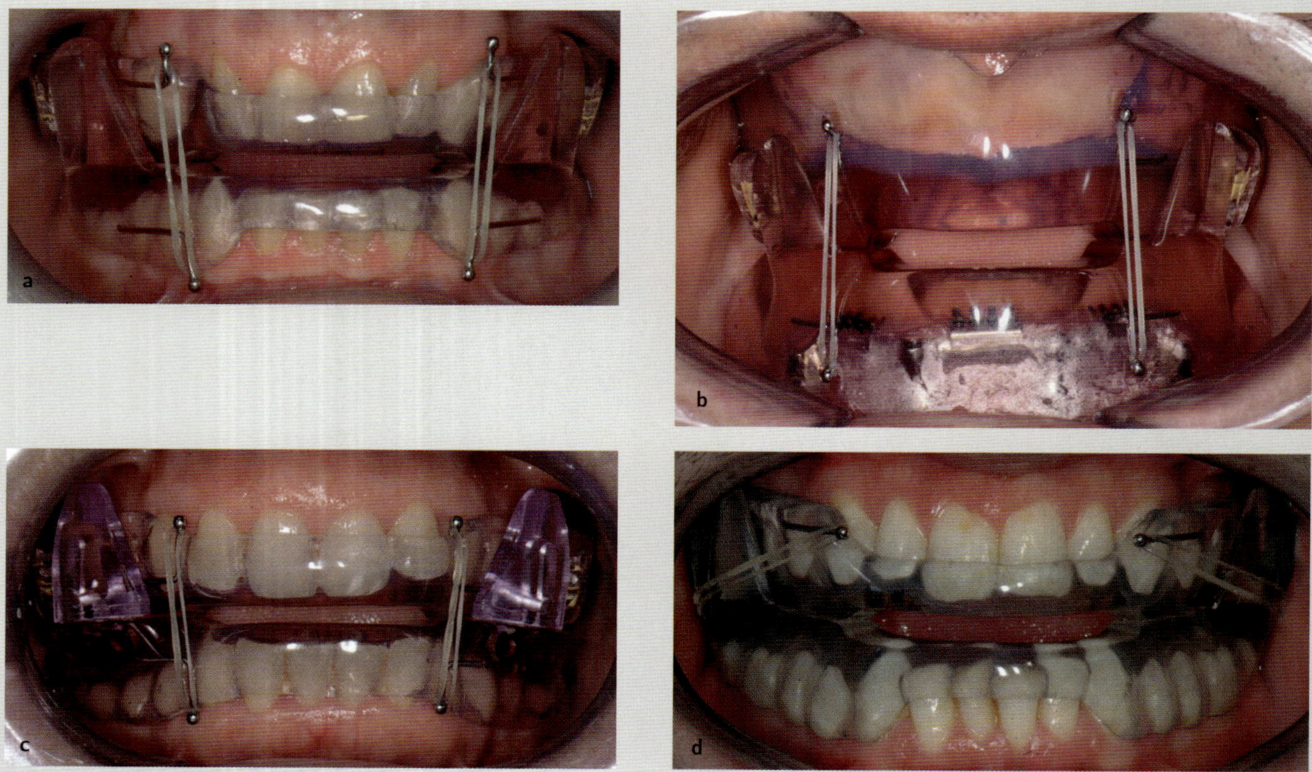

11.11 a. SomnoDent® with front mouth opening and hooks to attach vertical elastics. b. SomnoDent® Edentulous. c. SomnoDent® Fusion. d. Prosomnus® CA. e. Prosomnus® IA

With Somnodent® device is possible to advance the mandible using only a screw mechanism (SomnoDent® Flex; see 11.11a) or by exchanging the initial wings with thicker wings (SomnoDent® Fusion; see 11.11c). This may be very helpful for patients with severe OSAS, as it allows 3 mm of extra mandibular protrusion (in addition to the 6 mm allowed by the screw) compared to the chosen initial advancement. Another device that uses a fin/ramp mechanism is Prosomnus® IA (Iterative Advancement) (see 11.11d) and CA (Continuous Advancement) (see 11.11f): the difference is that is possible to prescribe to the patient a 30° inclined fin or a straight (90°) interface. The titration can be customized: it can be a stepwise advancement, with sequential trays (IA) or a continuous titration to achieve with a screw mechanism (CA).

The TAP® family devices (11.12) are bimaxillary appliances using an hook mechanism attached to a socket or to a bar positioned in the opposite tray. In front of a screw mechanism allows to titrate the device. Each full turn of the screw corresponds to 0.5 mm of advancement (Ghazal *et al.* 2009). Even if it allows a high degree of freedom for lateral mandibular movements (especially in the bar version), it allows only minimal freedom for vertical movement,

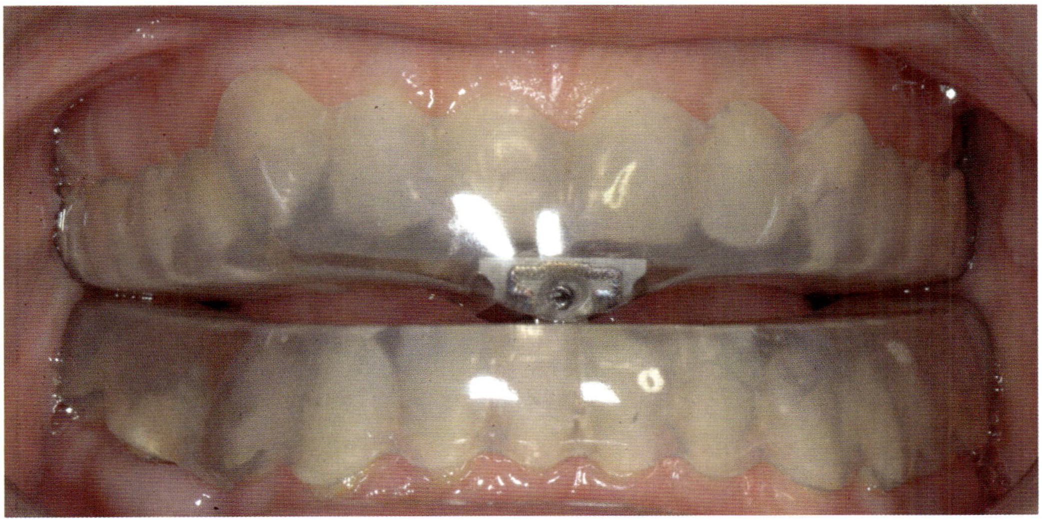

11.12 TAP® device.

and this may cause some discomfort during the adaptation stage. It requires a good inferior anchorage. Its efficacy is well documented and it is indicated for patients whose mouth opening must be strictly controlled.
Orthoapnea Classic device is a bimaxillary device using an inverse connecting rod system, attached to two bars positioned in the upper and in the lower trays. In the frontal part of the rod, a screw can be turned to increasethe advancement: 1 full turn correponds to 0,4 mm of advancement.

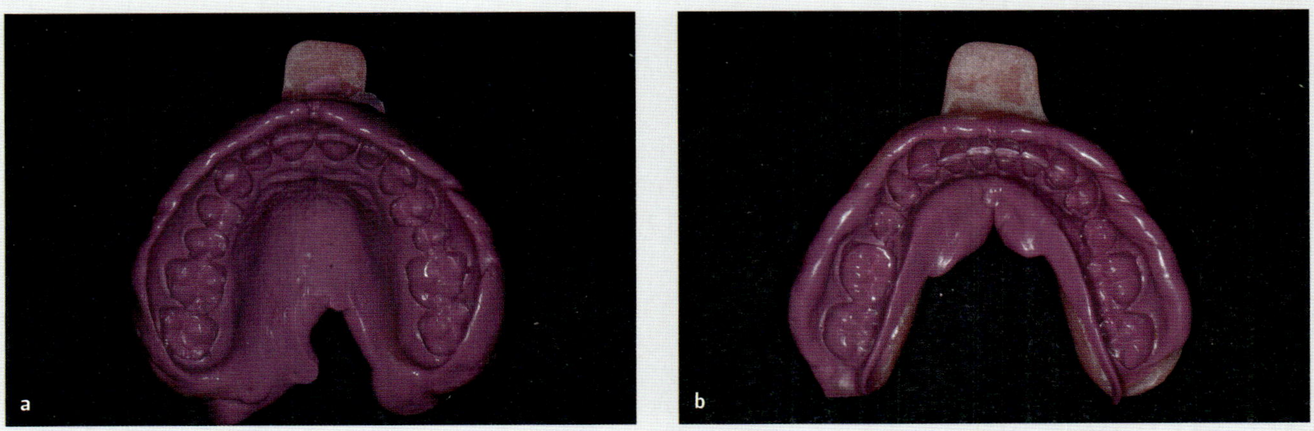

11.13 a. Silicone impression of the upper arch. b. Silicone impression of the lower arch.

Clinical phases

Recording of the impression

It is essential that the dental impressions (physical or digital) are very accurate and that all the elements are well represented: teeth, palate and arches (📷 11.13).

Recording must include the following:

- a centric occlusion wax rim;
- a construction bite that represents the anterior vertical dimension and the chosen initial advancement.

Choice of vertical dimension

There have been few studies on how the response to MAD therapy is affected by the degree of vertical distraction.

In 2002, Pitsis and coworkers published the results of a cross-over randomized trial on 23 patients who received an oral device with the same advancement and different interincisal openings: 4 mm (A) and 10 mm (B). The mean obtained advancement was 7.3 ± 0.5 mm (87% ± 4% of the maximal protrusive). The MADs were used with a randomized sequence (A/B-B/A) for two weeks, with a wash-out period of one week between them. The study did not show any statistically significant difference in the response to the therapy but did show a preference by patients for the smaller incisal distance (Pitsis *et al.* 2002; Ahrens *et al.* 2010). The rationale for keeping the vertical dimension to a minimum, aside from the patient's comfort, is the posterior direction that the jaw assumes while opening the mouth, which results in a posterior movement of the tongue and the hyoid bone (Johal and Battagel, 2001). The results of the study led by Pitsis and coworkers, together with the necessity to keep the lips aligned without effort, suggest the choice to keep a minimal vertical dimension. A minimal amount of Vertical anterior distraction is required to achieve enough space (at least a 3 mm) between the posterior teeth to build the posterior resin bites.

In bimaxillary devices it is essential to control mouth opening.

Vanderveken and Braem evaluated 40 patients in sleep endoscopy to investigate the effect of an increase in the interincisal distance from 4 mm to 2 cm. In 80% of the patients this maneuver worsened the patency of the airways (Vanderveken *et al.* 2012).

For this reason, it is advisable to design a device with a respiratory fissure that limits the need for opening of the mouth for patients with increased nasal resistance who refuse or are not candidates for ENT treatment (📷 11.14). To counteract the opening of the mouth with a dedicated frontal mechanisms or elastics, the devices must be well constructed and have good retention.

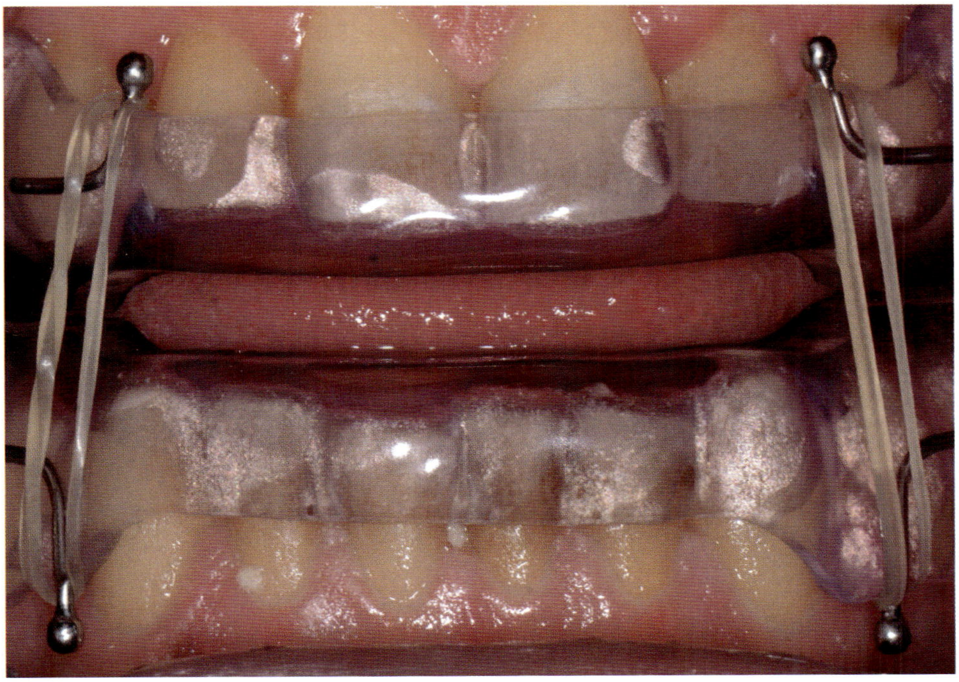

11.14 Front respiratory split.

Choices for advancement

Although the ideal advancement is considered to be equal to 70-80% of the maximal protrusive, the choice for the initial therapeutic position should correspond to the maximal comfortable protrusion (Aarab *et al.* 2010).

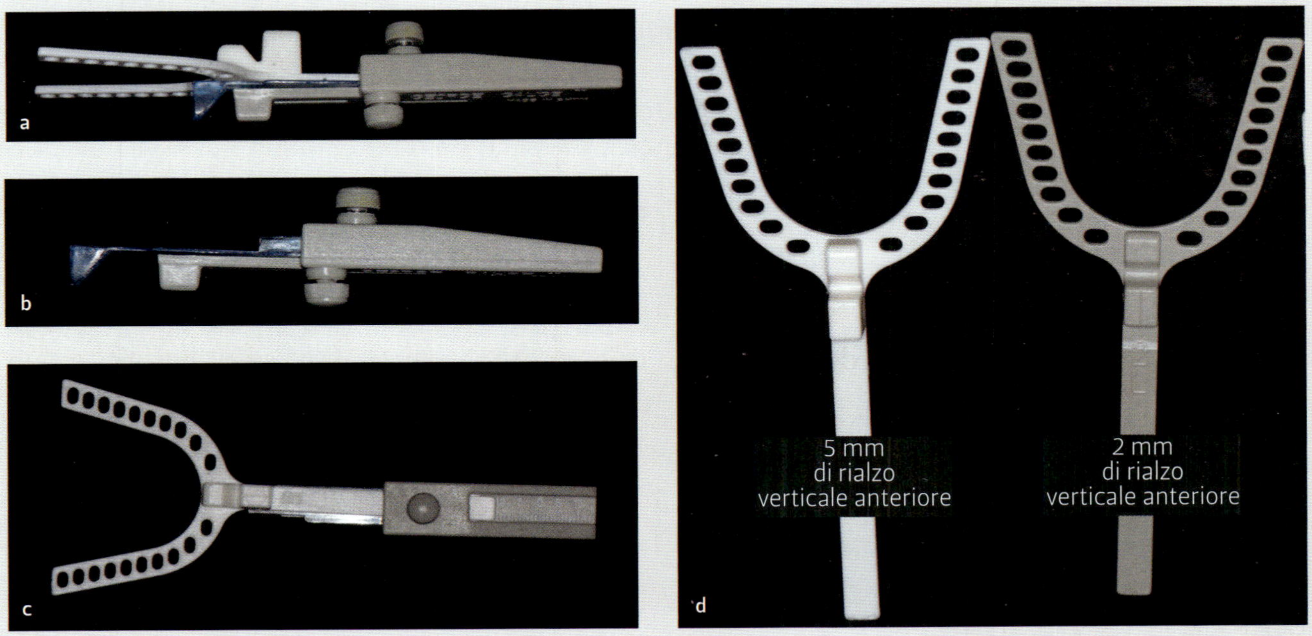

11.15 **a.** George Gauge. **b.** Body of George Gauge. **c.** George Gauge–millimeter scale. **d.** Forkbite with anterior vertical opening of 5 mm or 2 mm.

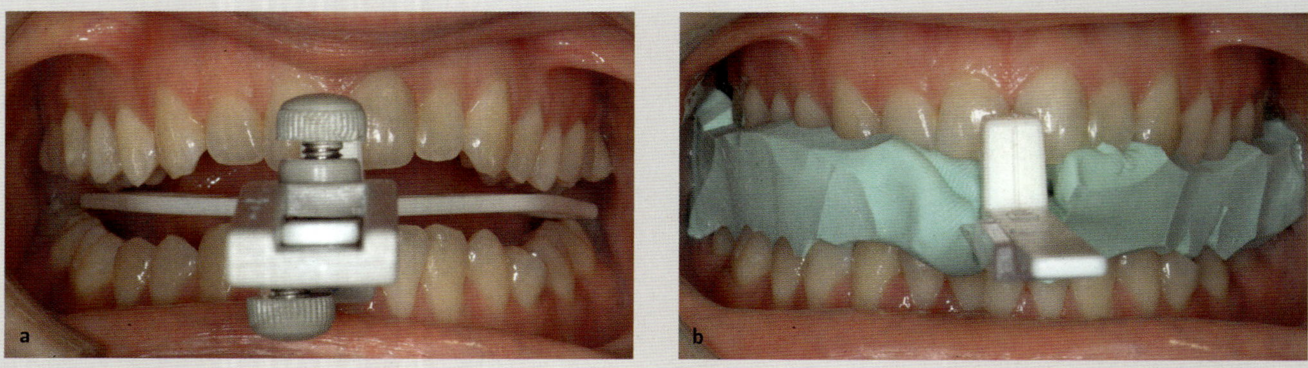

11.16 **a.** Rialzo verticale del George Gauge. **b.** Morso di costruzione con George Gauge – visione frontale.

One of the most accurate methods for determining the habitual position, the maximal protrusive and the initial advancement is the George Gauge bite (11.15a). The fork has a body (see 11.15b),) a millimeter scale (see 11.15c) and a removable fork with different dimensions and heights (see 11.15d). The height of the fork determines the anterior vertical dimension (11.16). The thickness of the lower incisor notch can be adjusted, the upper notch must be adapted to the form of the shape of the upper incisors.

The steps to make a construction bite are as follows:

- adapt the width of the lower incisal clamp that must be fixed by tightening the lower turn screw (11.17);
- use an acrylic bur to modify the upper incisor notch on the fork, taking care not to modify the thickness in the vertical direction (not to reduce the anterior vertical dimension) (11.18);
- insert the fork into the body, with a loosened upper screw, so that the fork can slide forward and backward), ask the patient to close the mouth in the habitual position and mark the position on the millimeter scale with a pencil (11.19);

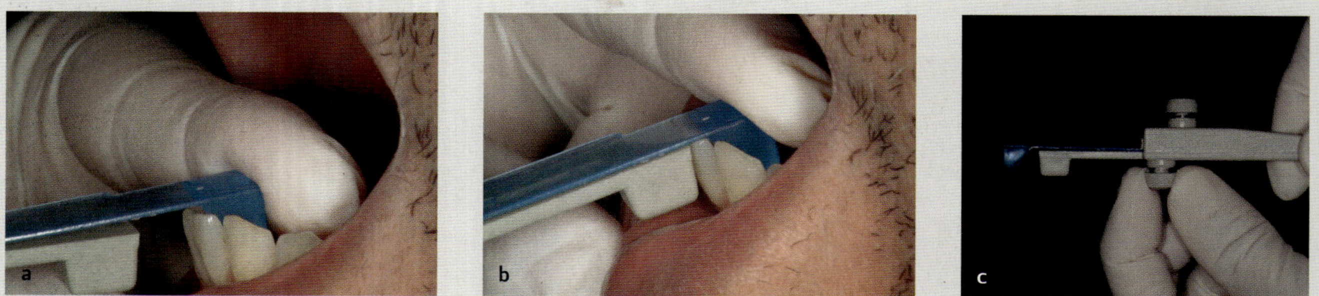

11.17 **a.** Adapting the width of the lower dental elements. **b.** The lower incisors must fit perfectly in the space between the body and the surface of the adjustable part. **c.** Tighten the lower screw to block the lower dental elements.

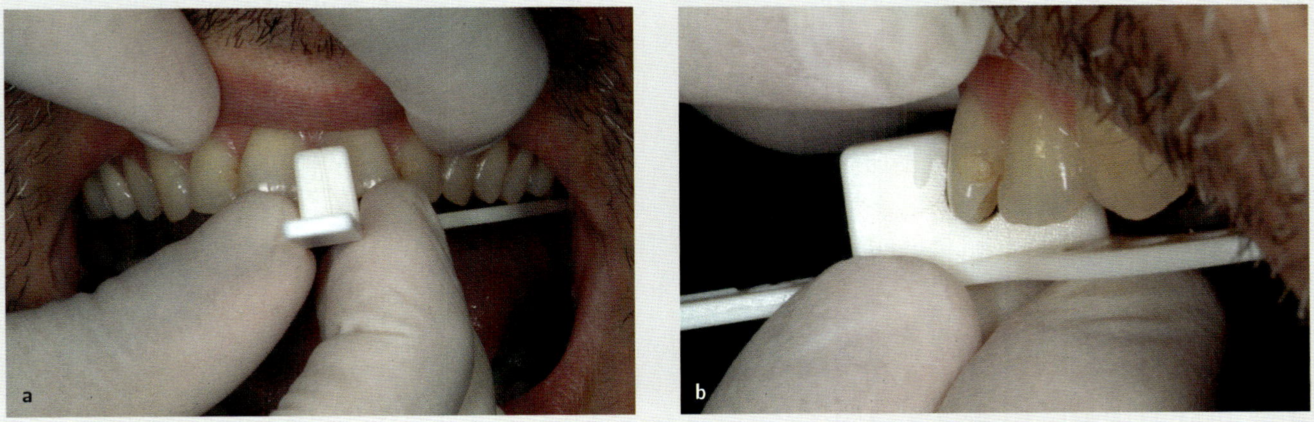

11.18 **a.** Inserting the fork in the upper part, **b.** the width of the lower dental elements must be adapted to the shape of the upper dental elements.

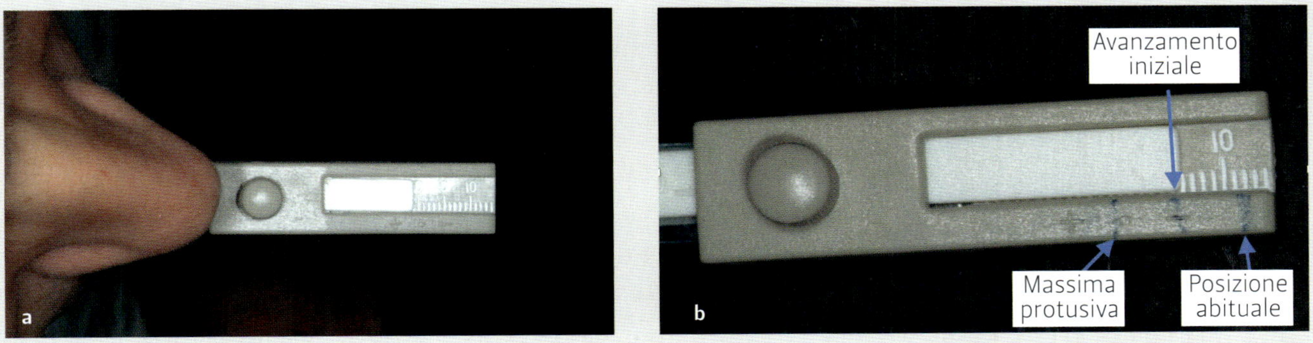

11.19 **a.** View from the top of the millimeter scale. **b.** Mark the habitual position, the maximal protrusion and the chosen initial position with a pencil.

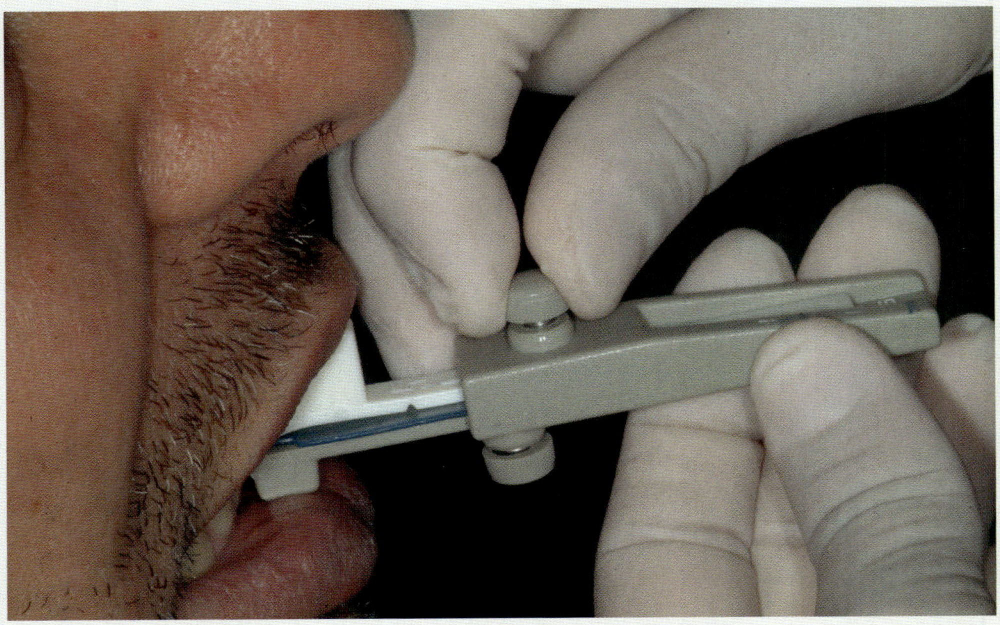

11.20 The chosen position is fixed by tightening the upper screw on the body of the George Gauge.

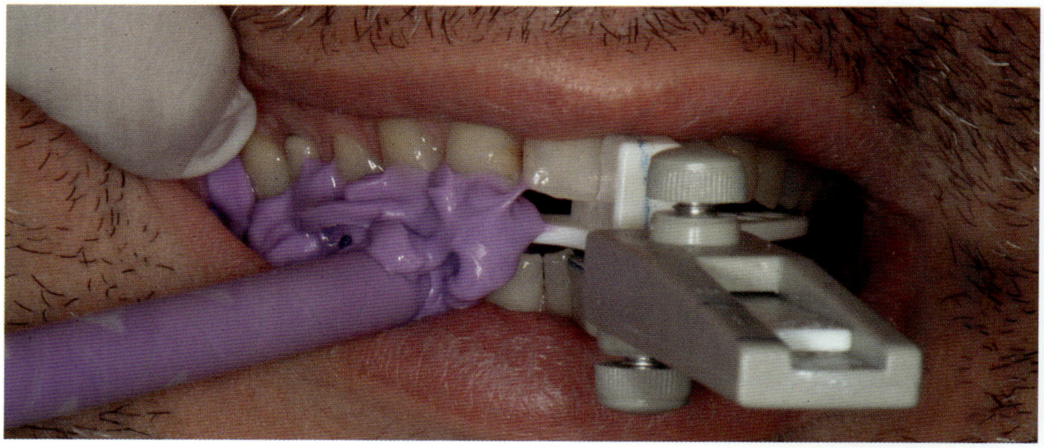

11.21 Silicone injection starting from the posterior area proceeding toward the mesial direction.

- ask the patient to advance the mandible as much as possible, sliding forward, and mark the maximal protrusive with a pencil on the scale
- choose the initial advancement (the maximal comfortable protrusion for the patient), mark the maximal protrusion on the scale with a pencil and tighten the upper screw; (11.20; see also 11.19b);
- inject the silicone for occlusal registration and wait for it to harden (11.21);
- remove the bite-fork and verify that there is an adequate number of contacts;
- try the construction bite again to verify that the symmetry presented by the patient during mandibular protrusion without the George Gauge is respected and that the patient does not feel pain in the chosen position.

If the patient does not have incisors or is edentulous, the construction bite with the George Gauge can be made with a wax rim well adapted to the fork and/or to the lower dental elements (11.22). Another solution may be to duplicate the total prosthesis by making a putty mold (11.23).

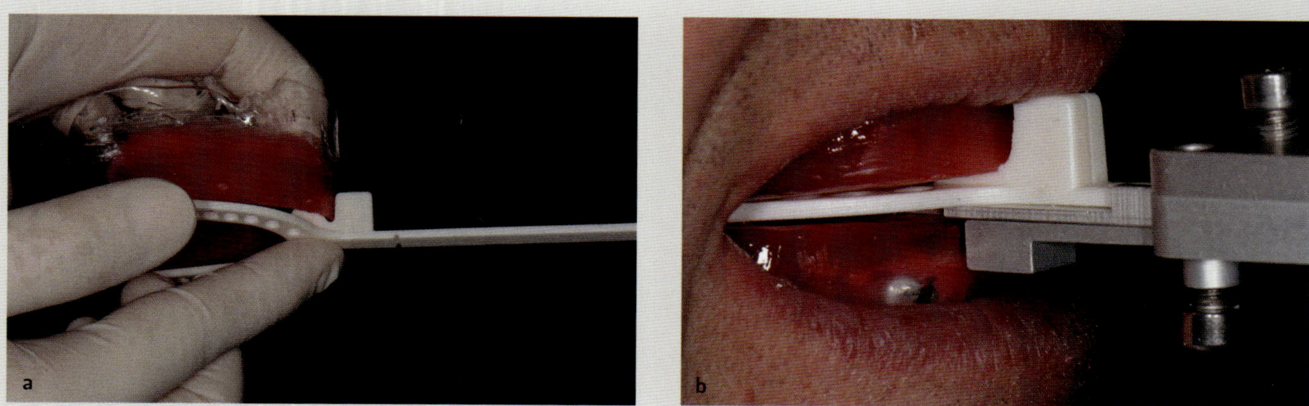

11.22 **a.** Bite wax to proceed with the construction bite making in a patient with one edentulous arch. **b.** George Gauge on bite wax.

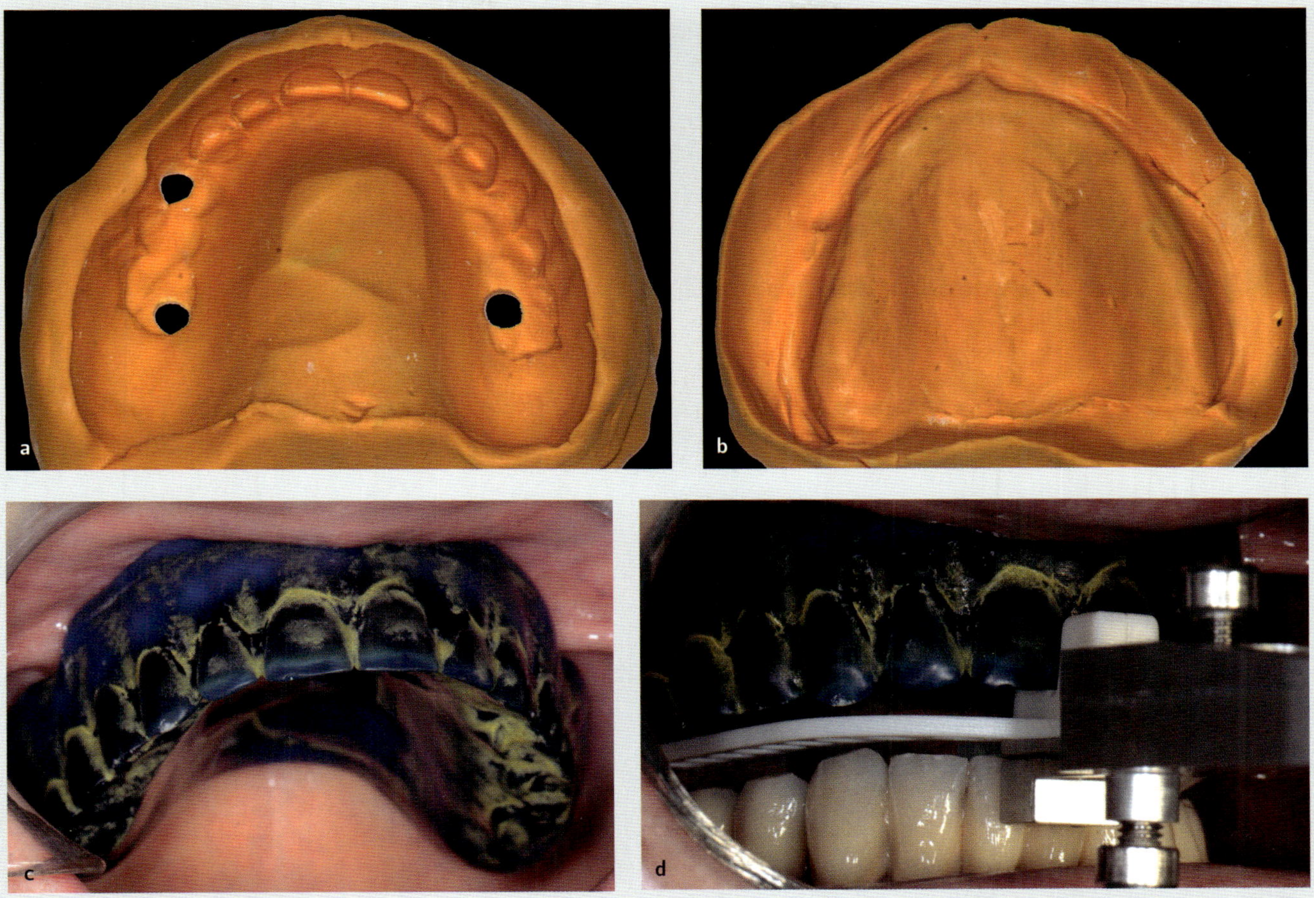

11.23 **a.** Putty mold of the exterior surface of a superior complete prosthesis. **b.** Mold of the interior surface of the prosthesis. **c.** Resin duplicate of the prosthesis. **d.** Bite registration with prosthesis duplication

Delivery of the device

On the day of delivery, it is essential to verify that the device fits perfectly in both dental arches, its adherence and retention and that it does not compress the periodontal tissues.

To evaluate the comfort of the device, it should be worn for at least five minutes before asking the patient about the presence of possible areas of compression and the tolerability of the protrusion.

If the patient expresses discomfort, it is useful to reduce the advancement in order to make initial adaptation easier. Possible areas of compression must be discharged, and the orientation of the hooks must be checked in order to avoid them touching the gum.

After these checks, the adverse effects that may occur in the short term should be reiterated to the patient and the exercises to be performed if the device is perceived to be different in the morning due to prolonged contraction of the lateral pterygoid muscle should be explained:

- open and close the mouth while placing the tongue as far back as possible on the palate;

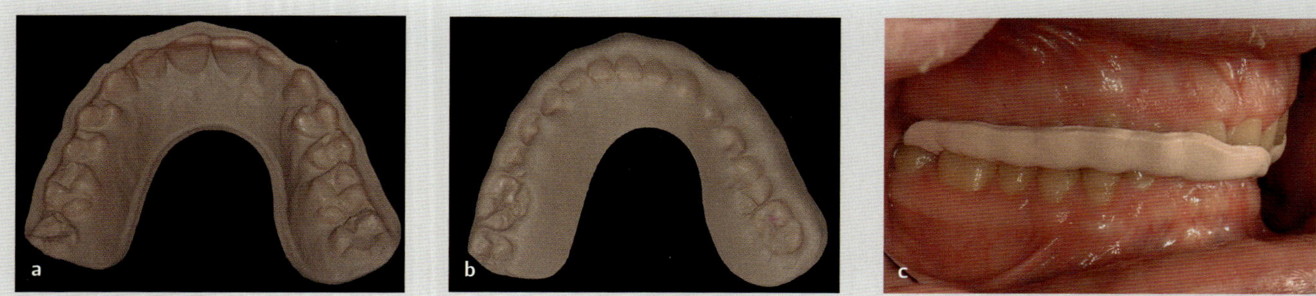

11.24 **a.** AM aligner. View from the top. **b.** AM aligner bottom view. **c.** AM aligner intraoral view.

- chew a bite trainer or an AM aligner for a few minutes (11.24), namely a bite or a bite recording made in soft thermoplastic material with the habitual closure.

In order to facilitate initial adaptation, the patient should be advised to wear the appliance for a few hours before going to sleep during the first few days and to practice advancing the mandible by sliding the lower teeth forward as much as possible and holding the position for some seconds.

The patient needs to be instructed on how to insert and remove the device and how to use the activation mechanism, if the appliance can be gradually activated.

If the device allows the mouth to be opened, it is useful to give the patient vertical elastics to control the opening. To determine the choice of the strength and diameter of the elastics, it is necessary to have the patient wearing the device with the elastics and opening the mouth. The strength of the elastic must not remove either of the two splints: if this happens, the choice will fall on a longer and less strong elastic.

Lastly, the patient should be instructed about the care and cleaning procedures for the device. It is important to teach the patient which products must be used in order to avoid damage (11.25).

Titration

The titration of the device is a gradual search for the therapeutic advancement needed to significantly reduce the number of obstructive events and to treat the symptoms.

All devices are now equipped with mechanisms that allow gradual advancement, but there is no "ideal" titration protocol.

During titration, the following must be taken into consideration:

- the severity of the pathology presented by the patient;
- the capacity of the patient to adapt to the first advancement.

Ideally, therefore, considering the patient's tolerance of the protrusion, the greater the risk represented by the ongoing pathology (high AHI, compromised oxygenation or comorbidities), the sooner the titration should be completed.

The final position is to be evaluated by cardiorespiratory monitoring or polysomnography recorded by a clinician expert in respiratory sleep disorders.

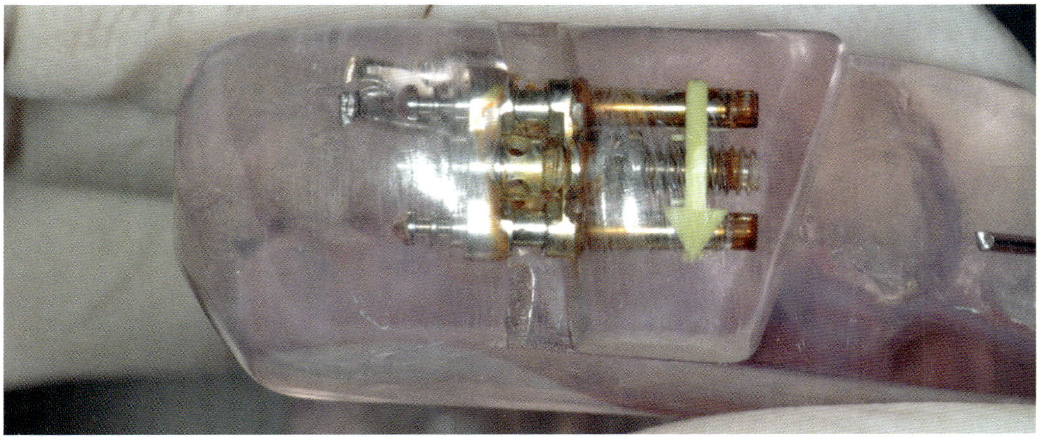

11.25 Oxidized expansion screw due to sodium hypochlorite washing.

The choice of such position can be led by the subjective symptoms of the patient (snoring, sleepiness, nocturia, apneas witnessed by the bed partner) or based upon objective evaluation with instrumental examinations. If the patient is given a monitor with two or more channels during titration, it should be kept in mind that the examination is valid only if it is interpreted by an operator who is expert in reading these records and that automatic analysis is not a reliable source.

Follow-up

The first control is scheduled two weeks after the delivery of the device and aims to discuss the subjective improvement and comfort with the patient.

The following visits must be planned according to each case. Their objective is to manage the titration protocol, evaluate the improvement of the subjective symptomatology and the patient's tolerance of the advancement and manage the onset of possible side effects.

Once these goals have been achieved, follow-up checks will be scheduled at six months and then yearly in order to evaluate the possible onset of occlusal changes and to verify that the symptoms are not worsening. In such cases, the patient must be referred to a sleep medicine clinician.

If there has not been any satisfactory result in terms of reduction in obstructive events and improvement of the symptomatology, it is up to the odontologist to evaluate the possibility of increasing the advancement or to treat the residual events by combining MAD therapy with another treatment.

In the event that the patient does not respond to the therapy, the case should be handled by a sleep medicine clinician, who will discuss a therapeutic alternative with the patient.

To complete this chapter, Fig. 11.26 illustrates a proposal for a clinical chart.

Name ______________________ **Surname** ______________________

Date of Birth __/__/__ **Weight** ____kg **Height** ____cm

What is the reason for this visit?

☒ Snoring
☒ Daytime sleepiness
☒ Apnea reported by the bed partner
☒ Awakening with choking sensation
☒ Non-restorative sleep
☒ Low use of CPAP
☒ Choice not to use CPAP
☒ Insufficient outcome after surgery
☒ Recommendation by Dr ______________________

Have you ever had or do you currently have:

☒ Hypertension
☒ Heart attack
☒ Stroke
☒ Atrial fibrillation/arrhythmia
☒ Diabetes
☒ Gastroesophageal reflux
☒ Cancer/chemotherapy/radiotherapy
☒ Stuffy nose

Do you consume regularly:

☒ Alcohol
☒ Sleeping pills or anxiolytics
☒ Cigarettes, cigars, pipe
☒ Narcotic drugs

Answer the following questions:

How do you consider the quality of your sleep: good, fair or poor? __________
Do you snore? ☒ Yes ☒ No
Do you wake up feeling tired? ☒ Yes ☒ No
Have you ever been tested for your sleep? ☒ Yes ☒ No
Have you ever fallen asleep while driving? ☒ Yes ☒ No

For female patients

Are you pregnant? ☒ Yes ☒ No
Are you in menopause? ☒ Yes ☒ No

Have you ever had orthodontic treatments? ☒ Yes ☒ No
Do you wear a removable dental prosthesis? ☒ Yes ☒ No
Do you have implants or a fixed prosthesis? ☒ Yes ☒ No
Do you clench your teeth during sleep? ☒ Yes ☒ No
Do you suffer from joint problems (arthrosis, arthritis etc.)? ☒ Yes ☒ No
Do you have pain in your neck? ☒ Yes ☒ No
Do you have pain in your shoulders? ☒ Yes ☒ No
Do you hear whistling in your ears? ☒ Yes ☒ No
Do you hear noises when you open and close your mouth? ☒ Yes ☒ No

Has your mouth ever locked while opening or closing? ☒ Yes ☒ No
Do you suffer from headaches? ☒ Yes ☒ No
If so, how often? __________
Do you have dental cleaning every six months? ☒ Yes ☒ No
Do your gums bleed when you brush your teeth? ☒ Yes ☒ No
Do you have toothache? ☒ Yes ☒ No
When was your last dental check? __________

11.26 Proposal for a clinical chart.

Cross the appropriate number (0-1-2-3) below to indicate how likely you are to doze off or fall asleep in the following situations:

EPWORTH SLEEPINESS SCALE

Sitting and reading	0-1-2-3
Watching TV	0-1-2-3
Sitting still in a public place (e.g., a theater, a meeting)	0-1-2-3
As a passenger in a car for an hour without a break	0-1-2-3
Lying down to rest in the afternoon when circumstances permit	0-1-2-3
Sitting and talking with someone	0-1-2-3
Sitting quietly after lunch without having consumed alcohol	0-1-2-3
In a car while stopped for a few minutes in traffic	0-1-2-3

SCORE ______

Significant anamnesis data

______

______

Polysomnographic data

______

______

ENT diagnosis

______

______

CLINICAL EXAMINATION

FACE: shape ______ symmetry ______
PROFILE: divergence ______ convexity ______
PALATE: shape ______ width ______
TRANSVERSAL RELATIONS: ______
TONSILLAR GRADING: ______ MALLAMPATI: ______
DENTAL CLASS: ______ SPEE: ______ OB: ______ OJ: ______
MEDIAN LINES ______ maximal opening ______
WEAR FACETS: ______

DENTAL FORMULA: ______ | ______ NUMBER OF TEETH: ______

DECAYED ELEMENTS: ______
MOBILE ELEMENTS: ______ BIOTYPE: ______
RECESSION: ______ PERIODONTAL POCKETS: ______
CONSERVATIVE, RESTORATIVE AND PROSTHETIC DENTISTRY: ______

______

MANDIBULAR MOVEMENT RANGE:
Maximal mouth opening ______ right laterality ______ left laterality ______ maximum protrusion ______
MUSCULAR PAIN and/or joint noises:

______

11.26

(to be continued)

BMI ____________ NECK CIRCUMFERENCE ____________________

Cephalometry

SNA (82 ± 2) ______ SNB (80 ± 2) ______ ANB (2 ± 2) ______ SN/PM ______ Hy/PM ______ PAS ______ Snp-P ______

Baseline polysomnography

AHI __________ sup AHI ________ nonsup AHI __________ ODI __________ min Sat O_2 ________ CT <90% ________

Therapeutic options

____

____

____

DEVICE ____

Anterior vertical opening ____________________________ Elastics ________________________________

Initial therapeutic advancement _____________________ Final therapeutic advancement _______________________

EVALUATION OF EFFICACY

Cross the appropriate number (0-1-2-3) below to indicate how likely you are to doze off or fall asleep in the following situations:

EPWORTH SLEEPINESS SCALE

Sitting and reading	0-1-2-3
Watching TV	0-1-2-3
Sitting still in a public place (e.g., a theater, a meeting)	0-1-2-3
As a passenger in a car for an hour without a break	0-1-2-3
Lying down to rest in the afternoon when circumstances permit	0-1-2-3
Sitting and talking with someone	0-1-2-3
Sitting quietly after lunch without having consumed alcohol	0-1-2-3
In a car while stopped for a few minutes in the traffic	0-1-2-3

SCORE

Polysomnography with MAD

AHI __________ sup AHI ________ nonsup AHI __________ ODI __________ min Sat O_2 ________ CT <90% ________

Adverse effects

____

____

____

____

11.26 (to be continued)

ACTIVATION PROGRAM

Name ______________________ **Surname** ______________________

DAY	ACTIVATIONS	COMFORT (0-5)	NUMBER OF HOURS	NOTES

INFORMED CONSENT

Snoring is sound produced due to the partial obstruction of the upper airways during sleep. On its own, it is not a dangerous condition unless it is the symptom of a more severe pathological condition: OSAS.

OSAS is a potentially serious condition due to the consequences of low oxygen saturation and sleep fragmentation.

This condition can lead to excessive daytime sleepiness, intermittent hypoxemia and increase arterial blood pressure, leading to a higher risk of heart attack and stroke.

For this reason, all the individuals with this syndrome should be examined by a specialist in sleep medicine in order to get an accurate diagnosis, carefully evaluate the associated comorbidities and ensure control of the therapy's efficacy.

Mandibular advancement devices represent one of the therapeutic options for snoring and sleep apnea and aim to increase the diameter of the airways by advancing the mandible.

A polysomnography with the device in situ is necessary to confirm the efficacy of the therapy.

Patients with mild and moderate OSAS are better candidates for this therapy than those with severe OSAS. However, it is not possible to guarantee the success of the treatment for any particular patient. Furthermore, it is not possible to predict an individual patient's tolerance to mandibular advancement, and some subjects may develop adverse effects such as hypersalivation, xerostomia, temporomandibular joint pain, tooth discomfort and occlusal changes.

These complications can be reversible or non-reversible.

The device must be checked every six months so the odontologist can verify that it continues to fit the dental arches as well as ensuring dental/periodontal health and joint comfort.

If painful symptoms occur, the patient should be examined by the odontologist and avoid wearing the device until after they have been examined.

11.26

REFERENCES

Aarab G, Lobbezoo F, Hamburger HL, Naeije M. Effects of an oral appliance with different mandibular protrusion positions at a constant vertical dimension on obstructive sleep apnea. *Clin Oral Investig.* 2010 Jun;14(3):339-345.

Ahrens A, McGrath C, Haeggc U. Subjective efficacy of oral appliance design features in the management of obstructive sleep apnea: A systematic review. *American Journal of Orthodontics and Dentofacial Orthopedics.* 2010 Nov;138(5):559-576.

Al-Saleh MA, Armijo-Olivo S, Flores-Mir C TN. Electromyography in diagnosing temporomandibular disorders. *J Am Dent Assoc.* 2012;143(4):351-362.

Battagel JM, L'Estrange PR. The cephalometric morphology of patients with obstructive sleep apnoea (OSA). *Eur J Orthod.* 1996 Dec;18(6):557-569.

Bloch KE, Iseli A, Zhang JN, et al. A randomized, controlled crossover trial of two oral appliances for sleep apnea treatment. *American Journal of Respiratory and Critical Care Medicine.* 2000;162:246-251.

Bucca C, Cicolin A, Brussino L, et al. Tooth loss and obstructive sleep apnoea. *Respiratory Research.* 2006 Jan 17;7:8.

Chen Y-H, Kang J-H, Lin C-C, et al. Obstructive sleep apnea and the risk of adverse pregnancy outcomes. *Am J Obstet Gynecol.* 2012;206:136:e1-e5.

de Leeuw R, Klasser G, eds. *Orofacial Pain. Guidelines for Assessment, Diagnosis and Management.* 5th ed. Hanover Park, IL: Quintessence; 2013.

Dommerholt J, Fernandez-de-las-Penas C, eds. *Trigger Point Dry Needling. An Evidenced and Clinical-Based Approach.* Elsevier Ltd; 2013.

Fleisher KE, Krieger AC. Current trends in treatment of obstructive sleep apnea. *J Oral Maxillofac Surg.* 2007;65:2056-2058.

Fransson A, Tegelberg A, Svenson B, Lennartsson B, Isacsson G. Influence of mandibular protruding device on airway passages and dentofacial characteristics in obstructive sleep apnea and snoring. *Am J Orthod Dentofacial Orthop.* 2002;122:371-379.

Friedman M, Hamilton C, Samuelson CG, et al. Compliance and efficacy of titratable thermoplastic versus custom mandibular advancement devices. *Otolaryngol Head Neck Surg.* 2012 Aug;147(2):379-386.

Friedman M, Landsberg R, Pryor S, et al. The occurrence of sleep disordered breathing among patients with head and neck cancer. *Laryngoscope.* 2001;111:1917-1919.

Fung AM, Wilson DL, Barnes M, Walker SP. Obstructive sleep apnea and pregnancy: the effect on perinatal outcomes. *J Perinatol.* 2012 Jun;32(6):399-406.

Gagnon Y, Mayer P, Morisson F, Rompré PH, Lavigne GJ. Aggravation of respiratory disturbances by the use of an occlusal splint in apneic patients: a pilot study. *Int J Prosthodont.* 2004 Jul-Aug;17(4):447-453.

Ghazal A, Sorichter S, Jonas I, Rose EC. A randomized prospective long-term study of two oral appliances for sleep apnoea treatment. *J Sleep Res.* 2009 Sep;18(3):321-328.

Hugentobler M, Scolozzi P. Severe dental malocclusion: a rare and insidious complication of mandibular advancement devices for obstructive sleep apnea syndrome treatment. *Oral Surg Oral Med Oral Pathol Oral Radiol Endod*-2010;109:e28-e32.

Johal A, Battagel JM. Current principles in the management of obstructive sleep apnoea with mandibular advancement appliances. *Br Dent J.* 2001;190:532-536.

Johal A, Conaghan C. Maxillary morphology in obstructive sleep apnea: a cephalometric and model study. *Angle Orthod.* 2004 Oct;74(5):648-656.

Kapsimalis F, Kryger MH. Gender and obstructive sleep apnea syndrome, part 2: mechanisms. *Sleep.* 2002 Aug 1;25(5):499-506. Review.

Kaynak H, Kaynak D , Oztura I. Does frequency of nocturnal urination reflect the severity of sleep-disordered breathing? *J Sleep Res.* 2004 Jun;13(2):173-176.

Klasser GD OJ. The clinical usefulness of surface electromyography in the diagnosis and treatment of temporomandibular disorders. *J Am Dent Assoc.* 2006;137(6):763-771.

Lawton HM, Battagel JM, Kotecha B. A comparison of the Twin Block and Herbst mandibular advancement splints in the treatment of patients with obstructive sleep apnoea: a prospective study. *Eur J Orthod.* 2005;27(1):82-90.

Lettieri CJ; Paolino N; Eliasson AH; Shah AA; Holley AB. Comparison of adjustable and fixed oral appliances for the treatment of obstructive sleep apnea. *J Clin Sleep Med.* 2011;7(5):439-445.

Levendowski DJ, Morgan T, Montague J, Melzer V, Berka C, Westbrook PR. Prevalence of probable obstructive sleep apnea risk and severity in a population of dental patients. *Sleep Breath.* 2008;12(4):303-309.

Lowe AA, Santamaria JD, Fleetham JA, Price C. Facial morphology and obstructive sleep apnea. *Am J Orthod Dentofacial Orthop.* 1986 Dec;90(6):484-491.

Manfredini D, Cocilovo F, Favero L, Ferronato G, Tonello S, Guarda-Nardini L. Surface electromyography of jaw muscles and kinesiographic recordings: diagnostic accuracy for myofascial pain. *J Oral Rehabil.* 2011;38(11):791-799.

Martínez-Gomis J, Willaert E, Nogues L, Pascual M, Somoza M, Monasterio C. Five years of sleep apnea treatment with a mandibular advancement device. Side effects and technical complications. *Angle Orthod.* 2010 Jan;80(1):30-36.

Mulla O, Agada F, Dawson D, Sood Sanjai. Obstructive sleep apnoea and snoring. Is examination necessary? *Australian Family Physician.* 2011;11(40):886-888.

Naeije M, Te Veldhuis AH, Te Veldhuis EC, Visscher CM, Lobbezoo F. Disc displacement within the human temporomandibular joint: a systematic review of a "noisy annoyance". *J Oral Rehabil.* 2013;40(2):139-158.

Nakano H, Mishima K, Matsushita A, et al. Efficacy Of The Silensor For Treating Obstructive Sleep Apnea Syndrome. *Oral Maxillofac Surg.* 2013 Jun;17(2):105-108.

Ng AT, Qian J, Cistulli PA. Oropharyngeal collapse predicts treatment response with oral appliance therapy in obstructive sleep apnea. *Sleep.* 2006 May;29(5):666-671.

Ohayon MM, Li KK, Guilleminault C. Risk factors for sleep bruxism in the general population. *Chest.* 2001 Jan;119(1):53-61.

Okeson J. *Management of Temporomandibular Disorders and Occlusion.* 7th ed. St. Louis, MO: Elsevier, Mosby; 2013.

Palla S. *Mioartropatie del sistema masticatorio e dolori orofacciali.* Milano: RC Libri; 2001.

Pitsis AJ, Darendeliler MA, Gotsopoulos H, Petocz P, Cistulli PA. Effect of vertical dimension on efficacy of oral appliance therapy in obstructive sleep apnea. *Am J Resp and Crit Care Med.* 2002 Sep;166(6):860-864.

Ramar K, Dort LC, Katz SG et al. Clinical Practice Guideline for the Treatment of Obstructive Sleep Apnea and Snoring with Oral Appliance Therapy: An Update for 2015. *J Clin Sleep Med.* 2015 Jul 15;11(7):773-827

Rose EC, Staats R, Virchow C, Jonas IE. A comparative study of two mandibular advancement appliances for the treatment of obstructive sleep apnoea. *Eur J Orthod.* 2002 Apr;24(2):191-198.

Rose EC, Staats R, Virchow C, Jonas IE. Occlusal and skeletal effects of an oral appliance in the treatment of obstructive sleep apnea. *Chest.* 2002 Sep;122(3):871-877.

Santos M, Laureano Filho, Campos JM, Ferraz EM. Dentofacial characteristics as indicator of obstructive sleep apnoea-hypopnea syndrome in patients with severe obesity. *Obes Rev.* 2011 Feb;12(2):105-113.

Schiffman E, Ohrbach R, Truelove E, et al. Diagnostic Criteria for Temporomandibular Disorders (DC/TMD) for Clinical and Research Applications: recommendations of the International RDC/TMD Consortium Network and Orofacial Pain Special Interest Group. *J Oral Facial Pain Headache.* 2014;28(1):6-27.

Seto BH, Gotsopoulos H, Sims MR, Cistulli PA. Maxillary morphology in obstructive sleep apnoea syndrome. *Eur J Orthod.* 2001 Dec;23(6):703-714.

Simons DG. *Travell & Simons' Myofascial Pain and Dysfunction : The Trigger Point Manual.* 2nd ed. Baltimore, MD: Williams & Wilkins; 1999.

Suvinen TI, Kemppainen P. Review of clinical EMG studies related to muscle and occlusal factors in healthy and TMD subjects. *J Oral Rehabil.* 2007;34(9):631-644.

Thomas CA, Okeson JP. Evaluation of lateral pterygoid muscle symptoms using a common palpation technique and a method of functional manipulation. *Cranio.* 1987;5(2):125-129.

Tsuda H, Almeida FR, Masumi S, Lowe AA. Side effects of boil and bite type oral appliance therapy in sleep apnea patients. *Sleep Breath.* 2010 Sep;14(3):227-232.

Vanderveken OM, Devolder A, Marklund M, et al. Comparison of a Custom-made and a Thermoplastic Oral Appliance for the Treatment of Mild Sleep Apnea. *Am J Respir Crit Care Med.* 2008 Jul;178(2):197-202.

Vanderveken OM, Van de Heyning PH, Braem MJ. Effects of vertical opening on pharyngeal dimensions in patients with obstructive sleep apnoea. *Sleep Med.* 2012 Mar;13(3):314-316.

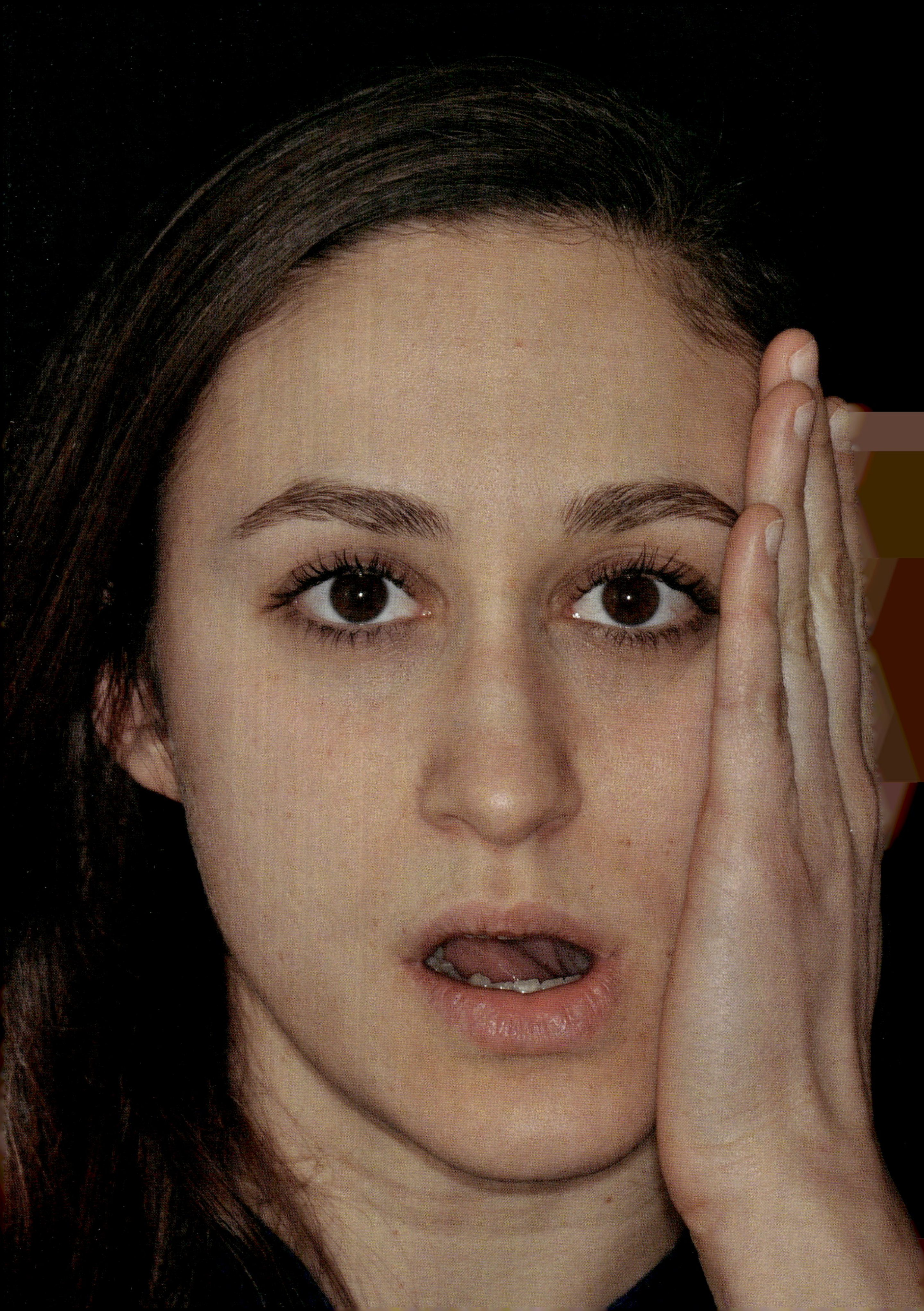

Side effects and management of oral device complications

Massimiliano Di Giosia ▪ Donald Falace

Objectives

- To describe the most common side effects that occur during therapy with MADs
- To understand the methods to manage side effects
- To understand the importance of educating patients about side effects

Introduction

There are two main types of oral devices (ODs): mandibular advancement devices (MADs) and tongue retainer devices (TRDs). The most commonly used devices are MADs, whose mechanism of action includes mandibular protrusion, which consequently maintains the tongue away from the pharynx, thereby enlarging the retropalatal and retrolingual airspace, particularly transversally.

TRDs increase the volume of the airways by anteriorly repositioning only the tongue and not the mandible. They can be used in patients who are not good candidates for MADs such as patients who are completely edentulous, and those with severe temporomandibular disorders or advanced periodontal disease.

Between the two types of appliances MADs are generally preferred and better tolerated. With both types of appliances, side effects are common, however, they are usually minor and transient and usually do not adversely affect their use. On occasion, side effects may become more problematic and may even prevent the use of the appliances.

With the use of MADs, side effects may include jaw pain, temporomandibular joint pain and/or dysfunction, sore teeth, loose teeth, tooth movement, dislodgement of dental restorations, posterior open bite, gingival or mucosal irritation, dry mouth, and drooling (de Almeida *et al.* 2005; Ferguson *et al.* 2006).

With TRDs, the most common reported side effects are tongue pain, tongue numbness, and excessive saliva with drooling. Tongue pain and numbness may be decreased by decreasing the degree of suction applied by the bulb. Drooling is inherent with the use of the TRD since the mouth must remain open.

Since side effects are common, it is important that patients be followed closely following delivery of the appliance and throughout the titration period, which may take several weeks or months. If side effects are experienced, patients can become discouraged quickly. Early recognition and treatment of side effects is key to ensuring a successful outcome.

Once an effective treatment position has been attained, patients should be seen on a recall basis to be sure that the appliance remains effective and that the patient is not experiencing any late onset side effects. Ideally, patients should be seen every six months to a year as long as they are using an appliance. Patients should also be encouraged to contact you if they have any problems or questions at any time between appointments.

This chapter describes the more frequent side effects, which are as follows:

- hypersalivation and dry mouth
- soft tissue trauma/irritation
- allergic reactions
- teeth pain and mobility
- dislodgement of dental restorations
- pain and/or dysfunction of the masticatory muscles and temporomandibular joints
- occlusal changes
- posterior open bite

Hypersalivation and xerostomia

Hypersalivation

According to the data available in the literature, the prevalence of this side effect varies from 7% to 68% (Fritsch *et al.* 2001; Ferguson *et al.* 2006; Gong *et al.* 2013).

Hypersalivation occurs quite frequently during the first week of device use, probably as a reaction to the adaptation to a "foreign body." For most patients, it gradually diminishes until it completely disappears. Moreover, it could be caused by an excessive vertical dimension of the device that prevents the patient from maintaining sealed lips. In such cases, it may be necessary to modify the device and reset it to a more physiological vertical dimension (Attanasio and Bailey 2010).

In severe and persistent cases of hypersalivation that cause social discomfort to the patients, it is possible to prescribe a scopolamine plaster. These plasters are used to prevent travel sickness (car, airplane, or boat), and their side effects include salivation reduction with consequential mouth dryness.

Dry mouth

Dry mouth is a rather frequent side effect with a prevalence of approximately 33% (Gong *et al.* 2013).

It could be caused by an excessive vertical dimension that prevents the sealing of the lips or by mouth breathing because of scarce nasal patency.

In persistent cases, it is possible to recommend some specific mouth rinses for dry mouth, such as Biotene®, or a medical tape, such as Micropore® tape, to be applied vertically for maintaining sealed lips and promoting nasal breathing (Parker 2014).

Some manufacturers of TAP® devices plan to add innovative changes, such as oral obturators applied to the device, to promote nasal breathing. In cases of devices that allow the patients to open their mouth, vertical elastics are recommended to limit the opening of the mouth.

Soft tissue trauma/irritation

Lesions or irritation of the oral mucosa can be initially caused by wrong maneuvers when inserting the device or by excessive "friction" of the advancement systems on the tongue, cheeks, and lips.

Typically, it is sufficient to discontinue wearing the device for a few days for healing these tissues. It is important to ensure that the metallic parts are polished and smooth.

In cases of persistent lesions in the area of the metallic parts, it might be necessary to change the type of device (Parker 2014).

Allergic reactions

Allergic reactions to the different materials of a device are rare, and these reactions may be caused by acrylic (methyl methacrylate acrylic) and some metallic parts (nickel) or by the latex orthodontic elastics that are used to limit the mouth from opening (Ferguson *et al.* 2006).

It is crucial to collect a detailed history to identify the patient's possible allergies before fabricating the MAD.

Dental pain and mobility

Previous studies have reported that the prevalence of dental pain caused by the use of device varies from 13% to 60% (Ferguson *et al.* 2006; Martinez-Gomis *et al.* 2010). It may be caused by dental crowding or rotation.

In such cases, the device may excessively compress the interproximal areas. Other causes can include a hyperextension of the vestibular and/or linguopalatal margins of the device or imprecise impressions with consequent technical flaws.

Typically, it is sufficient to internally modify the device in the areas of hypercompression and/or shorten the edges. The most comfortable devices are those in which the internal parts that are in contact with the teeth are prepared with soft materials.

An increase in dental mobility may be generated by the traction forces exerted by the device on the teeth or by occlusal trauma secondary to a malocclusion because of an extended use of a MAD.

As a remedy, a temporary mandibular trainer may be employed in the morning (AM Aligner) to reduce the occlusal changes or an Essix-type retainer may be used during the day to stabilize the teeth position (Parker 2014).

Dislodgement of dental restorations (bridges and crowns)

Dislodgement of dental restorations is often caused by a device that is extremely retentive, by prosthesis that was inadequately cemented, or by the presence of advanced decay in the dental pillars.

A Careful evaluation of dental health and state of the prosthesis is paramount before starting therapy with a MAD (Parker 2014).

Muscular and/or articular pain (temporomandibular disorders–TMDs)

The onset of joint noises and/or temporomandibular joints is often a source of concern for dentists. According to the data reported in the literature, the prevalence of pain related to masticatory muscles and temporomandibular joints during therapy with a MAD varies from 13% to 67%, and it is typically a transient side effect (Ferguson et al. 2006).

The American Academy of Orofacial Pain defines temporomandibular disorders as "a pathology involving the masticatory muscles, temporomandibular joints, and their associated structures." Fundamentally, they are musculoskeletal disorders of the masticatory system whose most frequent symptoms are as follows:

- masticatory muscle pain and/or temporomandibular joint pain
- limitations and/or changes in mandibular movements
- joint sounds.

Several studies have demonstrated that temporomandibular disorders due to therapy with MADs are often transient and rarely cause patients to discontinue the treatment permanently (de Almeida *et al.* 2002; Giannasi et al. 2009; Doff *et al.* 2011; Chen 2013; Lowe 2013). If the disorders exist before therapy, they do not typically represent an absolute contraindication to the treatment. In 2011, Cunali and collaborators demonstrated that some mandibular exercises may increase the compliance of patients with a temporomandibular disorder already present before the beginning of therapy with a MAD (Cunali *et al.* 2011).

An absolute contraindication can be the presence of a painful disc displacement without reduction (articular lock) or an extremely painful osteoarthritis of the temporomandibular joint. In such cases, the issues pertaining to the joint must be treated before starting therapy with a MAD.

In cases of monolateral pain occurring after beginning the therapy with a MAD, a possible cause could be the forced asymmetric position of the jaw due to a bad construction bite or an asymmetric advancement of a MAD. In such cases, it is sufficient to "reset" MAD by drawing backward the advancement screw on the painful side. In some cases, it may be necessary a new construction bite to reset the device in the laboratory.

In a device with posterior contacts (Somnodent, Herbst®), it is crucial to exclude pre-contacts that cause device instability. A conservative approach is often sufficient to manage the muscular and/or articular pain (Ueda *et al.* 2009; Sheats *et al.* 2017):

- undergoing self-treatment is recommended, and it includes thermotherapy, heat or cold application in the masticatory muscle areas, followed by stretching exercises

- adopting a soft diet for a few days
- applying a short pharmacological therapy with non-steroidal anti-inflammatory drugs (i.e., Naproxen 550 mg, one tablet twice a day for 5–7 days, or Ibuprofen 600 mg, one tablet three times a day a day for 5–7 days) or, if necessary, temporary discontinuation of a MAD
- controlling and managing the daytime parafunction (clenching) that could worsen the muscular pain. In such cases, patients should be instructed to avoid the diurnal dental contacts

The onset of joint noises during therapy with a MAD is rare. More frequently there is a temporary reduction or disappearance of the joint noises that existed before beginning therapy (Perez *et al.* 2013).

It is crucial to execute a thorough screening of the masticatory muscles and temporomandibular joints before initiating therapy with a MAD, document the signs/symptoms found during the visit, and to inform the patient regarding the possible side effects.

Data in the literature indicate that these side effects are mild and transient; however, in some cases, pain and dysfunction may become chronic. Therefore, it is important that the dentist responsible for the dental sleep medicine acquires good preparation for diagnosing and managing temporomandibular disorders (Spencer *et al.* 2013).

Dental movements and occlusal changes

The long-term use of a MAD may cause undesired mild dental movements (Marklund *et al.* 2001; Robertson 2001; Rose *et al.* 2002; Marklund 2006; Hammond *et al.* 2007; Ghazal *et al.* 2008). They occur in most patients despite being rarely perceived.

Occlusal changes were observed in >80% of the investigated participants in a study conducted in Vancouver on dental casts of patients undergoing treatment with MADs for 7 years (de Almeida *et al.* 2006). The more frequent occlusal changes include the reduction of the overjet and reduction of an overbite (due to the retroclination of the superior incisors and proclination of the inferior incisors).

The mean variation in the overjet is 1.4 mm, whereas it is 1.3 mm for the overjet. Moreover, previous studies have reported the distal tipping of superior molars and mesial tipping of inferior molars (Ferguson *et al.* 2003).

According to a recent study, the entity of occlusal changes may vary depending on the design and fabrication material of the MAD, adherence to treatment, and duration of therapy (Venema *et al.* 2018).

In a wide percentage of cases (patients with dental class II with an increased overbite and overjet), dental movements can be considered favorable under the viewpoint of the occlusal improvement (Tsuda *et al.* 2010; Pliska *et al.* 2014).

Posterior open bite

The posterior open bite is characterized by the lack of occlusal contacts between the posterior teeth as well as by more marked contact between the anterior teeth. It is often perceived in the morning after the MAD is removed, and it typically lasts for a few minutes, following which the occlusion normalizes and the patients are able to close their mouth in their habitual position. Occasionally, it persists for more than a few minutes to some hours, and in some cases, the condition may become permanent.

In a recent study, it has been reported that there is a presence of a persistent posterior open bite in 17% of the analyzed patients. According to the authors, this happens particularly in individuals who did not participate in follow-up for months or years. These data highlight the importance of regular follow-ups every 6 months-1 year for patients undergoing therapy with MADs.

Posterior open bite purportedly occurs due to the contracture of the lateral pterygoid muscles after being in a shortened or contracted position overnight. It is unclear why some patients experience this effect while others do not, although empirically it appears to be more common in patients who require greater amounts of mandibular protrusion. It is interesting to note that most patients with posterior open bite are unaware of the presence of the condition and do not report any chewing or biting difficulties (Perez *et al.* 2013).

It is important that the presence of or tendency for the development of posterior open bite be recognized early and that treatment and/or prevention be initiated as soon as possible

The morning use of a bite repositioner (AM aligner) after the removal of a MAD is considered a good method to prevent the development of a posterior open bite (see Chapter 10).

The device, which is made in the patient's normal maximum intercuspal position, guides the teeth into their normal occlusal relationship upon biting . The appliance can be fabricated by the laboratory or it can be fabricated by the dentist at chairside prior to delivery of the MAD.

Another treatment/preventive approach is to prescribe jaw exercises that encourage retrognathic movement of the jaw to re-lengthen the lateral pterygoids (Ueda *et al.* 2009). Other measures that have been used include the use of chewing gum, use of a leaf gauge, and forced retrognathic jaw movement by manually pushing on the jaw.

As is typically the case when multiple treatment approaches are advocated, none are uniformly effective, therefore, it may be necessary to try several until success is achieved..

At a skeletal level, previous studies have described the tendency to develop a mild mandibular post-rotation and an increase in the vertical dimension that are statistically (but not clinically) significant (Bondemark 1999; Robertson 2001; Fransson *et al.* 2002; de Almeida *et al.* 2006; Doff *et al.* 2010).

REFERENCES

ATTANASIO R, BAILEY DR. *Dental Mangement of Sleep Disorders*. Wiley-Blackwell; 2010.

BONDEMARK L. Does 2 years' nocturnal treatment with a mandibular advancement splint in adult patients with snoring and OSAS cause a change in the posture of the mandible? *Am J Orthod Dentofacial Orthop*. 1999;116:621-628.

CHEN H, LOWE AA. Updates in oral appliance therapy for snoring and obstructive sleep apnea. *Sleep Breath*. 2013;17 (2):473-486.

COHEN-LEVY J, PÉTELLE B, PINGUET J, LIMERAT E, FLEURY B. Forces created by mandibular advancement devices in OSAS patients: a pilot study during sleep. *Sleep Breath*. 2013;17(2):781-789.

CUNALI PA, ALMEIDA FR, SANTOS CD, ET AL. Mandibular exercises improve mandibular advancement device therapy for obstructive sleep apnea. *Sleep Breath*. 2011;15(4):717-727.

DE ALMEIDA FR, BITTENCOURT LR, DE ALMEIDA CIR, TSUIKI S, LOWE AA, TUFIK S. Effects of mandibular posture on obstructive sleep apnea severity and the temporomandibular joint in patients fitted with an oral appliance. *Sleep*. 2002;25(5):507-513.

DE ALMEIDA FR, LOWE AA, OTSUKA R, FASTLICHT S, FARBOOD M, TSUIKI S. Long-term sequellae of oral appliance therapy in obstructive sleep apnea patients: Part 2. Study-model analysis. *Am J Orthod Dentofacial Orthop*. 2006;129(2):205-213.

DE ALMEIDA FR, LOWE AA, TSUIKI S, ET AL. Long-term compliance and side effects of oral appliances used for the treatment of snoring and obstructive sleep apnea syndrome. *J Clin Sleep Med*. 2005;1(2):143-152.

DOFF MH, HOEKEMA A, PRUIM GJ, HUDDLESTON SLATER JJ, STEGENGA B. Long-term oral-appliance therapy in obstructive sleep apnea: a cephalometric study of craniofacial changes. *J Dent*. 2010 Dec;38(12):1010-1018.

DOFF MHJ, VELDHUIS SKB, HOEKEMA A, ET AL. Long-term oral appliance therapy in obstructive sleep apnea syndrome: a controlled study on temporomandibular side effects. *Clin Oral Investig*. 2011;16(3):689-697.

FERGUSON KA, CARTWRIGHT R, ROGERS R, SCHMIDT-NOWARA W. Oral appliances for snoring and obstructive sleep apnea: a review. *Sleep*. 2006;29(2):244-262.

FERGUSON KA. The role of oral appliance therapy in the treatment of obstructive sleep apnea. *Clin Chest Med*. 2003 Jun;24(2):355-364.

FRANSSON AM, SVENSON BA, ISACSSON G. The effect of posture and a mandibular protruding device on pharyngeal dimensions: a cephalometric study. *Sleep and Breathing*. 2002;6:55-68.

FRITSCH KM, ISELI A, RUSSI EW, BLOCH KE. Side effects of mandibular advancement devices for sleep apnea treatment. *Am J Respir Crit Care Med*. 2001;164(5):813-818.

GHAZAL A, JONAS IE, ROSE EC. Dental side effects of mandibular advancement appliances - a 2-year follow-up. *J Orofac Orthop*. 2008;69(6):437-447.

GIANNASI LC, ALMEIDA FR, MAGINI M, ET AL. Systematic assessment of the impact of oral appliance therapy on the temporomandibular joint during treatment of obstructive sleep apnea: long-term evaluation. *Sleep Breath*. 2009;13(4):375-381.

GONG X, ZHANG J, ZHAO Y, GAO X. Long-term therapeutic efficacy of oral appliances in treatment of obstructive sleep apnea-hypopnea syndrome. *Angle Orthod*. 2013;83(4):653-658.

HAMMOND RJ1, GOTSOPOULOS H, SHEN G, PETOCZ P, CISTULLI PA DM. A follow-up study of dental and skeletal changes associated with mandibular advancement splint use in obstructive sleep apnea. *Am J Orthod Dentofac Orthop*. 2007;132(6):806-814.

MARKLUND M, SAHLIN C, STENLUND H, PERSSON M FK. Mandibular advancement device in patients with obstructive sleep apnea: long-term effects on apnea and sleep. *Chest*. 2001;120(1):162-169.

MARKLUND M. Predictors of long-term orthodontic side effects from mandibular advancement devices in patients with snoring and obstructive sleep apnea. *Am J Orthod Dentofac Orthop*. 2006;129(2):214-221.

MARTÍNEZ-GOMIS J, WILLAERT E, NOGUES L, PASCUAL M, SOMOZA M, MONASTERIO C. Five years of sleep apnea treatment with a mandibular advancement device. Side effects and technical complications. *Angle Orthod*. 2010;80(1):30-36.

PARKER J. Side effects and management. AADSM webinar. 2014. www.aadsm.org

PEREZ CV, DE LEEUW R, OKESON JP, ET AL. The incidence and prevalence of temporomandibular disorders and posterior open bite in patients receiving mandibular advancement device therapy for obstructive sleep apnea. *Sleep Breath*. 2013;17(1):323-332.

PLISKA BT, NAM H, CHEN H, LOWE AA, ALMEIDA FR. Obstructive sleep apnea and mandibular advancement splints: occlusal effects and progression of changes associated with a decade of treatment. *J Clin Sleep Med*. 2014;10(12):1285-1291.

ROBERTSON CJ. Dental and skeletal changes associated with long-term mandibular advancement. *Sleep*. 2001;24(5):531-537.

ROSE EC, STAATS R, VIRCHOW C JR JI. Occlusal and skeletal effects of an oral appliance in the treatment of obstructive sleep apnea. *Chest*. 2002;122(3):871-877.

SHEATS RD, SCHELL TG, BLANTON AO, ET AL. Management of side e ects of oral appliance therapy for sleep-disordered breathing. *J Dent Sleep Med*. 2017;4(4):111-125.

Spencer J, Patel M, Mehta N, et al. Special consideration regarding the assessment and management of patients being treated with mandibular advancement oral appliance therapy for snoring and obstructive sleep apnea. *Cranio.* 2013;31(1):10-13.

Tsuda H, Almeida FR, Tsuda T, Moritsuchi Y, Lowe AA. Craniofacial changes after 2 years of nasal continuous positive airway pressure use in patients with obstructive sleep apnea *Chest.* 2010;138(4):870-874.

Ueda H, de Almeida FR, Chen H LA. Effect of 2 jaw exercises on occlusal function in patients with obstructive sleep apnea during oral appliance therapy: a randomized controlled trial. *Am J Orthod Dentofac Orthop.* 2009;135(4).

Venema JA, Stellingsma C, Do MH, Hoekema A. Dental side e ects of long-term obstructive sleep apnea therapy: a comparison of three therapeutic modalities. *J Dent Sleep Medi.* 2018;5(2):39-46.

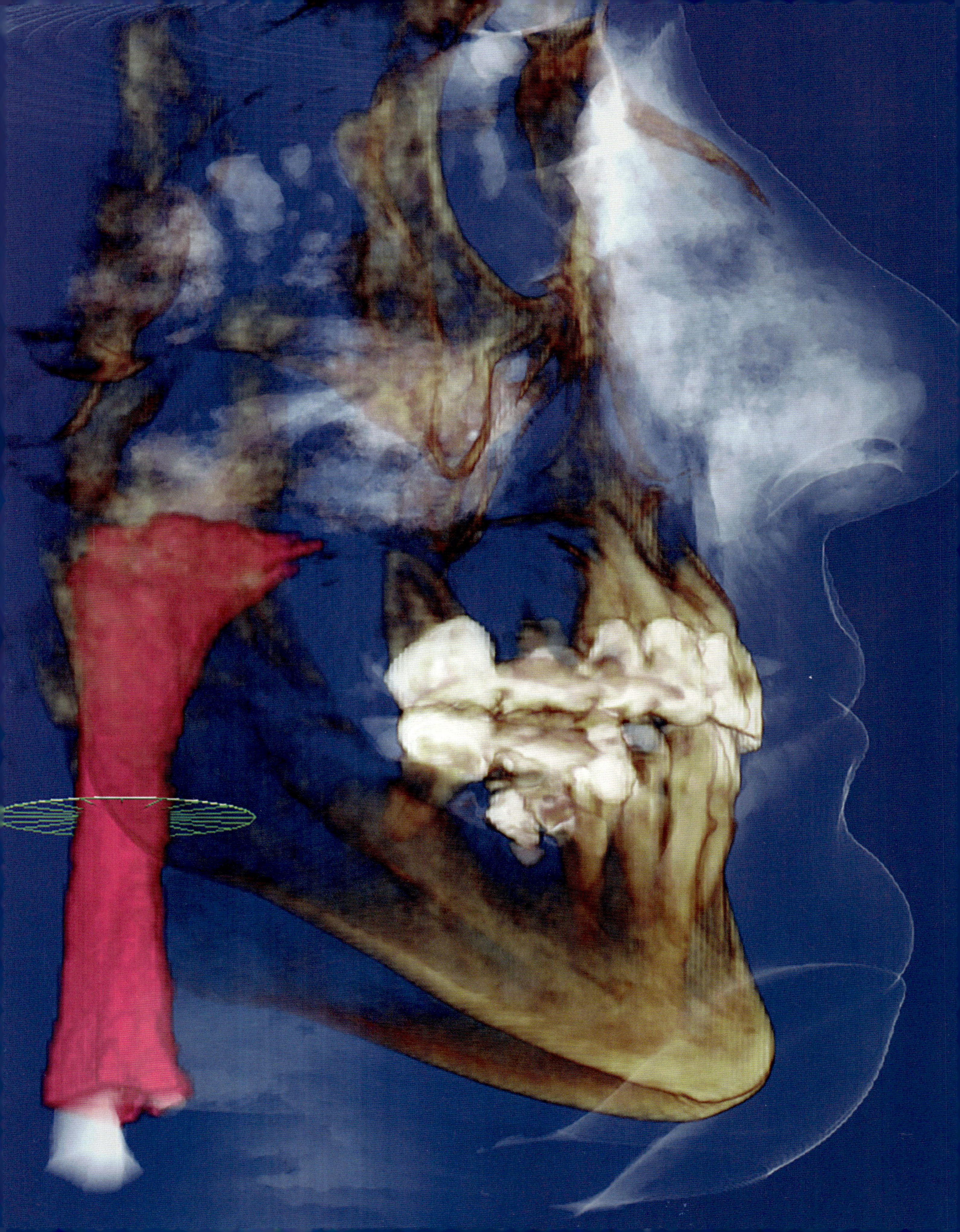

Clinical cases

Francesca Milano · Antonio L. Gracco

Case 1

Male patient 45 y.o.; body mass index (BMI) = 28 kg/m^2

History of habitual and persistent snoring since childhood. The patient experienced unsatisfactory sleep at night, daytime sleepiness under relaxed conditions, and motor inactivity. Apneas were witnessed by his wife. No state of sleepiness while driving was reported. The patient was never involved in road accidents. Epworth sleepiness scale (ESS): 12

Significant anamnesis elements: the patient was a nonsmoker but reported occasional alcohol consumption and mild hypertension under good pharmacological control.

The patient was subjected to full *cardiorespiratory monitoring* highlighting the presence of severe obstructive sleep apnea syndrome (OSAS) [apnea-hypopnea index (AHI) = 52; supine AHI = 52; nonsupine AHI = 51; oxygen desaturation index (ODI) = 51; minimum oxygen saturation (SaO_2) = 88; < 90% = 14], which was independent of the sleeping position.

Ear, nose, and throat (ENT) objectivity: Deviated nasal septum, hypertrophic turbinates, tonsillar hypertrophy, tonsillar grading 3; Mallampati 3

Nasal endoscopy with Müller's maneuver: RL+ 3AP; RP+ 3C

Dental clinical and radiographic evaluation:

- oval-shaped face with chin asymmetry toward the right (13.1a);
- bimaxillary retrusion profile with increased length of the lower third and short neck-chin distance (13.1b);
- high-arched and deep palate, contracted upper arch, overcrowded and contracted lower arch with missing dental elements, migrations, and residual spaces (13.2a);
- right posterior crossbite and lower midline deviated by 2 mm toward the right (13.2b);
- dental Class II, I division in a patient with deep bite, 9 mm overjet, 5 mm overbite, i.e., excessive vertical overlapping of the mandibular incisors by the maxillary incisors in centric occlusion (13.2c and d);
- skeletal biretrusion due to retrodisplaced superior maxillary bone and retrodisplaced and postrotated mandible, increased distance between the hyoid bone and mandibular plane, reduced PAS, and elongated soft palate (13.3);
- asymmetric condyles with missing elements: 18-28-36-38-46-48, multiple direct restoration, dental treatment with prosthesis at 24 and prosthetic restoration at 46 (13.4);
- multiple gingival recessions in an otherwise stable and healthy periodontal state (13.5a and b).

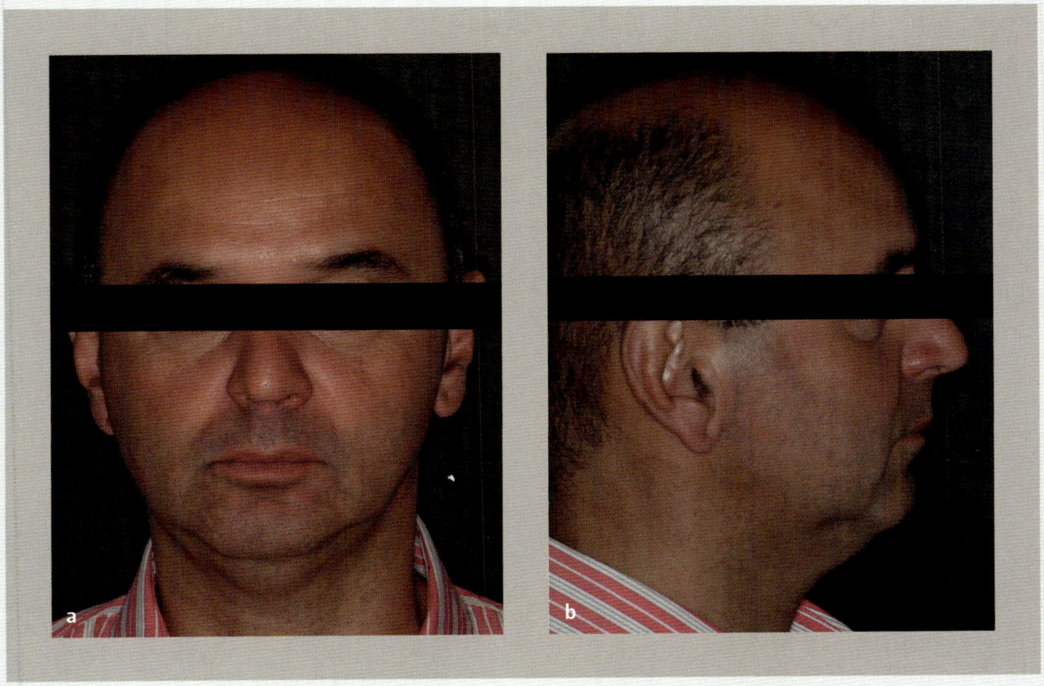

13.1 **a–b)** Frontal and lateral view of the face.

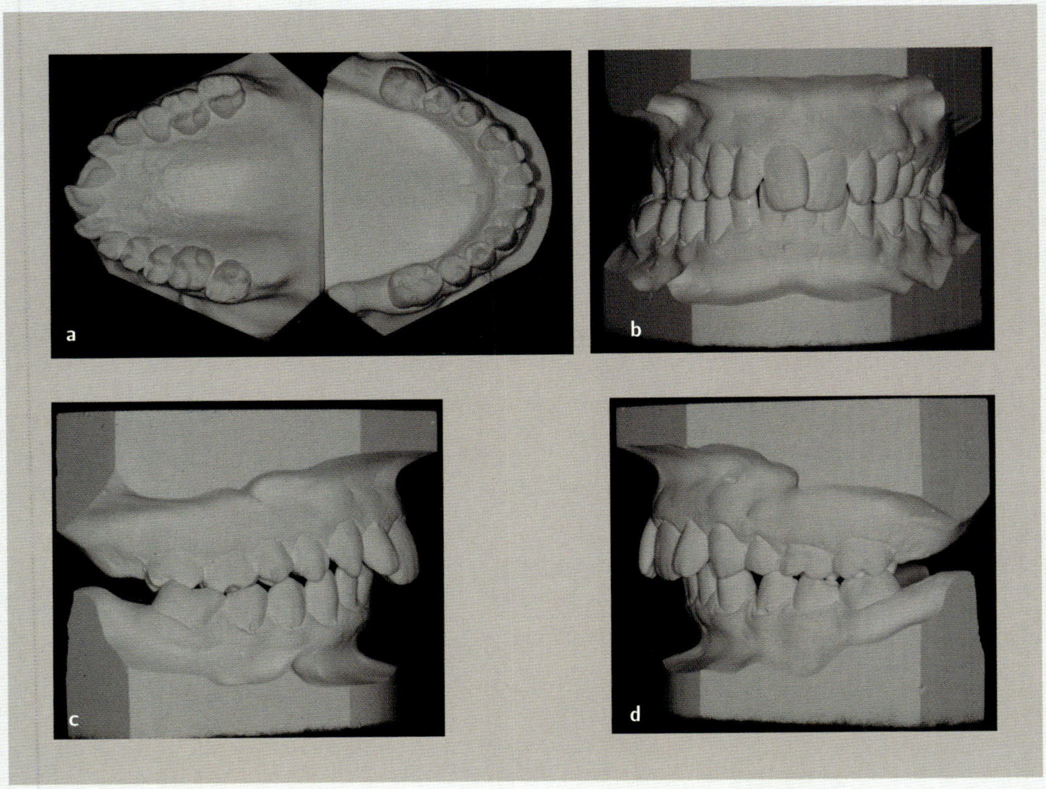

13.2 **a–d)** Plaster model used in this study. Frontal and lateral occlusal view.

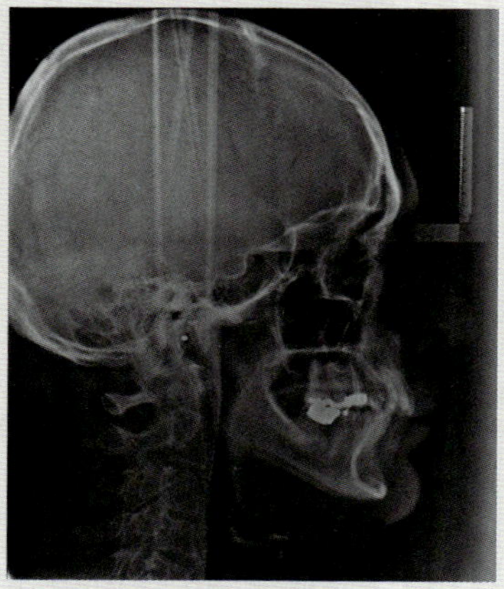

13.3 Teleradiography. Lateral projection of the skull.

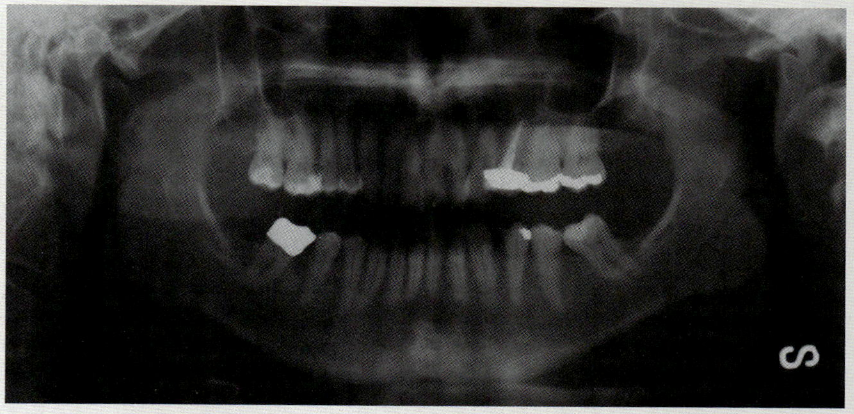

13.4 Panoramic radiography.

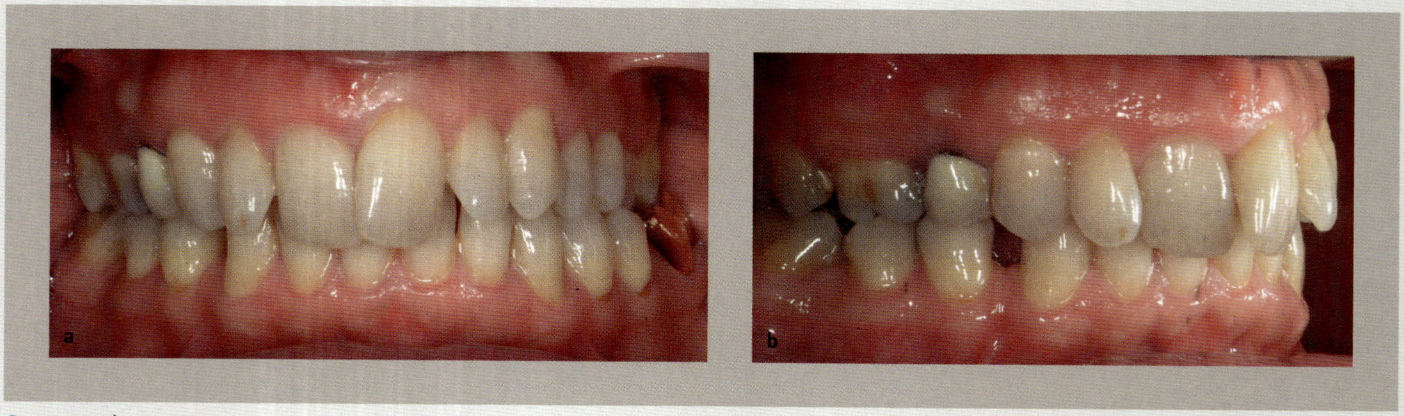

13.5 a–b) Intraoral images. Frontal and lateral view.

Temporomandibular joint (TMJ) evaluation: good range of motion. Maximum protrusion :11 mm.Pain upon palpation of the right masseter muscle. No pain upon palpation of the TMJs.No joint noises were identified.

Considering the severity of OSAS, continuous positive airway pressure (CPAP) therapy was initially suggested as a therapeutic treatment.
However, the patient stated that he preferred to undergo surgical treatment. Therefore, the patient was subjected to drug-induced sleep endoscopy (DISE) with a previous construction of a mandibular advancement device (MAD) simulator to evaluate the airways and his response to the mandibular advancement during induced sleep (13.6).

The mandibular advancement simulator was constructed using a George Gauge with a vertical opening of 5 mm and and a mandibular advancement of 7.5 mm (maximal comfortable advancement).
During sleep endoscopy with and without the simulator, circumferential obstruction was observed in the retropalatal and retrolingual regions. The obstruc-

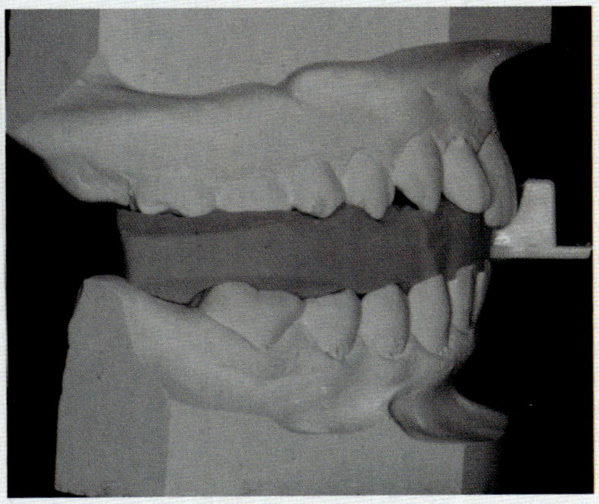

13.6 Construction bite.

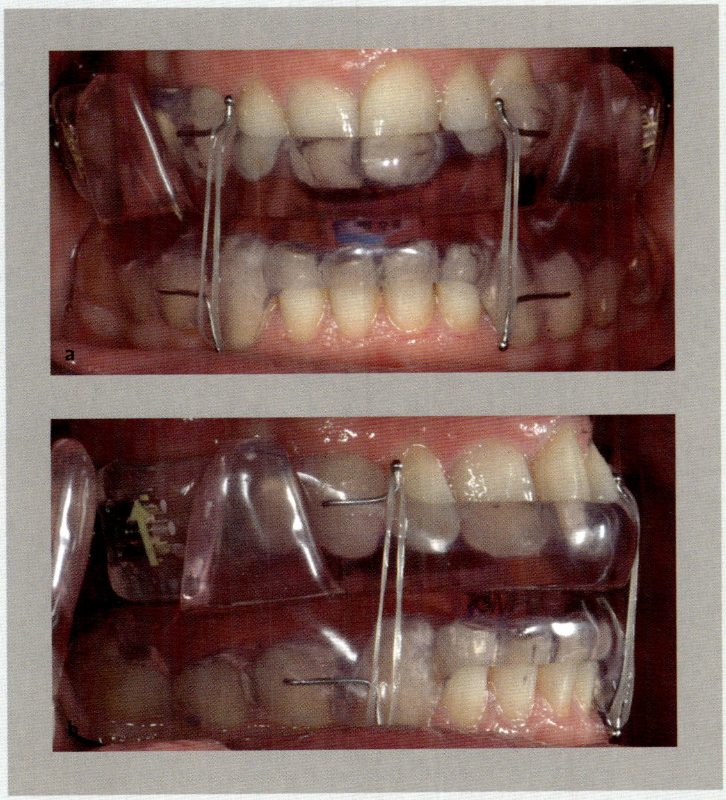

13.7 a–b) Intraoral images with MAD and vertical elastics. Frontal and lateral view.

tion was partially resolved with the application of the mandibular advancement simulator (particularly in the retrolingual region).

Treatment plan: after completing the diagnosis with DISE, the patient was suggested to undergo lateral pharyngoplasty and tonsillectomy followed by a subsequent treatment with MAD (Somnodent Flex® fabricated with the construction bite used during DISE and delivered 4 weeks after the surgery) (13.7a e b).

Delivery: Instructions for use and selection of vertical elastics (85 g-1/4").

Titration: Two weeks after the delivery, the patient reported hypersalivation. However, this patient did not register or experience any pain. A titration program was initiated with a planned activation of 0.1 mm every 3 days until resolution of patient's symptoms (snoring and sleepiness). Four weeks after the delivery, the patient reported that his prior discomfort due to hypersalivation was mitigated, whereas the achieved advancement was 8 mm. Therefore and because of the profound perceived improvement, the therapeutic plan was discontinued.

During polygraphic follow-up 4 months after the surgery and MAD implementation, the patient reported subjective improvement in snoring and sleepiness symptoms (ESS = 3).

At PG without MAD (result of the surgical treatment) a moderate residual OSAS (AHI = 29; supine AHI = 53; nonsupine AHI = 22; ODI = 29; minimum SaO_2 = 89; CT < 90% = 2.1).

PG with MAD (result of the surgical treatment and MAD) reported excellent control of the respiratory events was observed (AHI = 0.7; supine AHI = 1; nonsupine AHI = 0; ODI = 1.2; minimum SaO_2 = 91; CT < 90% = 0).

Long-term follow-up with MAD (3 years) exhibited excellent adherence to the therapy (the patient is wearing this device every night and throughout the entire night).

Symptoms: Mild snoring in the supine position, nondisturbing snoring, and lack of daytime sleepiness (ESS = 4)

Case 2

Male patient. 62 y.o. BMI = 32.5 kg/m^2

History of habitual and persistent snoring; the patient exhibits moderate daytime sleepiness that becomes more prominent after meals. He reported two episodes of nocturia per night and no cases of sleepiness while driving. ESS: 11

Full *cardiorespiratory monitoring* underlined the presence of a moderate positional OSAS (AHI = 24; supine AHI = 39; nonsupine AHI = 10; ODI = 26; minimum SaO_2 = 74; CT < 90% = 9).

Significant anamnesis elements: The patient was a nonsmoker, but he admitted occasional alcohol consumption. He was diagnosed with hypertension that was under good pharmacological control. Furthermore, the patient has also developed dyslipidemia that is being pharmacologically treated.

ENT objectivity: the patient exhibits hypertrophic lower turbinates, tongue base hypertrophy, elongated soft palate and uvula, and Mallampati 4. The patient has also undergone tonsillectomy (performed during childhood).

Nasal endoscopy with Müller's maneuver: obstruction RL + 3AP; RP + 2L

Dental clinical and radiographic evaluation:

- square-shaped face (🔍 13.8a);
- straight and hypodivergent profile and short neck-chin distance (🔍 13.8b);
- upper and lower arches have a normal width with an absence of dental elements (🔍 13.9a);
- left posterior crossbite and lower midline deviated by 2 mm toward the left (🔍 13.9b);
- dental Class II, 3 mm overjet, and 2 mm overbite (🔍 13.9c and d);
- bimaxillary retrusion profile and inferior retroalveolia that were facilitated by the early loss of 3.6, 3.7, and 4.6, hypodivergent, increased distance between the hyoid bone and mandibular plane, reduced PAS, and elongated soft palate (🔍 13.10);
- 1.8 -1.6 -2.4 -2.8 -3.7-3.6 -4.6 -2.5 are missing, multiple direct restoration, dental prosthesis on 2.6, and partial fixed prosthesis on 1.4 and 1.5 with 1.6 for distal extension (🔍 13.11);
- mild/moderate attachment loss, generalized horizontal bone loss, angular mesial bony defect at 4.7 and 2.7, tooth mobility grade I on 4.7; furcation defects of grade I on 4.7; multiple noncarious lesions (abfractions), and multiple gingival recessions (🔍 13.11, 13.12a and b).

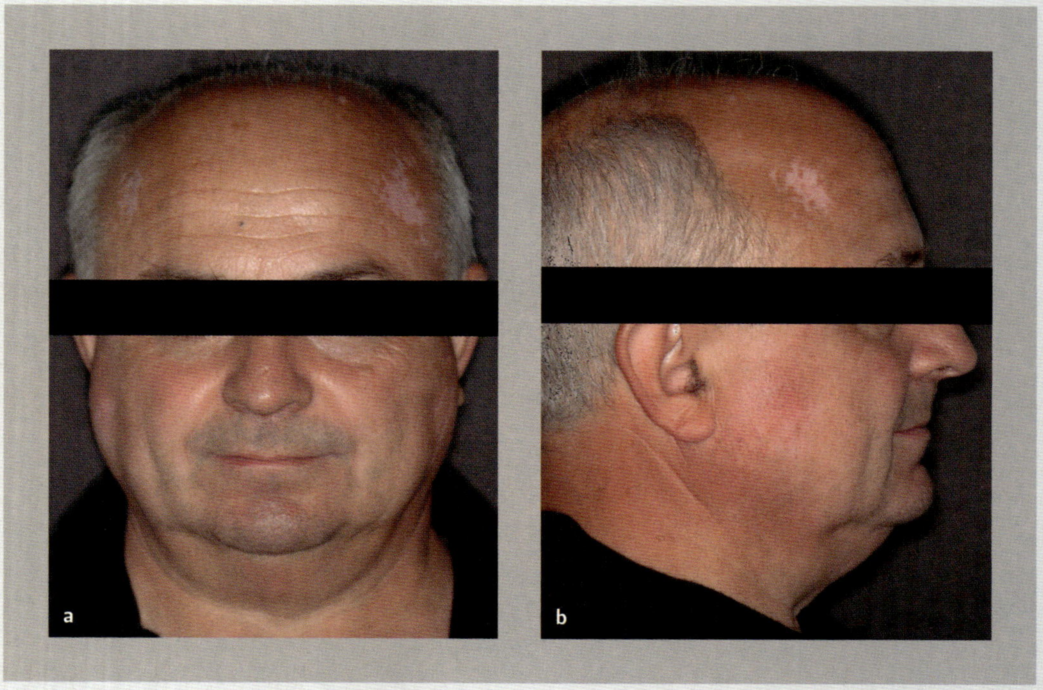

13.8 a–b) Frontal and lateral view of the face.

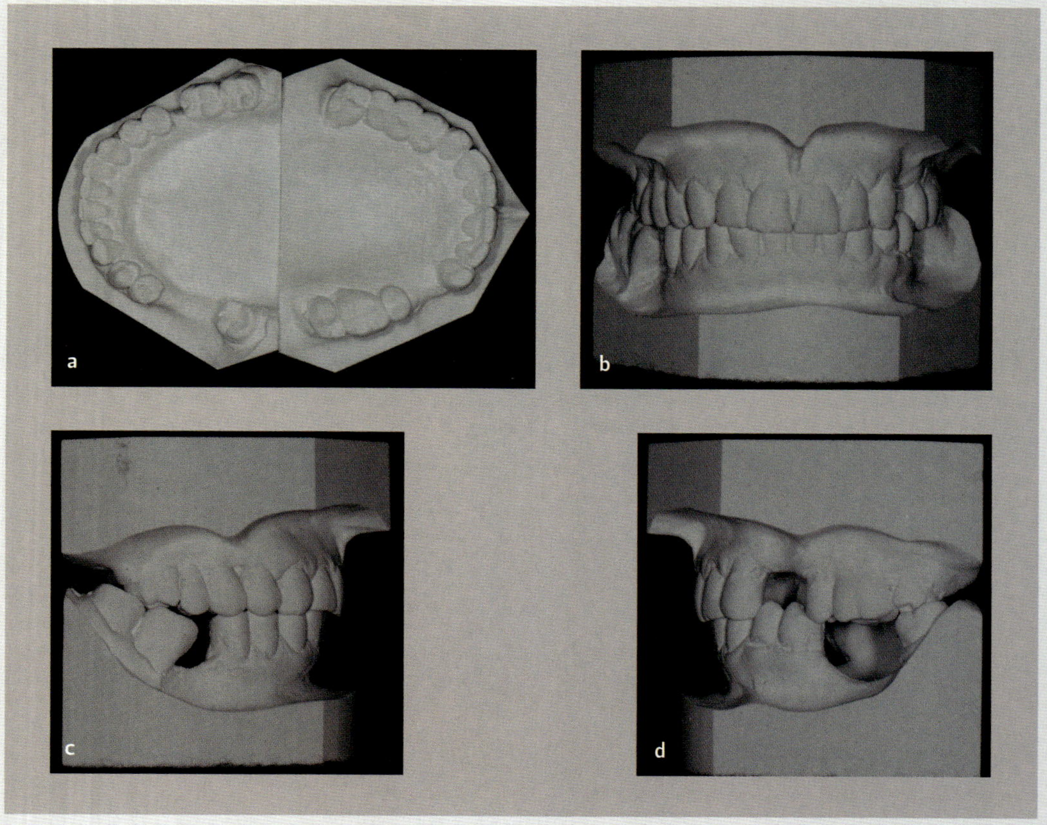

13.9 a–d) Frontal and lateral occlusal view of the plaster study models.

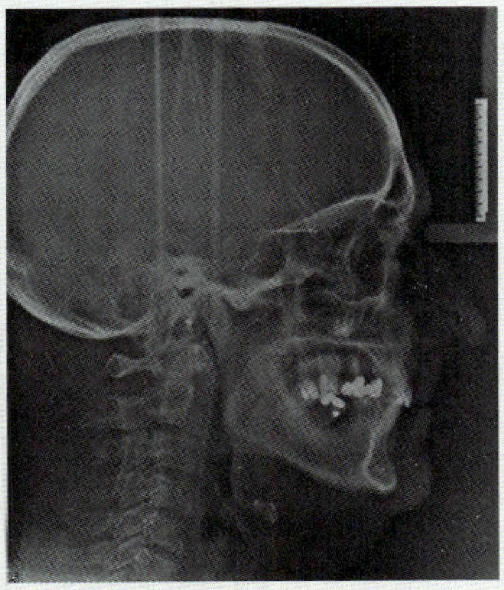

13.10 Teleradiography. Lateral projection.

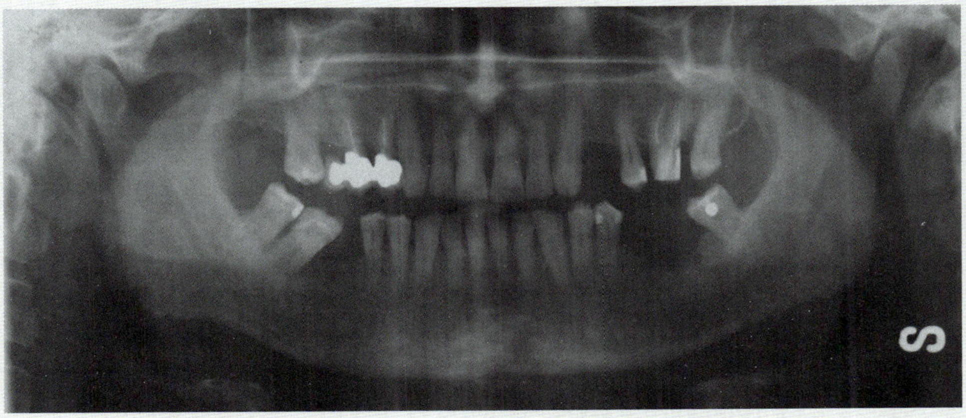

13.11 Panoramic radiography.

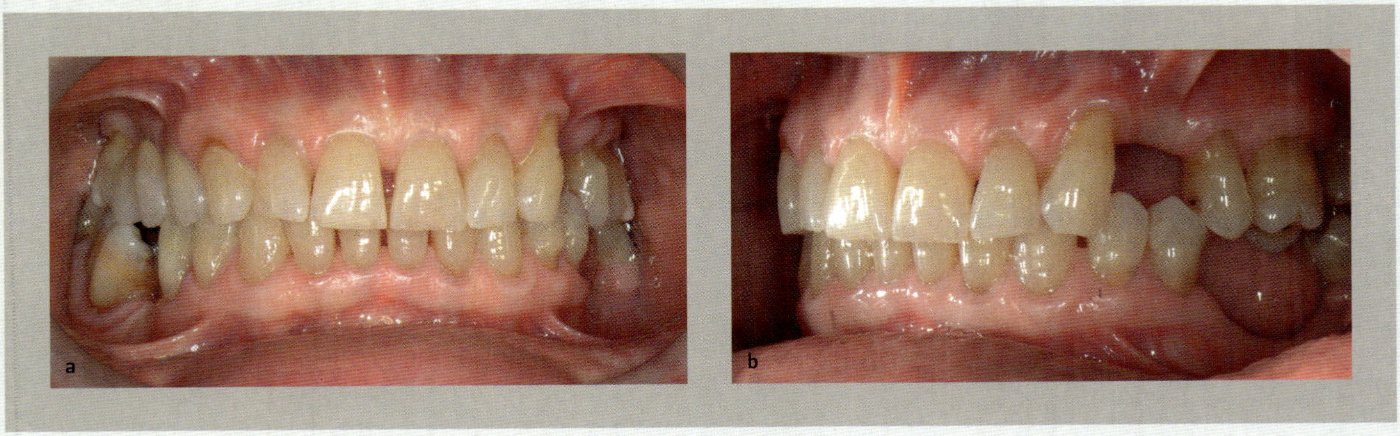

13.12 a–b) Intraoral images. Frontal and lateral view.

Despite the clinical and radiographical signs of the previous chronic periodontal disease, the subsequent treatment facilitated a stable and healthy periodontal state [full mouth bleeding score (FMBS) = 15%; full mouth plaque score (FMPS) = <20%].

TMJ evaluation: the maximal protrusive range was 10 mm. Pain was observed when palpating the masseter and temporal muscles. No pain was recorded during TMJ palpation. Absence of joint sounds and functional limitations and deviations in the opening and advancement.

Current therapy: the patient is receiving CPAP therapy with a full face mask (effective pressure = 10 cmH2O) for 1 year. CPAP has optimally controlled the number of obstructive events, but the patient reports low adherence to the therapy because of the manifestation of abdominal bloating. The patient is interested in trying an alternative therapy to CPAP.

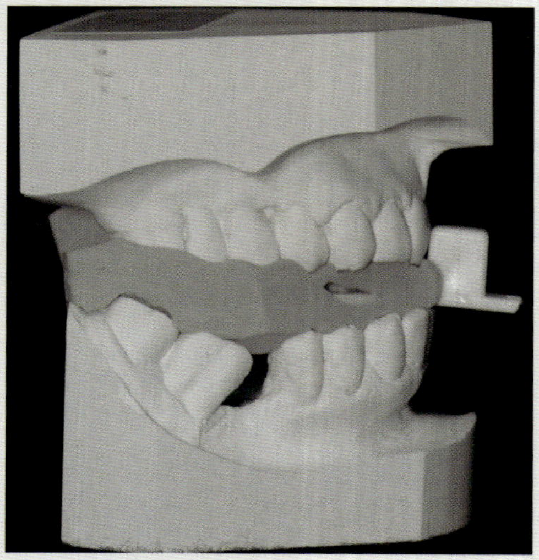

13.13 Construction bite.

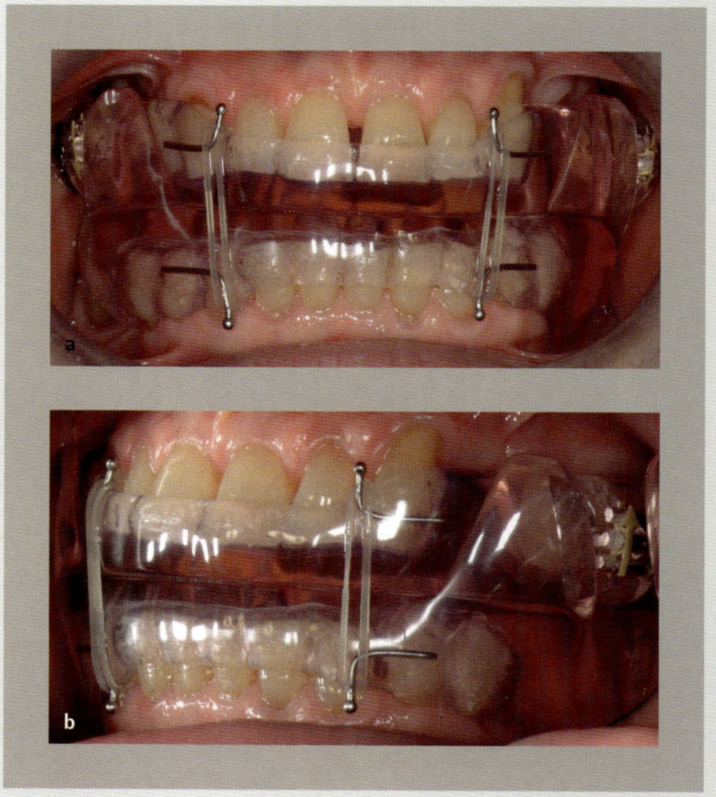

13.14 a–b) Intraoral images with MAD and vertical elastics. Frontal and lateral view.

Treatment plan: We decided to treat this patient with an MAD (Somnodent Flex®).

Construction bite: George Gauge with a vertical opening of 5 mm and advancement of 6 mm (13.13 e 13.14a and b).

Delivery: Instructions for use and selection of vertical elastics (170 g/3/16").

Titration: The patient reported an improvement in snoring and daytime sleepiness and a reduction in nocturia episodes 2 weeks after the application of the device. Titration was postponed because of mild muscular soreness at awakening. The patient was educated to perform muscle stretching exercises every morning after awakening.

Four weeks after delivery of the device, the patient's muscular soreness was spontaneously resolved.

The titration program involves an activation every 3 days until complete resolution of all related symptoms. The patient is instructed to quit this program in case of severe pain.

Three months after delivery of the device, an advancement of 8 mm was achieved. The patient was very satisfied about its efficacy in terms of his sleepiness and snoring. He reported the elimination of nocturia episodes. Therefore, we decided to stall the advancement.

During *follow-up*, the patient reported a subjective improvement in snoring and sleepiness (ESS = 5) at *6 months after the delivery of MAD*. No episodes of nocturia were reported.

PG with MAD highlights its efficient capacity to control the obstructive events. However, there were 10 residual events/hour in the supine position (AHI = 5; supine AHI = 10; nonsupine AHI = 0; minimum Sa2O = 82; CT 90% = 1). Therefore, the patient was recommended to control his sleeping position by means of bumper belts or positional trainers.

The patient reported adherence (subjective evaluation) to MAD: Six nights per week for at least 6 hours during each night.

Long-term follow-up of MAD: The patient wears the device every night and throughout the entire night; he did not use positional therapy.

Symptoms: Five years after delivery of the device, the patient reported mild snoring, absence of daytime sleepiness (ESS = 5), and absence of nocturia episodes.

Case 3

Male patient. 52 y.o. BMI = 22 kg/m^2

This patient has a history of snoring since early childhood and is susceptible to fatigue. However, he had recently exhibited a sudden onset of sleepiness while driving concurrent with intense daytime sleepiness during the last months.

Significant anamnesis elements: The patient was a nonsmoker, and he does not consume alcohol in the evening hours. He had undergone radiotherapy and chemotherapy treatment (approximately 6 months before) for right tonsillar carcinoma.

Evaluation of the sleep clinician and instrumental diagnosis (full cardiorespiratory monitoring with 6 channels): Severe OSAS (AHI = 55.1; supine AHI = 55; non-supine AHI = 55.1; ODI = 48.8; minimum Sa2O = 0.84; CT < 90% = 4.1%; ESS = 15)

ENT clinical evaluation: Rest of excision of the residual right tonsil tissue in a patient who has undergone tonsillectomy during early childhood, hypertrophic turbinates, and deviated nasal septum elongated soft palate, Mallampati 2

DISE: Complete collapse RP (circumferential) and obstruction in the RL area in the anteroposterior direction that is temporarily and partially resolved by a (partial) pull-up maneuver

Dental clinical and radiographic evaluation (no radiography was performed to avoid radiation exposure to the patient):

- oval-shaped elongated face (🔍 13.15a);
- bimaxillary retrusion and hypodivergent profile, short neck-chin distance (🔍 13.15b);
- high arch and deep palate, upper and lower arches were extremely contracted and crowded, missing elements: 1.8-2-4-4.4 (🔍 13.16a);
- lateral crossbite and upper midline slightly deviated toward the right (🔍 13.16b);
- dental Class I on the right side, dental Class II on the left side, 7 mm overjet, and 1.3 mm overbite (🔍 13.16c and d);
- skeletal biretrusion due to superior maxillary retrusion and retrodisplaced and postrotated mandible, hyperdivergent, increased distance between the hyoid bone and mandibular plane, reduced PAS, and elongated soft palate (🔍 13.17);
- multiple direct dental restoration, multiple noncarious lesions due to changes in the saliva content and quality after radiotherapy, and multiple gingival recessions (🔍 13.18a and b);
- current periodontal state is stable and healthy;
- the patient is being treated by his general dentist with a patient-tailored prevention program employed for individuals who have undergone radiotherapy in the head-neck area.

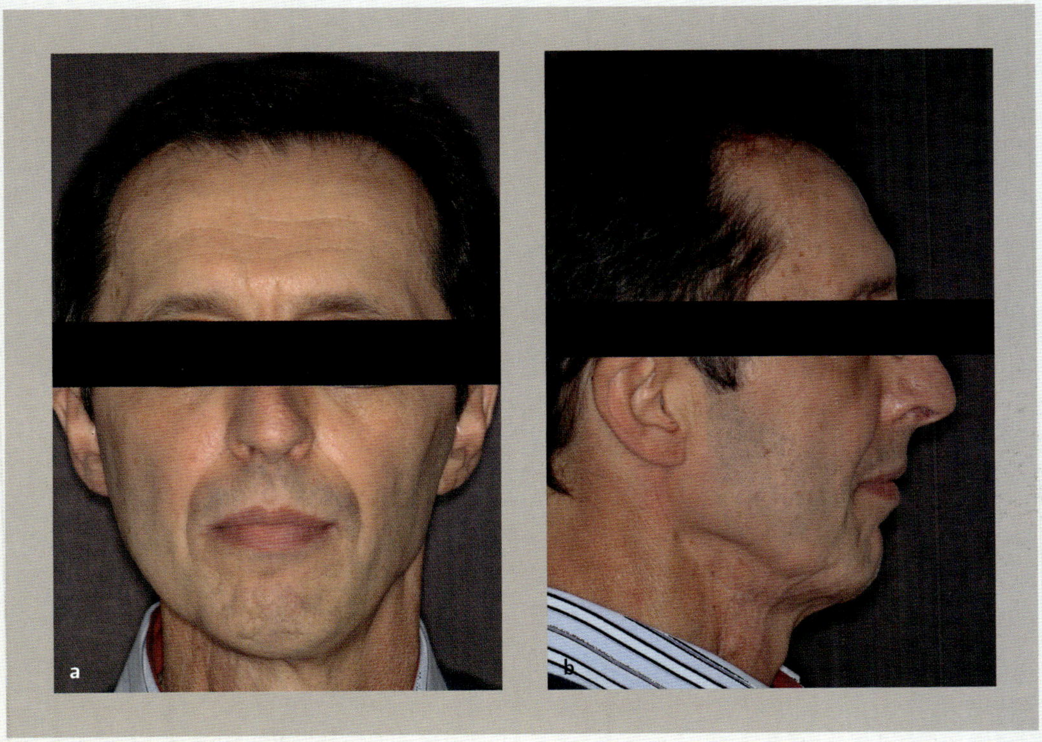

13.15 **a–b)** Frontal and lateral view of the face.

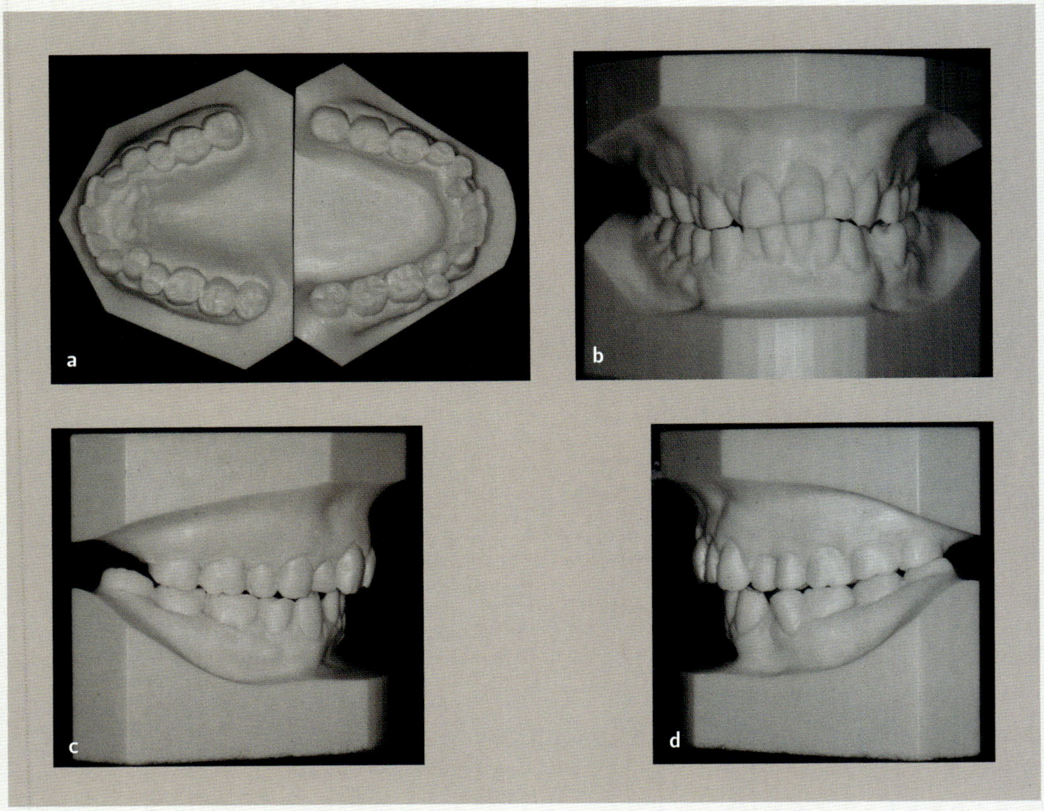

13.16 **a–d)** Frontal and lateral occlusal view of the study models.

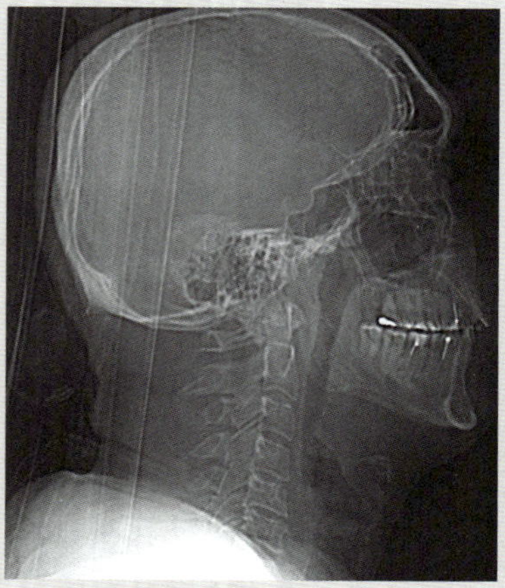

13.17 Teleradiography. Lateral projection.

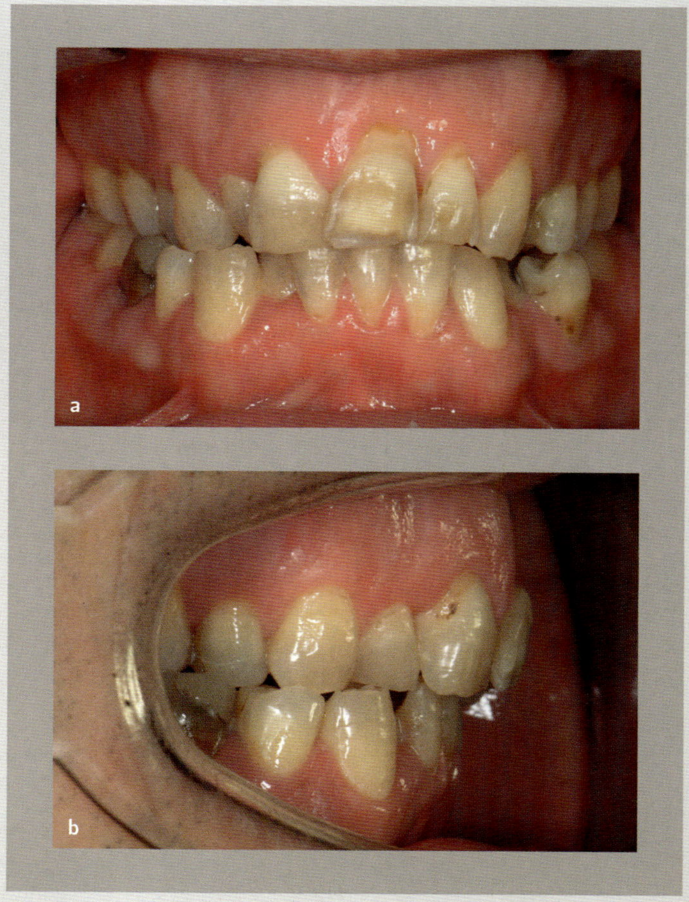

13.18 a–b) Intraoral image. Frontal and lateral view.

TMJ evaluation: The maximal protrusive range was 11 mm, anamnesis was independent of any previous muscular and articular pain, no pain was recorded when palpating the muscles and/or TMJ, and absence of functional limitations and of deviations in opening and advancement was observed.

Treatment plan: MAD (due to the severe xerostomia reported by the patient and his response to mandibular advancement during DISE)

Construction bite: George Gauge with a vertical opening of 5 mm and advancement of 6.5 mm for the TAP 3 design (13.19, 13.20a and b).

Delivery: Instructions for using this device and managing subsequent the side effects.

Titration: two weeks after delivery of the device, the patient did not report any pain or undesired effects. However, he underlined excellent therapeutic outcomes with respect to his sleepiness and susceptibility to fatigue. It was then decided to commence the following titration protocol: 0.5 mm/week [1 complete clockwise screw turn (360°) of the anterior screw].

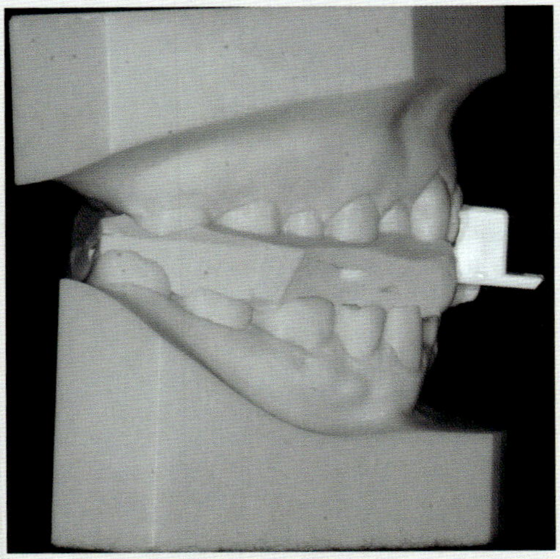

13.19 Construction bite.

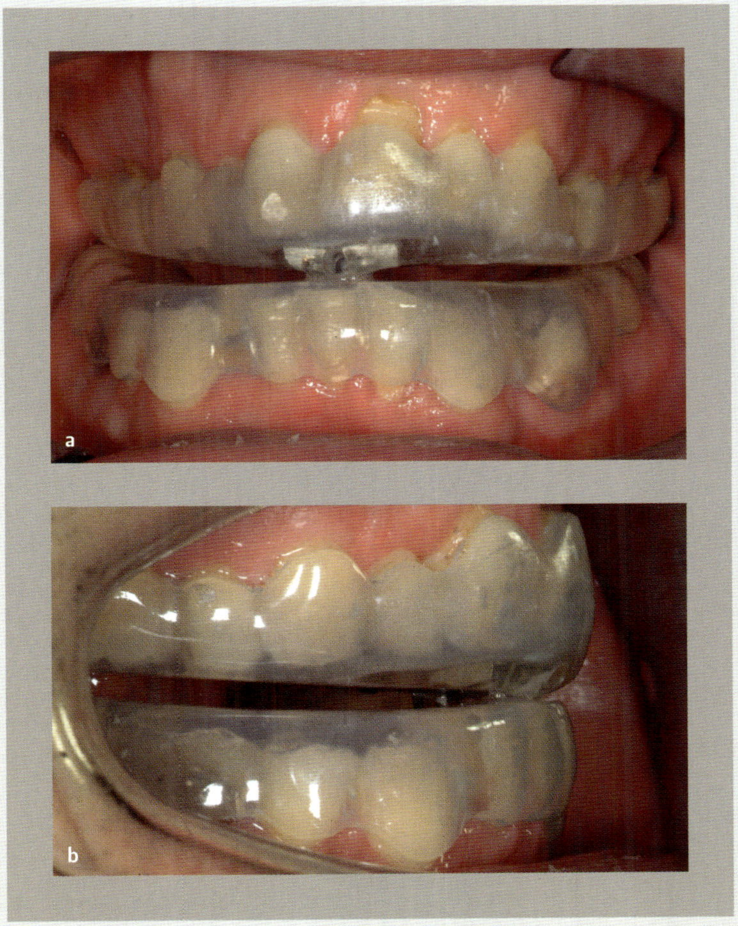

13.20 a–b) Intraoral images with MAD. Frontal and lateral view.

End of titration: Eight weeks after delivery of the device, the patient achieved an advancement of 8.5 mm that allowed him to feel comfortable and fine. We then decided to plan his first polygraphic follow-up.

Follow-up at 3 months after MAD delivery: the patient exhibited significant improvement in his snoring and daytime sleepiness symptoms (ESS = 7). He reported adherence to the MAD (subjective evaluation): The patient used the device for six nights a week and throughout the entire night.

Short-term side effects: Pain at upper incisors and transient xerostomia

At PG with MAD: AHI = 20; supine AHI = 43; nonsupine AHI = 15; ODI = 18; minimum Sa2O = 0 84; CT < 90% = 5%

We decided to retitrate CPAP with a nasal mask and MAD in situ.

After 1 week, the patient reported positive and efficient tolerance of the CPAP; the effective pressure was 7.5 cm H2O.

At PG with MAD and CPAP: AHI = 3; supine AHI = 5; nonsupine AHI = 2; ODI = 2; minimum Sa2O = 91; CT < 90% = 0%.

ESS = 6

Case 4

Female patient. 54 y.o. BMI = 28.3 kg/m^2.

Symptoms correlated to nocturnal respiratory disorders: Snoring, nocturnal respiratory pauses, sudden awakenings with a choking sensation, and daytime sleepiness (ESS = 10).

Significant anamnesis elements: The patient had undergone hysterectomy, left adnexectomy and partial right oophorectomy for endometriosis and left laparoscopic andrenalectomy for aldesteronoma. The patient was also suffering from arterial hypertension, gastroesophageal disorder and lumbar and cervical disc disease. The patient was overweight (BMI: 28.3 kg/m^2).

Instrumental examination:

- ECG: Results were found to be well within the predefined healthy limits
- spirometry: Normal values
- polysomnography: Normal cycle of sleep; presence of sleep fragmentation due to arousals primarily as a result of spontaneous obstructive events/desaturation/PLM (Periodic Leg Movements during sleep); presence of nocturnal respiratory events represented mainly by obstructive apneas and hypopneas with index/hour 19; flow analysis underlines signs of flow limitation; normal mean oxygen saturation values and periodic leg movements; snoring was recorded during 49.4% of the monitoring time

The patient was subjected to a trial of ventilation with auto-adjusting CPAP to identify the suitable pressure, and hence overcome the nocturnal respiratory events. A pressure of 10 cmH_2O was identified to be optimum.

Recommended therapy:

- nocturnal ventilation with CPAP full mask pressure of 10 cm H_2O and a starting ramp pressure of 5 cm H_2O.
- therapy focused on behavioral changes such as losing weight, following anti-reflux rules, sleeping on the side or in prone position, light dinner so as not to interfere with the subsequent bedtime and avoiding alcohol and sedative-hypnotic drugs.

The patient reported scarce tolerance to CPAP. She was subjected to a second consultation by specialists (2 months following the first one), which demonstrated the following:

- The patient was still overweight (BMI: 27.6 kg/m^2). The patient reported that she had started a diet with a weight loss of approximately 3 kg within the last 2 months.
- The patient's oral cavity parameters were within the limit; Mallampati/Friedman class IV, hypertrophic tonsils grade 2; intact/retro velar space.

- Video laryngoscopy: modest hypertrophy of the lower turbinates, free nasopharynx, hypertrophy of the lingual base, mobile larynx with signs of pharyngolaryngeal reflux.
- Müller test revealed the presence of a grade IV velopharyngeal circular collapse, a grade III oropharyngeal transversal collapse and a grade III anteroposterior hypopharyngeal collapse.
- *Nose and oral snoring endoscopy* indicated the development of a velar flutter (snorting sound) with efficient airway re-opening at the retrolingual level with the mandibular protrusion maneuver.

Recommended therapy:

- sleeping on one side
- antireflux measures
- esomeprazole 20 mg, 2 tablets a day for 1 month
- Mandibular Advancement Device (MAD)

Dental clinical and radiographic evaluation:

- adequate face proportion, absence of mandibular asymmetry (13.21a);
- class III profile with excessive projection, increased length of the inferior third and short chin-neck distance (13.21b);

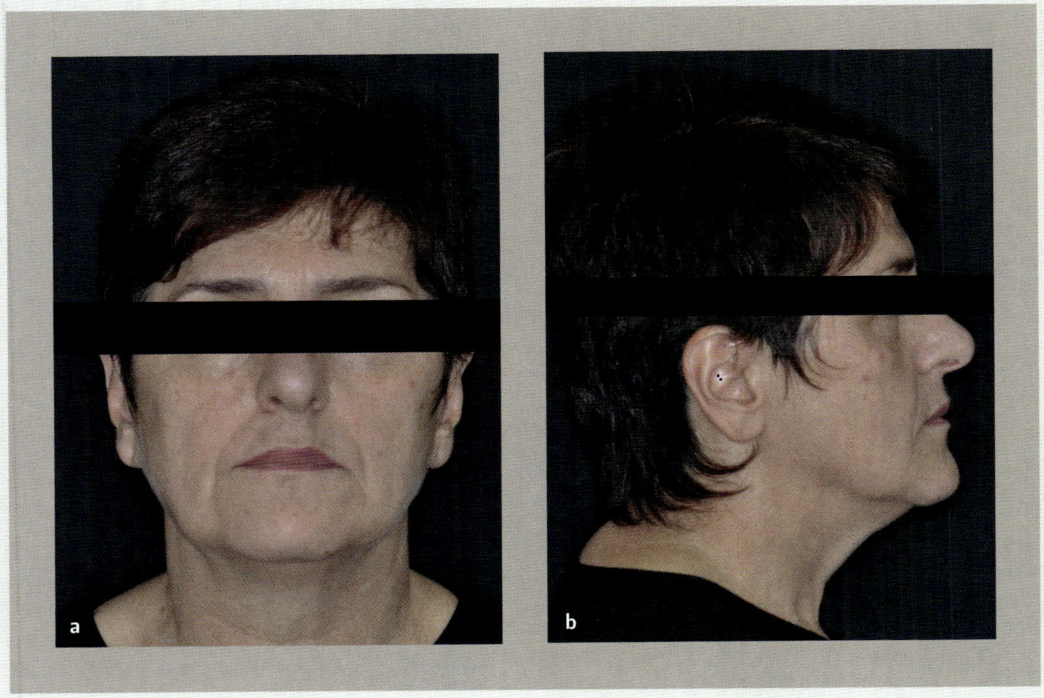

13.21 a–b) Frontal and lateral view of the face.

- spatially adequate arch with moderate anterior-inferior crowding and presence of superior and inferior dental implant rehabilitation, multiple gingival recessions with a satisfactory periodontal state (13.22a and b);
- posterior crossbite on the right and coincident midlines (13.22c);

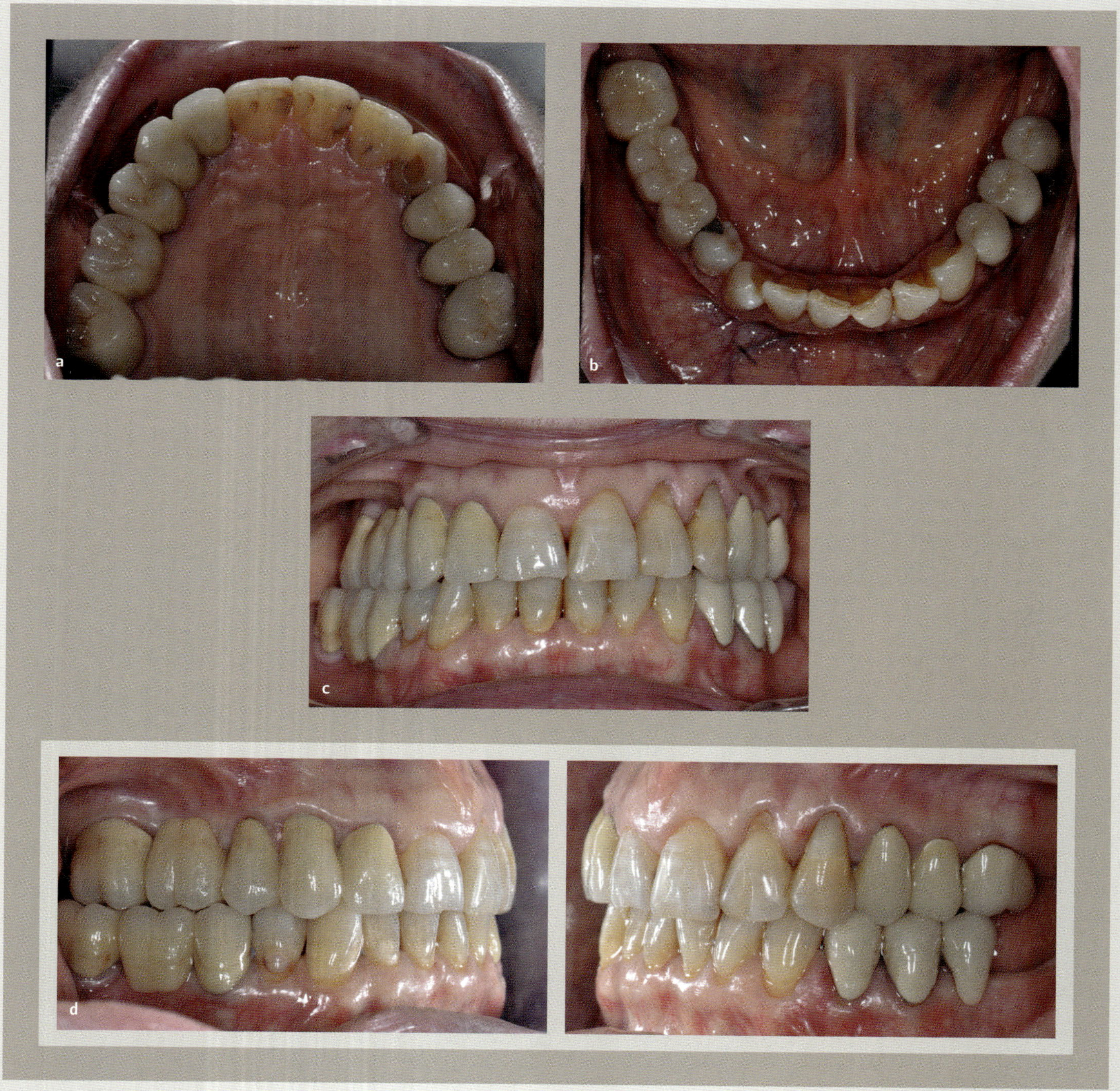

13.22 a–d) Intraoral images. Frontal and lateral occlusal view.

- bilateral canine class I with inferior incisors in class III compensation position and lingual crown torque, gingival recessions in both the arches (13.22d);
- class III skeletal pattern with increased sagittal projection of the chin; upper incisors adequate to the anterior nasal spine, retroposition of lower incisors in relation to pogonion; normal distance between hyoid bone and mandibular plane; reduced PAS and elongated soft palate (13.23a and b);
- missing elements: 15-16-18-27-28-36-37-47-48, multiple prosthetic restorations; endoscopic treatment with prosthetic restoration of nr.12-23-24 (13.24).

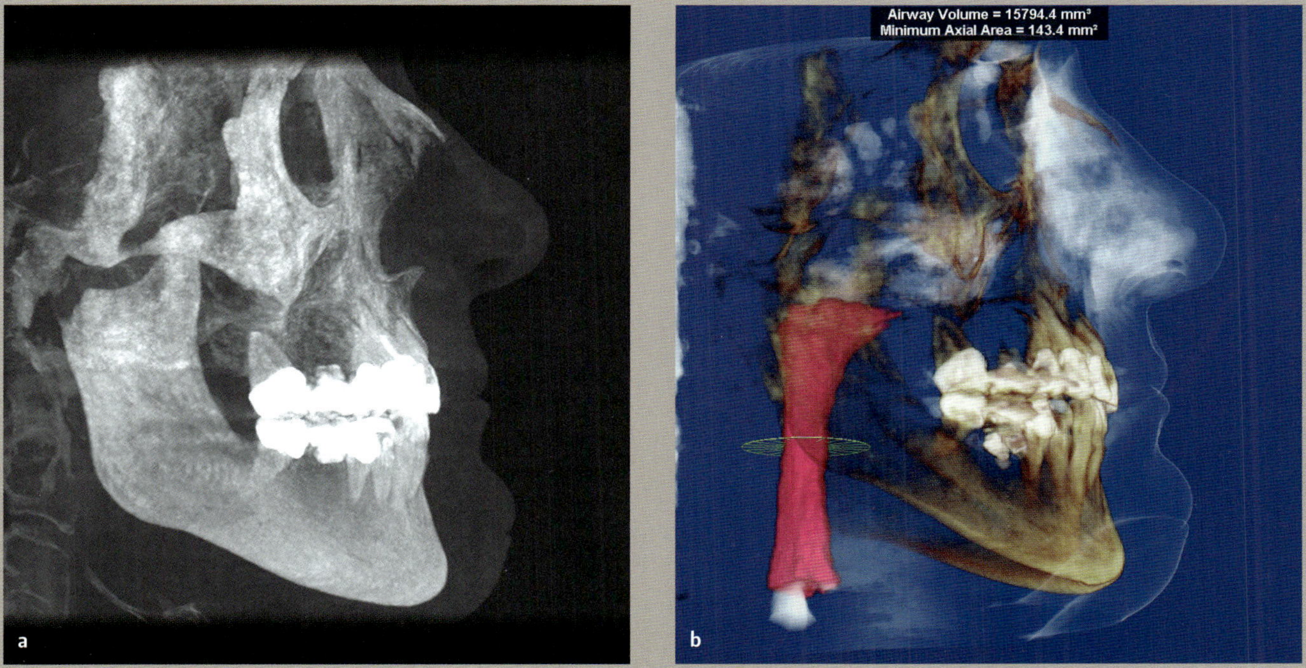

13.23 a–b) Teleradiography in lateral projection from cone beam computed tomography (CBCT); 3D rendering of the craniofacial complex identified the pharyngeal volume and the narrowest area.

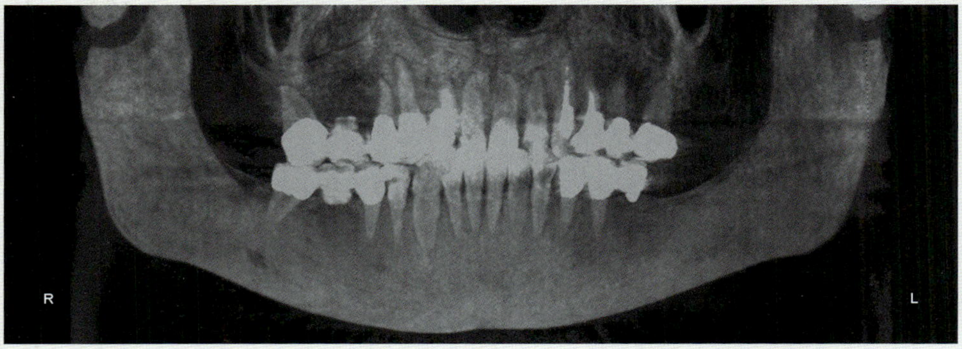

13.24 Panoramic radiograph from CBCT.

TMJ evaluation: the patient reported occasional TMJ soreness: no pain at palpation, absence of limitations and deviations in eccentric movements. The maximal protrusive range was 11 mm.

Treatment plan: the therapeutic approach was to treat this patient with a MAD (Somnodent Flex® with bilateral anterior hooks for vertical elastics use). Construction bite: George Gauge with a vertical opening of 5 mm and advancement of 7 mm (13.25).

Delivery: Instructions for use and delivery of vertical elastics (170g-3/16") (13.26a and b).

Titration: three weeks following the delivery of MAD, the patient reported

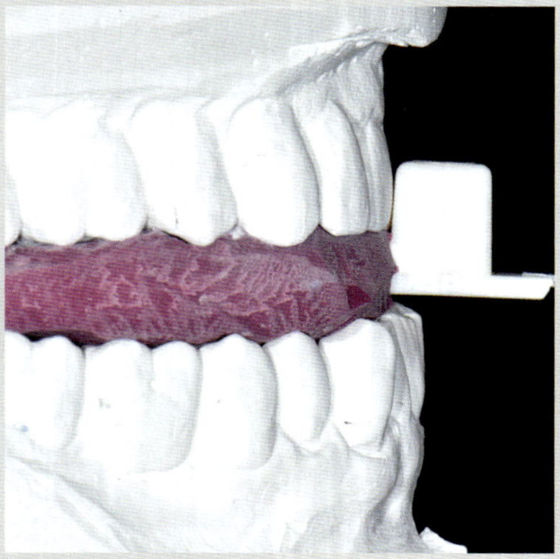

13.25 Construction bite.

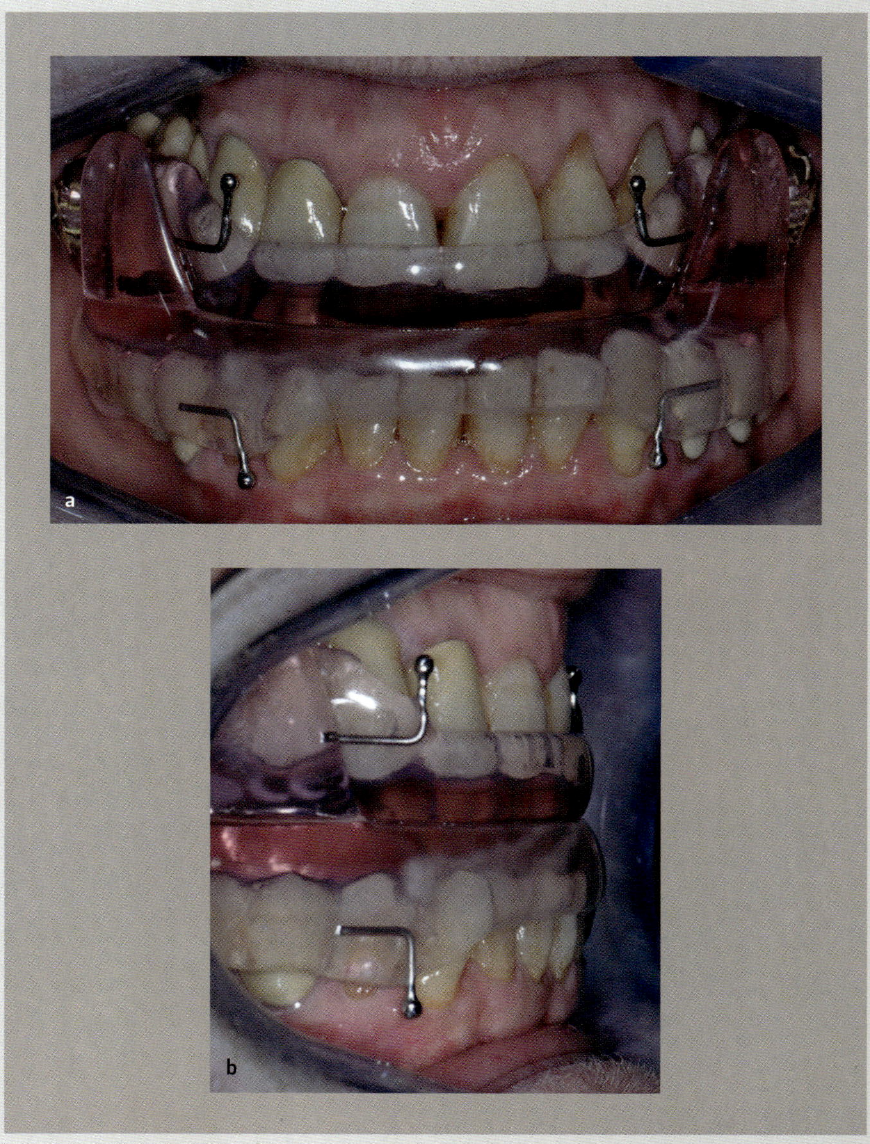

13.26 a–b) Intraoral images with MAD. Overjet frontal view.

good adherence to the device and absence of pain. Furthermore, the partner underlined that her nocturnal snoring symptoms were resolved. However, a slight daytime sleepiness still persisted.

A titration program commenced with an activation of 0.1 mm every two days until resolution of sleepiness. The final advancement achieved by the patient was 7.6 mm.

Two months after the delivery of the mandibular advancement device, the patient was subjected to PG with MAD: the sleep phases were normally represented with rare nocturnal respiratory events with index/hour of 1.1. Patient exhibited normal mean oxygen saturation (96), no periodic leg movements, whereas snoring was present in 29% of the monitored time.

The patient reported adherence to MAD (subjective evaluation): the device was worn 7 nights a week for the whole night (approximately 6 hours per night).

Long-term follow-up with MAD (3 years): Excellent therapeutic adherence (the patient wears the device every night and throughout the entire night).

Symptoms: Moderate snoring in the supine position persists; absence of daytime sleepiness (ESS = 5). The patient is still experiencing difficulties maintaining a healthy diet and controlling her weight.

Case 5

Male patient. 49 y.o. BMI = 23.2 kg/m^2, neck circumference = 37 cm.

Symptoms correlated to nocturnal respiratory disorders: the patient's partner reported snoring with manifestation of nocturnal respiratory pauses. The patient reported normal daytime sleepiness (ESS = 9), and efficient nighttime sleeping quality. The Stop Bang questionnaire did not detect a high risk for the manifestation of OSAS.

Significant anamnesis elements: good general state of health, mild hypertension.

Instrumental examination:

- polygraphy: AHI was 15.7/hour with 22.2/hour in the supine position (desaturation was evaluated according to the AIPO/American Academy of Sleep Medicine (AASM) 1999 criteria, se > 4%); normal mean oxygen saturation values (95.6%), nadir 87.0% with ODI 17/hour; sleep phases were normally represented; presence of fragmentation as a result of arousals primarily from obstructive events/desaturation induced by mixed and central obstructive events; flow exhibited signs of flow limitations; snoring was present in 56.6% of the monitored time
- sleep nose endoscopy: grade III anteroposterior collapse in velum-pharynx and oropharynx, grade IV in the hypopharynx (13.27a, b and c); collapse in all the subareas was improved following a mandibular pull-up; the lower nasal turbinates were decongested during that session
- polygraphy performed one month after the turbinates decongestion: AHI of 31.2/hour (desaturation was evaluated according to the AIPO/AASM 1999 criteria, se > 3%); normal mean oxygen saturation values (94.8%), nadir 78.0% with ODI 3/hour.

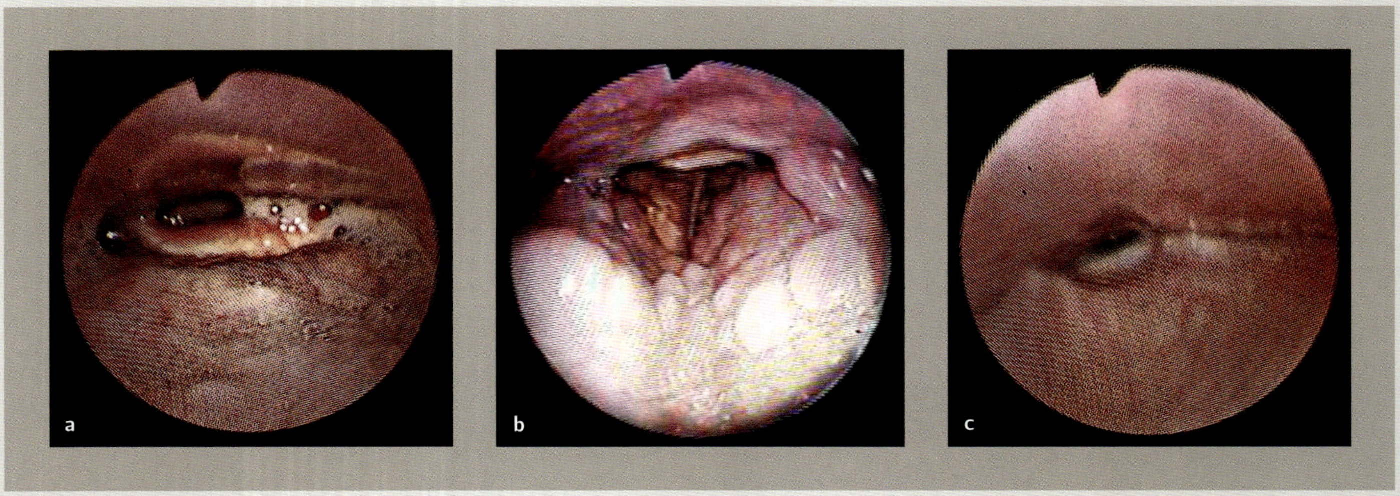

13.27 a–c) Images of sleep endoscopy highlight velum-pharyngeal, oropharyngeal and hypopharyngeal collapse.

The observed deterioration between the first two polygraphs (pre-intervention polygraph and the polygraph performed following the decongestion of turbinates) is relative. Numbers should not be misleading because the scoring criteria used in the first two examinations were in fact different: in the first case, desaturation events were only considered if > 4% according to the criteria of AASM 1999 and AIPO, whereas in the second examination (which was more restrictive), the criterion was exceeding 3% according to the 2012 AASM guidelines.

The patient inquired for an alternative approach to ronchopathy surgery, suggesting a lateral pharyngoplasty associated with adenotonsillectomy. Furthermore, he asked for a treatment other than CPAP.

Recommended therapy:
- MAD;
- behavioral changes: enhanced sleep hygiene, positional therapy, sleeping on one side or in a prone position.

Dental clinical and radiographic evaluation:
- satisfactory face proportion, mandibular asymmetry toward the right (13.28a and b);
- flat facial profile with normal cheekbones, straight tip of the nose (13.28c);
- slightly closed nasolabial angle with reduced thickness of the upper lip (13.28c);
- retruding anteroposterior position of the upper incisors with normal vertical exposition (13.28c);

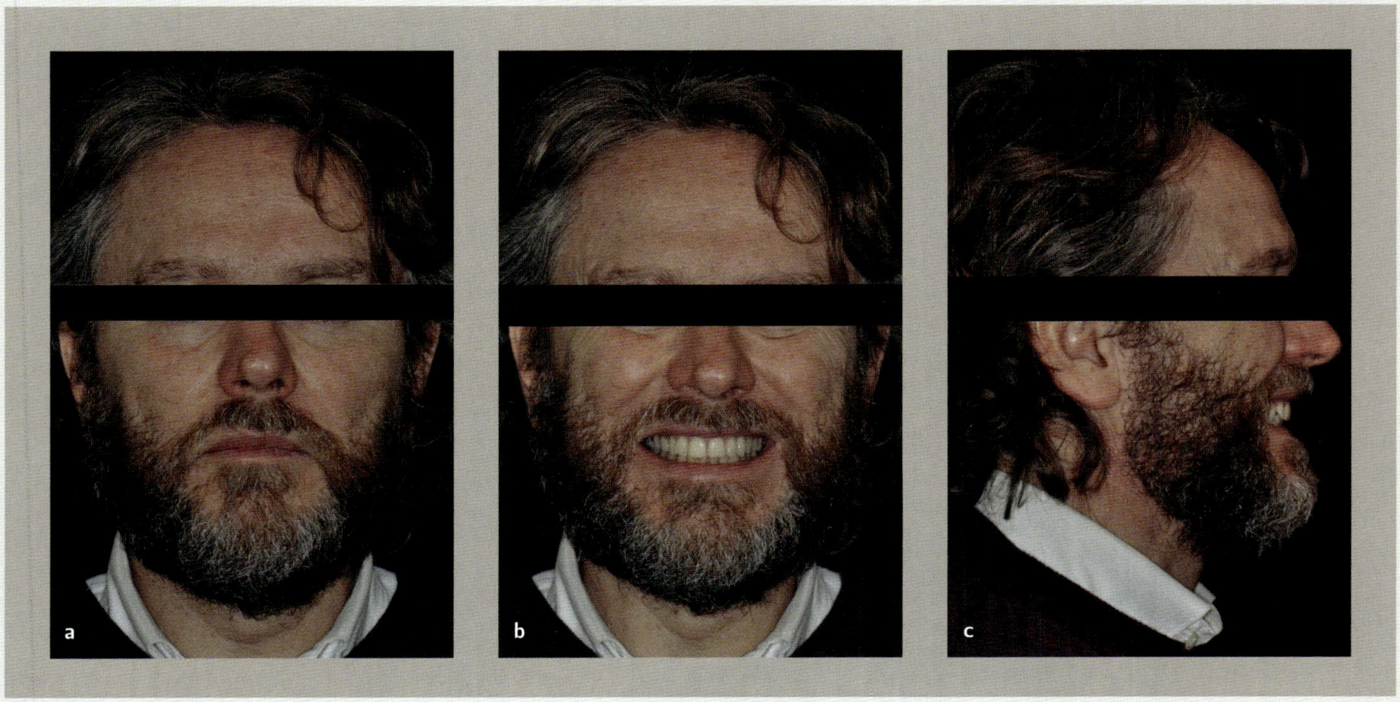

13.28 a–c) Frontal view of the face with closed mouth with a smile. Lateral view of the face with a smile.

- the arches are dimensionally adequate with mild anterosuperior crowding and moderate inferior crowding; satisfactory periodontal state (13.29a and b);
- coincident midlines (13.29c and d);
- bilateral Class I canine and molar relationship (13.29e and f);

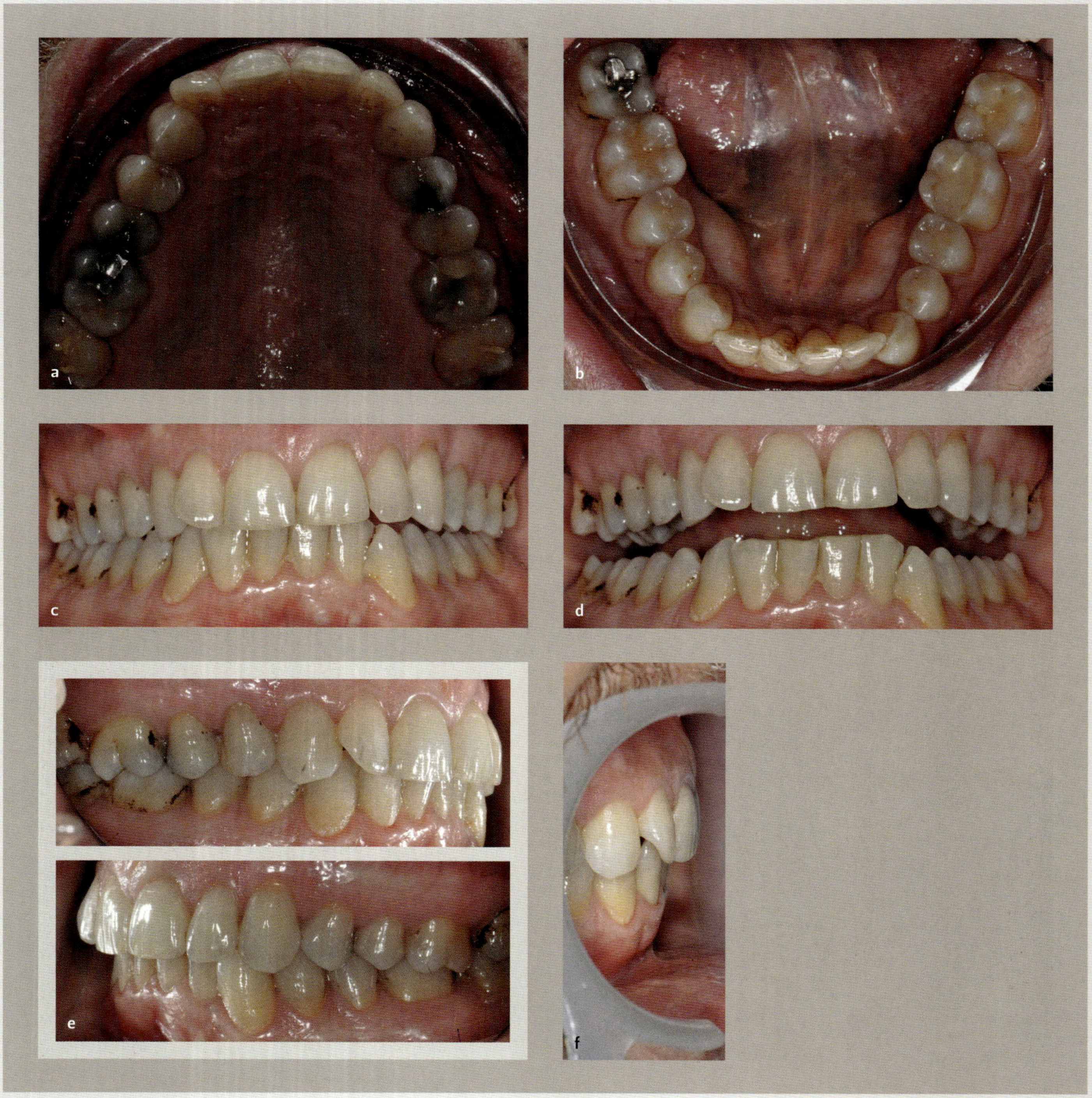

13.29 a–f) Intraoral images. Frontal and lateral view with closed mouth and half-open mouth and overjet.

- class I skeletal pattern with reduced anterior cranial base, anterior and posterior facial height; upper incisors adequate in relation to the anterior nasal spine; lower incisors are retropositioned in relation with the pogonion (13.30a, b, c and d);
- development of tartar, mouth hygiene needs to be improved (13.31).

TMJ evaluation: the patient did not report TMJ disorders; no pain at palpation, absence of limitations and deviations in eccentric movements.
The maximal protrusive was 12 mm.

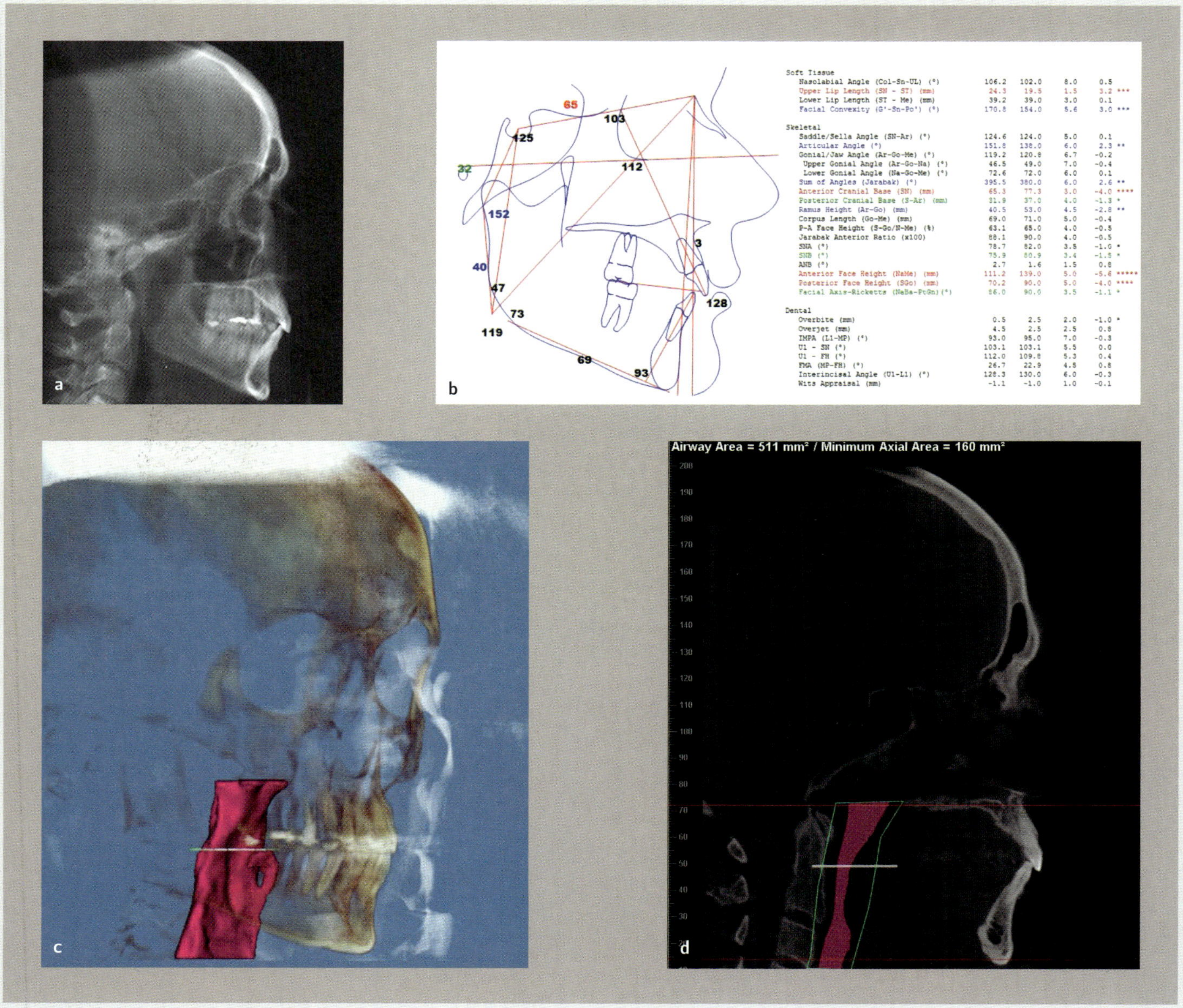

13.30 a–d) Teleradiography in lateral projection from CBCT. Cephalometric analysis. 3D rendering highlighted the pharyngeal volume. Median sagittal section of the skull from CBCT with pharyngeal volume and the narrowest posteroanterior area.

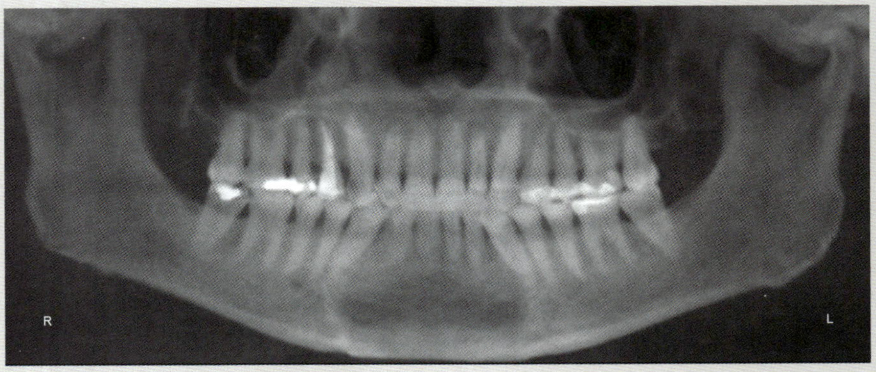

13.31 Panoramic radiography from CBCT.

Treatment plan: we decided to treat the patient with a MAD (Somnodent Flex® with bilateral anterior hooks for vertical elastics use).

Construction bite: George Gauge with a vertical opening of 5 mm and advancement of 9 mm (13.32).

Delivery: instructions for use and delivery of vertical elastics to keep the teeth together (170 g, 3/16") (13.33a, b e c).

Titration: Four weeks after the delivery of MAD, the patient reported good tolerance to the device, a mild pain in the TMJ left side and a general improvement of daytime life quality. Furthermore, his bed partner reported a significant decrease in nocturnal snoring.

Titration program required an activation of 0.1 mm every three consecutive days until the elimination of all related symptoms.

The final advancement achieved by the patient was 13 mm with concurrent absence of pain.

One year after delivery of the device, the patient was subjected to a polygraph with MAD: 7.9 is in the supine position; normal mean oxygen saturation values (96.3%), nadir 92.0% with ODI 0/hour; sleep stages were normally represented; sleep fragmentation by recurrent brief arousals, exclusively

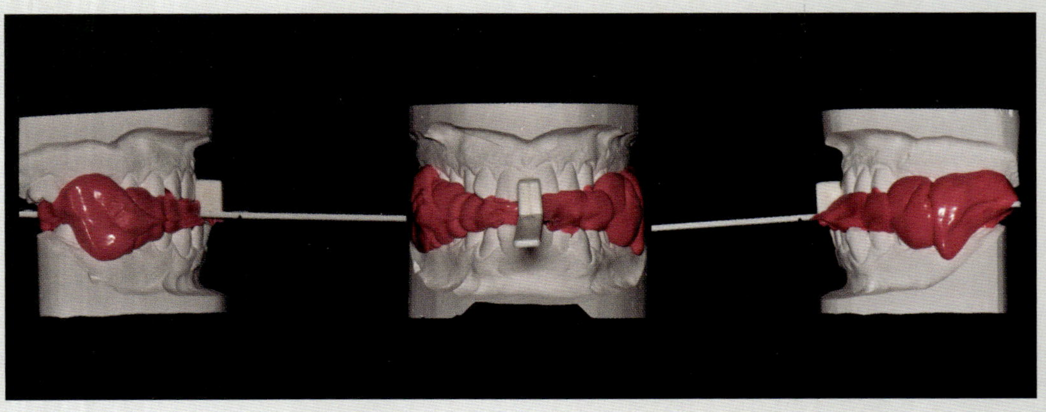

13.32 Construction bite. Frontal and lateral view.

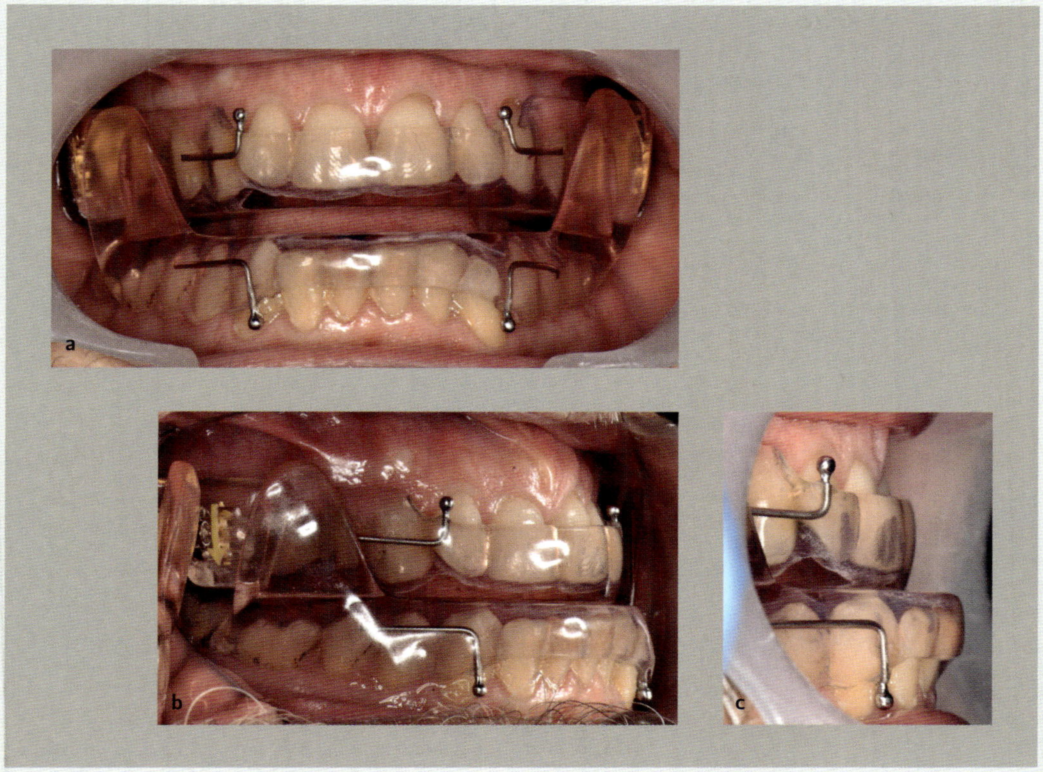

13.33 a–c) Intraoral image with MAD. Frontal and lateral view of the overjet.

obstructive events/desaturation events; snoring presented 18.2% of the monitored time.

Follow-up performed with a MAD polygraphy at 1.5 years after delivery: AHI was 0.9/hour with 1.4/hour in the supine position; normal mean oxygen saturation (98%), nadir 94%, ODI 0/hour; the patient did not change his lifestyle with respect to increasing physical exercise or enhancing sleep hygiene.

The patient reported adherence to MAD (subjective evaluation) seven nights a week (approximately 6 hours per night).

Case 6

Male patient. 56 y.o. BMI = 30.1 kg/m^2, neck circumference = 43 cm.

Symptoms correlated to nocturnal respiratory disorders: snoring; nocturnal respiratory pauses: (ESS = 11)

Significant anamnesis elements: the patient was subjected to septoturbinoplasty surgery and lateral pharyngoplasty; asthma; parietaria allergy; subjective hypoacusis; overweight.

Instrumental examination: initial polygraph test demonstrated mixed nature apnea-hypopnea respiratory events, mainly obstructive events of severe degree (AHI = 61.0), remarkable oxygen desaturation values (mean saturation = 88%, nadir = 74%), an extremely high number of snoring events (519,2 events/hour), presence of rare arrhythmic events.

The patient was subjected to a ventilation trial with CPAP to identify how to solve these nocturnal respiratory events. Pressure identified as effective was 9 cm H_20.

Recommended therapy:

- nocturnal ventilation with continuous positive pressure (CPAP with full mask)
- therapy focusing on behavioral changes: weight loss, sleeping on one side or in prone position; light dinners, avoiding late-night eating, avoiding alcohol consumption and sedative-hypnotic drugs
- surgical therapy: pharyngoplasty and septoturbinoplasty
- cardiological evaluation if needed.

Müller's test highlighted grade III collapse in all the subareas. A circular type collapse in the velopharyngeal region and a transversal collapse in oropharyngeal and hypopharyngeal region were identified.

Sleep nose endoscopy detected IV grade circular collapse in the velopharyngeal region with grade III transversal velar flutter in oropharynx. The mandibular traction maneuver managed to improve the hypopharyngeal occlusion, which was turned into grade III, although not in the remaining subareas. During the same session, lateral pharyngoplasty and septoturbinoplasty were performed.

The patency of the nasal passages was improved after septoturbinoplasty surgery.

Post ENT surgery polygraph: reduction in AHI to 29.0; supine AHI = 40.6, nonsupine AHI = 4.5; improvement in the level of oxygen saturation values (mean saturation = 92.7%, nadir = 78%); snoring was present in 42.3% of the monitored time.

Due to a scarce compliance to CPAP, the patient required for an alternative treatment. Considering the good state of health of the patient's oral cavity, we considered the use of MAD with an enhanced sleep hygiene.

Recommended therapy: orthodontic consultation for the construction of a mandibular advancement device.

Dental clinical and radiographic evaluation:

- flat facial profile/slightly convex, absence of mandibular asymmetry (13.34a);
- good chin projection but with reduced chin-throat distance (13.34b);
- dimensionally adequate arches with missing elements 3.6 and 4.6, satisfactory periodontal state; absence of dental mobility (13.35b);
- right posterior bite and coincident midlines (13.35c);
- bilateral canine class I (13.35d and e);
- class I skeletal pattern; upper incisors were adequate in relation to the anterior nasal spine; lower incisors were retropositioned in relation to the pogonion (13.36a and b);
- multiple dental conservative restoration at elements 14, 15, 16, 22, 23, 24, and 47; prosthetic restoration at element 27 (13.37).

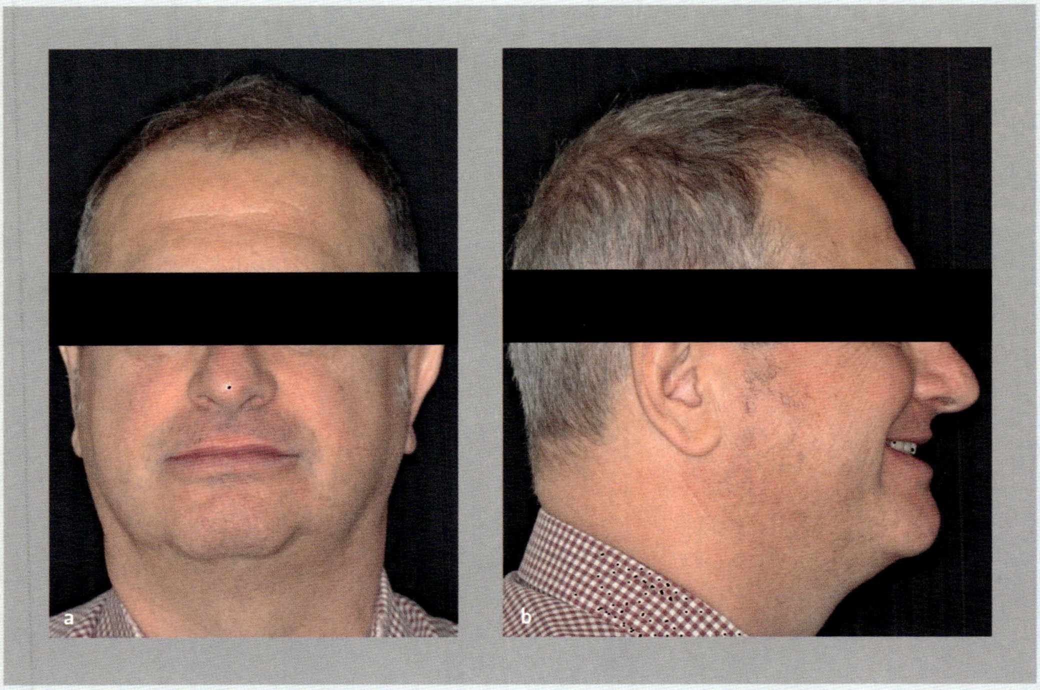

13.34 a–b) Frontal and lateral view of the face.

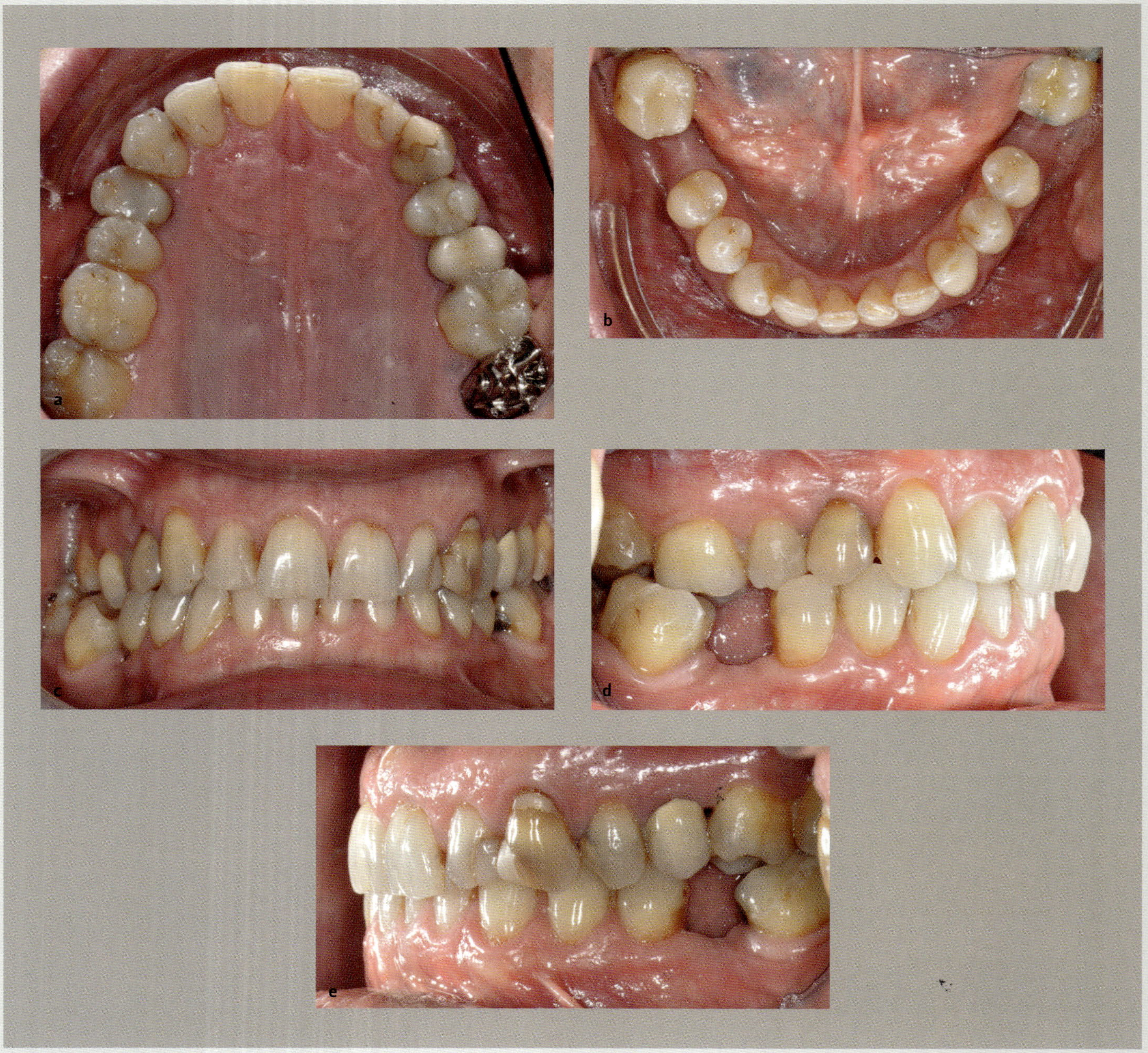

13.35 a–e) Intraoral images. Frontal and lateral occlusal view.

TMJ evaluation: Absence of pain at palpation, absence of articular clicking, absence of limitations and deviations in eccentric movements. The maximal protrusive range was 13 mm.

Treatment plan: we decided to treat this patient with a MAD (Somnodent Flex® with bilateral anterior hooks for the use of vertical elastics).

Construction bite: George Gauge with a vertical opening of 5 mm and advancement of 9 mm (13.38).

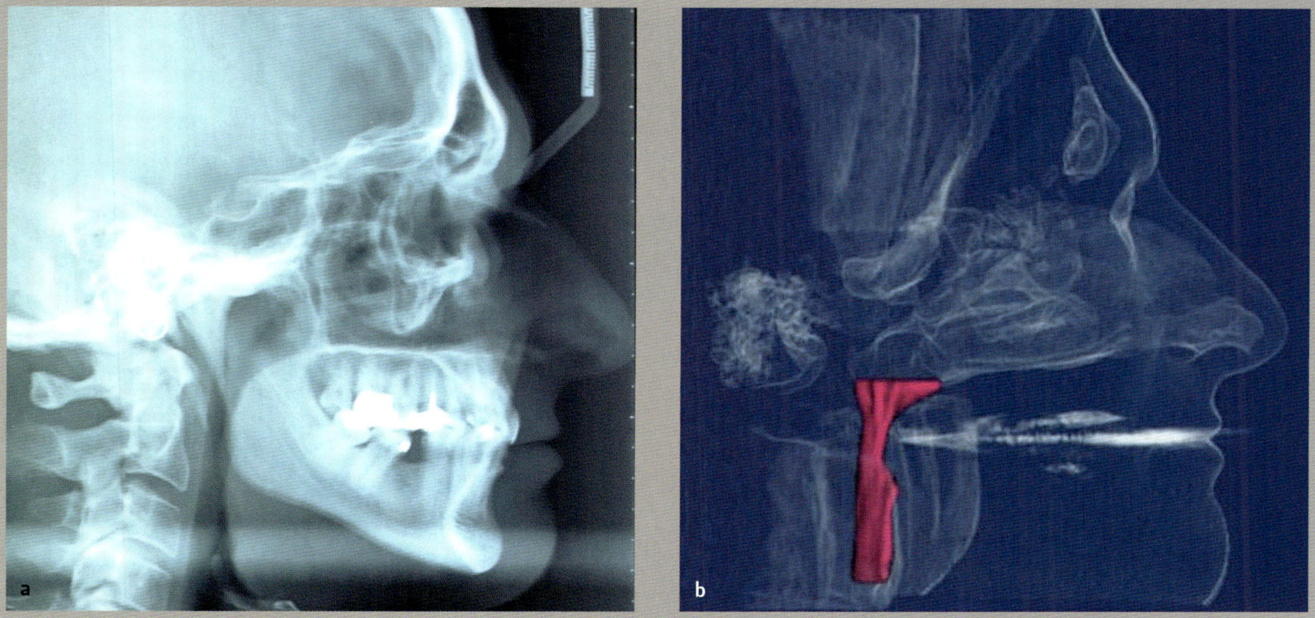

13.36 a–b) Teleradiography in lateral projection. 3D Rendering of the craniofacial complex. The airways are highlighted.

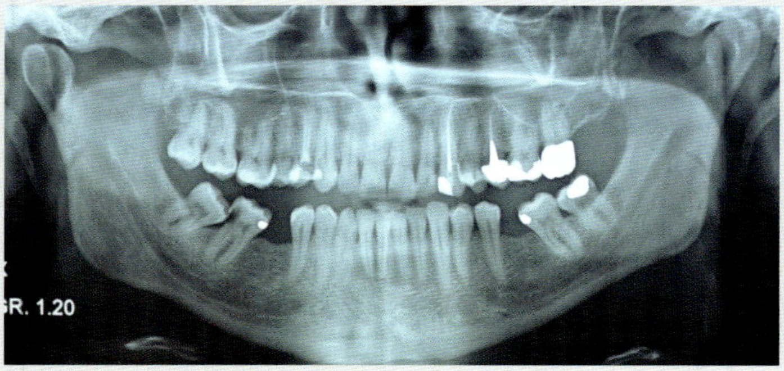

13.37 Panoramic radiography.

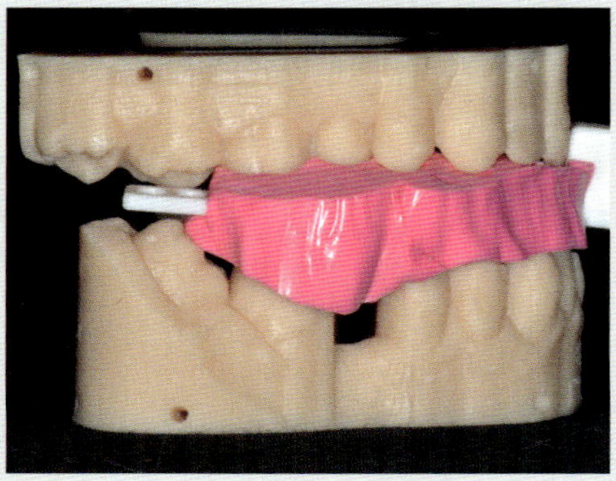

13.38 Construction bite.

Deliver: instructions on using the device but also on its activations and cleaning procedures, delivery of vertical elastics (99 g-5/16” [CLIFF®]) on anterior hooks, educating the patient on muscle stretching (13.39a e b).

Titration: Overall, 70% of the protrusive range of the initial advancement. Two weeks following the delivery, 10 activations were prescribed to the patient. Two months following the last control the patient reported a distinct decrease in snoring and daytime sleepiness. During the same consultation, the patient was prescribed 10 additional activations and a control polysomnography.

At the following appointment 2 months later, the polysomnographic reports were evaluated and demonstrated that the apneas had been decreased

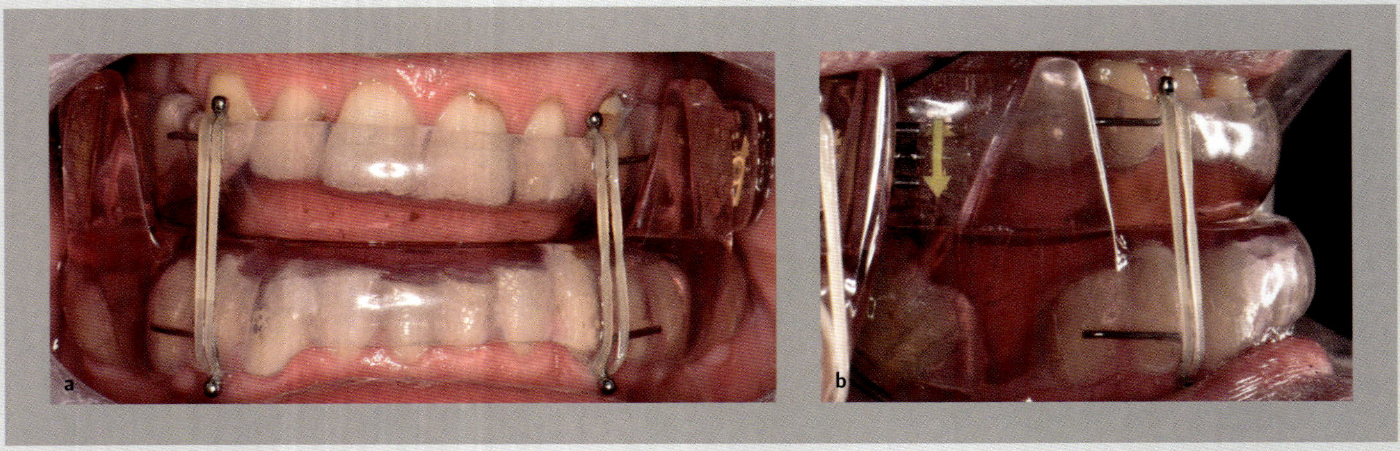

13.39 a–b) Intraoral images with MAD. Frontal and lateral view.

from moderate to mild (AHI = 14.2; supine AHI = 17.9; nonsupine AHI = 3.3) with an additional improvement of the levels of oxygen saturation rates (mean saturation = 93.7%, nadir = 83%). Snoring was present in 39.5% of the monitored time and the patient was prescribed 10 additional activations (one activation per week).

Long-term follow-up with MAD: one year after delivery of the device, the patient continued to report a progressive decrease in daytime sleepiness and a drastic reduction in snoring. Five additional activations and a polysomnography control were prescribed. This last control reported the following: AHI = 8.5; supine AHI = 12.8; nonsupine AHI = 0.4; mean Sa2O = 93% (nadir = 83%); snoring was present in 0% of the monitored time. The patient reported once again a progressive decrease in daytime tiredness and almost disappearance of snoring episodes.

A total of 35 activations (0.1 mm of advancement per activation) have been implemented since the delivery.

Symptoms: No other symptoms except for mild hypersalivation were identified.

Case 7

Female patient. 56 y.o. BMI = 25 kg/m^2, neck circumference = 39 cm.

Significant anamnesis elements: Chronic disturbing snoring and respiratory pauses were reported by the patient's son, negative Epworth for daytime sleepiness (ESS = 9).

Significant anamnesis elements: the patient is suffering from hypertension, which is well controlled by an appropriate pharmacological therapy. She presented a nasal septum deviation and hypertrophic turbinates. Therefore, the patient reported nasal congestion during the night and awakening with a dry mouth. The patient had normal weight.

Instrumental examination: the initial polygraph test reported obstructive apnea-hypoapnea events of moderate degree and position related (AHI = 27.0; supine AHI = 35; nonsupine AHI = 11) with a mildly compromised nocturnal oxygenation (CT > 90% = 2).

Recommended therapy:

- Behavioral changes: avoiding the supine position, losing weight, and quitting unhealthy habits such as smoking and alcohol consumption in the evening)
- MAD
- Surgical therapy: septoturbinoplasty

Müller's maneuver highlighted a grade II collapse at the retropalatal level with lateral pattern and a grade III anteroposterior collapse at the retrolingual level.

Dental clinical and radiographic evaluation:

- Straight profile in normal divergent patient;
- Contracted upper arch, missing elements: 1.4, 1.8, 3.5, 3.6 and 3.8; gingival recessions; absence of dental mobility (13.40);
- Lower midline slightly deviated toward the left (13.41a);
- Class I bilateral canine (13.41b and c);

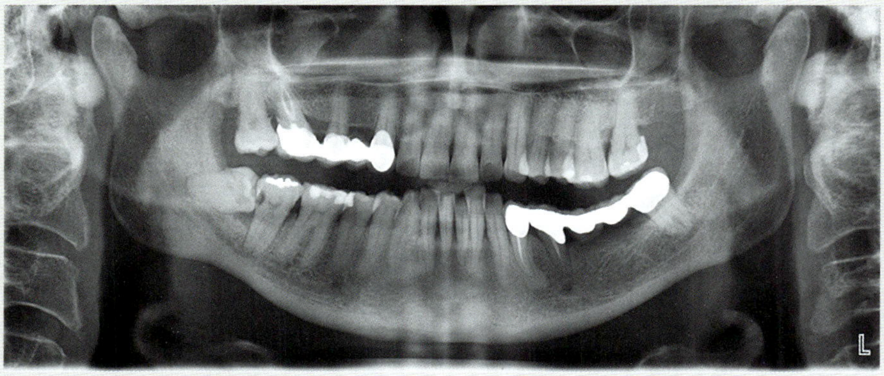

13.40 Panoramic radiography.

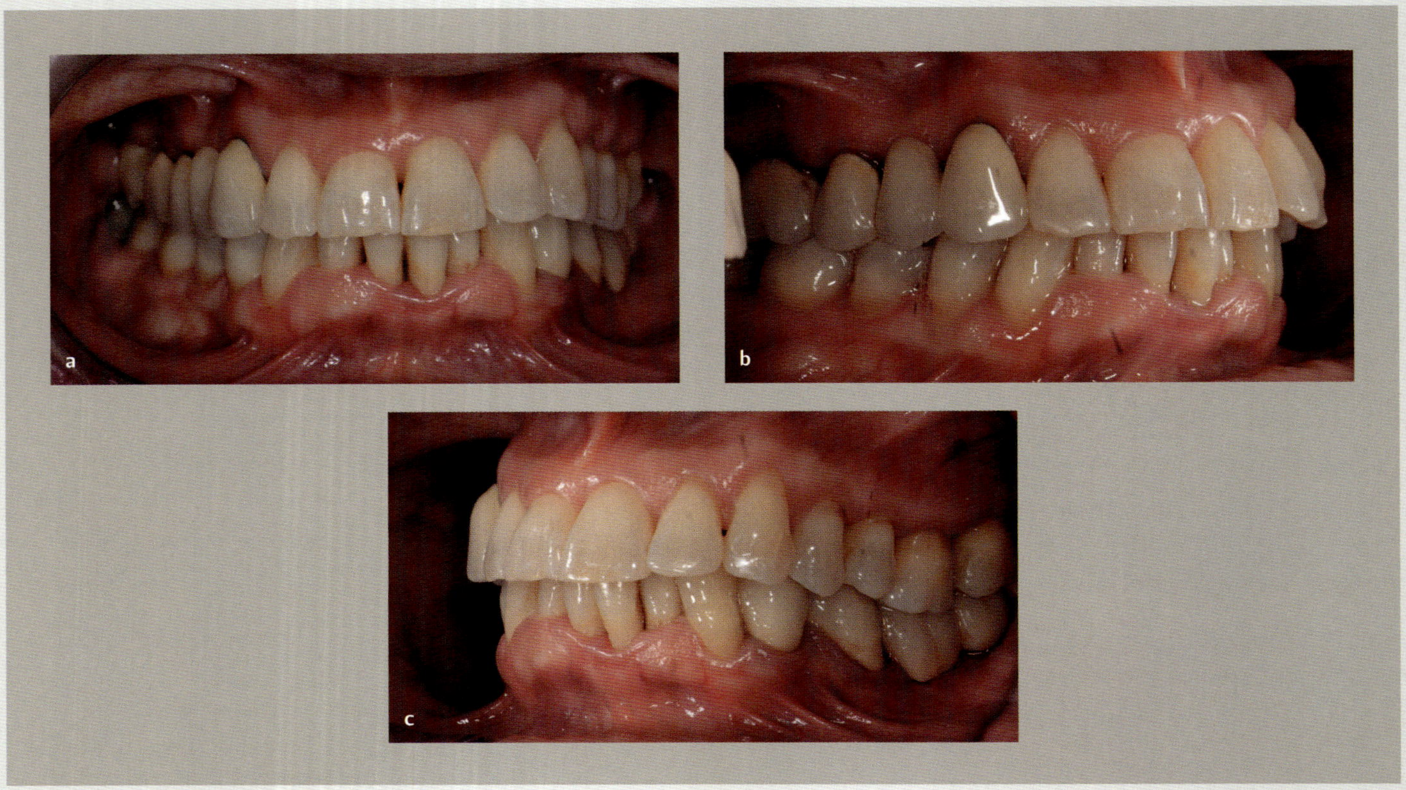

13.41 a–c) Intraoral images. Frontal and lateral view.

- Skeletal class I, normal divergence, proclined upper incisors (13.42);
- Multiple dental restoration and dental implants in the first and third quadrant (13.41b and c).

TMJ evaluation: pain was experienced when palpating the masseter muscle, absence of joint clicking, absence of limitations and deviations during eccentric movements. The maximal protrusive range was 11 mm.

Treatment plan: we decided to treat this patient with a MAD (Orthoapnea®).
Construction bite: George Gauge with a vertical opening of 7 mm and advancement of 8 mm (13.43).

Delivery: instructions to use, activate, and clean the device as well as educate the patient on muscle stretching exercises (13.44 a–c).

Titration: two weeks following the delivery, 10 activations were prescribed (one every three days). Two months following the last control, the patient reported a reduction of snoring and daytime sleepiness. Control by polygraph was prescribed during the same consultation.

PG control: resolution of the clinical condition (AHI = 4; supine AHI = 5; non-supine AHI = 2) with improvement in oxygen saturation levels (CT > 90% = 0).

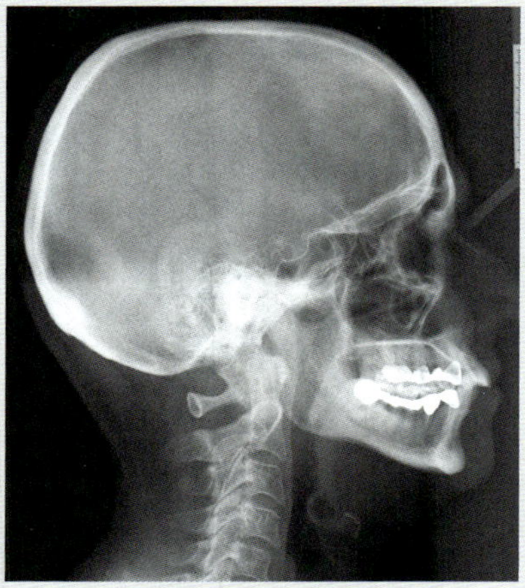

13.42 Teleradiography in lateral projection

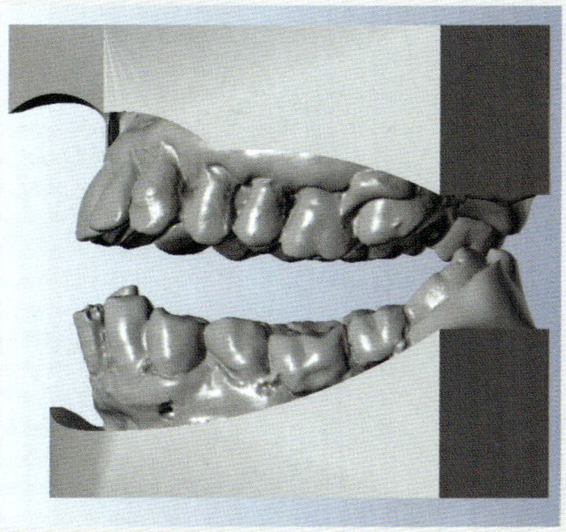

13.43 Scan of the dental arches with construction bite. Isolation of single images exhibiting the relation between the arches.

The patient reported a distinct improvement in snoring, which was not disturbing her anymore.

Long-term follow-up with MAD: one year after delivery of the device, the patient reported a drastic improvement in snoring again.

Symptom: none

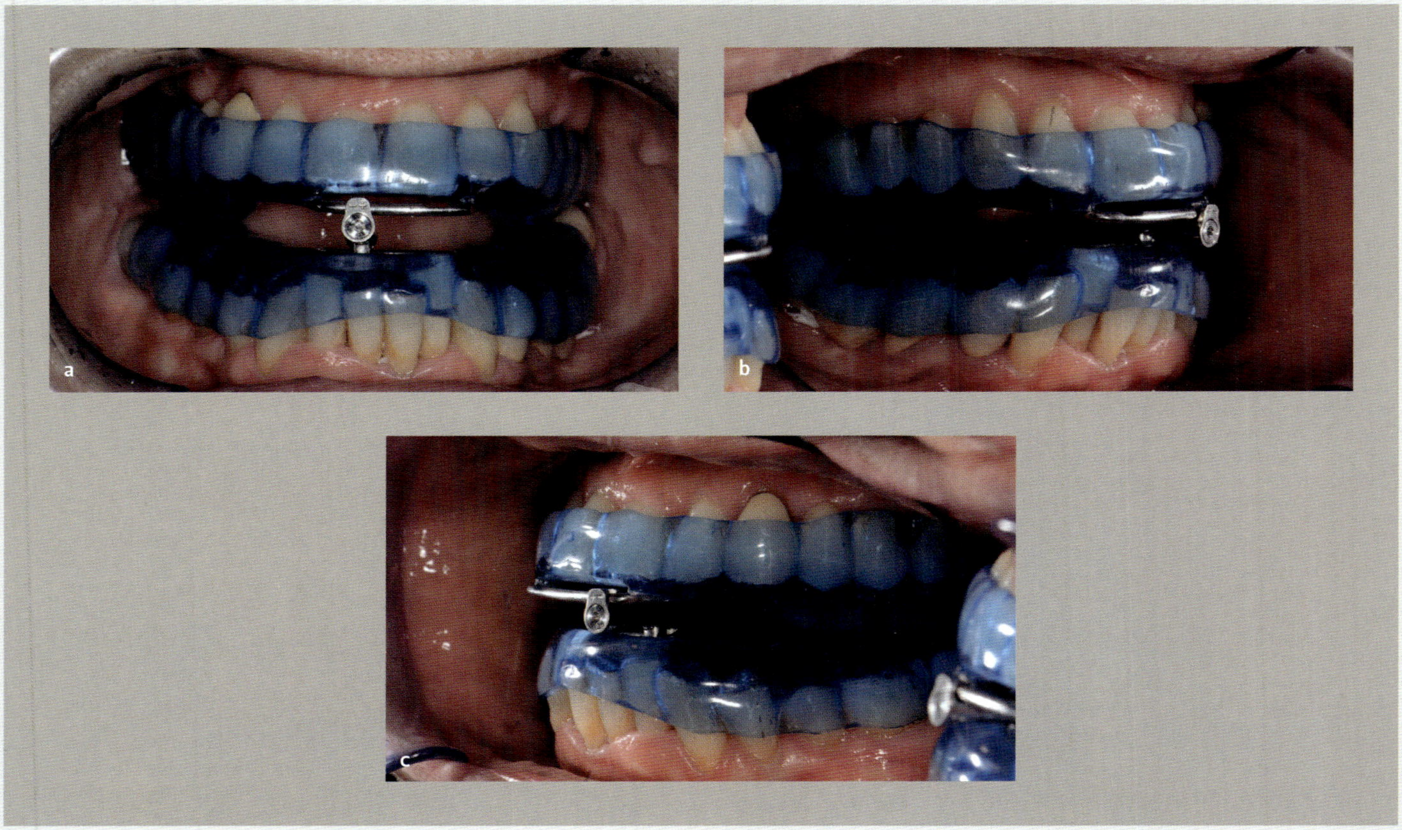

13.44 a–c) Intraoral images with MAD. Frontal and lateral view.

Index

f and *t* denote figures and tables

M

N

O

P